José Uberos Fernández

Pediatrics and occupational therapy

José Uberos Fernández

Pediatrics and occupational therapy

Pediatrics in Health Sciences

ScienciaScripts

This book is a translation from the original published under ISBN 978-620-2-09765-9.

Publisher:
Sciencia Scripts
is a trademark of
Dodo Books Indian Ocean Ltd. and OmniScriptum S.R.L publishing group

120 High Road, East Finchley, London, N2 9ED, United Kingdom
Str. Armeneasca 28/1, office 1, Chisinau MD-2012, Republic of Moldova, Europe
Printed at: see last page
ISBN: 978-620-6-44291-2

Contents

Authors 2

PART I 3

PART II 74

PART III 154

PART IV 246

Authors

Blanca Jover, Enrique - Collaborating Professor of Paediatrics, University of Granada. Paediatric Cardiologist, Facultativo especialista de area, Hospital Universitario San Cecilio de Granada.

Campoy Folgoso, Cristina - Professor of Paediatrics, University of Granada.

Dieguez Castillo, Estefania - Department of Paediatrics. University of Granada.

Fernandez Lopez, Maria Luisa - Early Childhood Care Centre, Granada Health District.

Fernandez Marin, Elisabeth - Specialist in Neonatology, Hospital Universitario San Cecilio de Granada.

Garcia Santos, Jose Antonio - Department of Paediatrics. University of Granada.

Machado Casas, Irene - Child Neurology, Hospital Universitario San Cecilio de Granada.

Molina Carballo, Antonio - Professor of Paediatrics, University of Granada. Child Neurology, Hospital Universitario San Cecilio de Granada.

Moreno Madrid, Francisco - Associate Professor of Paediatrics, University of Granada. Head of Section of Paediatrics, Hospital Universitario San Cecilio de Granada.

Ocete Hita, Esther - Associate Professor of Paediatrics, University of Granada. Head of Section of Paediatrics, Hospital Universitario Virgen de las Nieves de Granada.

Uberos Fernandez, Jose - Professor of Paediatrics, University of Granada. Head of Neonatology Section, Hospital Universitario San Cecilio de Granada.

PART I

1.From the dawn of paediatrics to the present day

Dr. Jose Uberos Fernandez

Depending on the level of cultural evolution, various peoples achieved important advances in the knowledge and treatment of diseases. In Egypt, some 1500 years before Christ, the art of healing was practically in the hands of the priests. Circumcision was practised, and newborn babies received immediate care from women dedicated to childbirth. The Ebers papyrus refers to infant diseases, and contains numerous prescriptions, as well as their preparation and administration. It also describes means of observing and measuring the quality of the wet-nurse's milk, and it may be assumed that the people in charge of carrying out this control were trained in this respect.

The Sumerians, Babylonians and Assyrians show a clearly theurgic and demomac medicine. The goddess Labarta was responsible for making women and children sick. While the goddess Ishtar exercised a protective and caring action towards the child. The Hebrews also practiced circumcision, and from the Talmud and the Bible it is known that breastfeeding lasted from 2 to 3 years.

The Hindus were able to imagine the repercussions that processes suffered by the mother could have on the unborn child: The violent and bad-tempered pregnant woman would have an epileptic child. An alcoholic mother will have a child with a weak memory. The one with a dissolute life will have a depraved or effeminate child. However, we find in this culture and for the first time a reasoned and consistent body of paediatric medicine. We refer to the Sushruta Samhita. In it we find a chapter on Paediatrics included in the section on pregnancy, dedicated to the care of the umbilical cord and its diseases.

The Incas and Aztecs had an evolution very similar to that of the Eastern peoples, initially theurgic and later empirical. The care of the sick was exercised by physicians, priests and sorcerers who maintained botanical gardens, where they cultivated plants with curative effects. Children did not receive much attention and often the children of enemy tribes were sacrificed to the gods. Breast-feeding was maintained until the eighth month. In the Homeric penode of classical Greece children are generally raised by their mothers, with reference to the use of wet nurses, usually female captives. Toys of various kinds are also described in these works. In Sparta the harshness of their education is well known. In Hellenistic Athens children were often brought up by wet nurses as well. We can point out, as one of the first rules of modern mental hygiene, the advice given by authors such as Aristotle, Plutarch or Plato against telling mythological stories to children because of their danger to mental health.

Rome was a nation of legislators, among other things, and laws concerning children were a must. It is indeed from Rome that the first laws for the protection of children originated. But from then until now, between the law and its actual execution there is a long way: it was a constant struggle against the practice of infanticide, the systematic destruction of children and the inhumanity of "patria potestas". Antoninus Pius (138-

161), founded for the first time and in honour of his wife Faustina, an institution for the protection of the child destined to save it from destruction. Later Marcus Aurelius (161-180) placed this food institution under the supervision of a praetorian of consular rank. The last edict before the fall of the Empire was that of Gratian, punishing parents who abandoned their children.

During the Middle Ages there were many people who dedicated themselves to the care of the sick, generally religious people who responded to the social situation of the time, satisfying more the basic needs of sustenance, clothing and shelter, than the health needs themselves, with the elevation of their souls being more important than that of their bodies. It can be said that the advance in the care of the sick was not important, although the so-called "enfermenas" or "hospitals" proliferated, institutions generally attached to convents.

a)   St. Basil and St. John Chrysostom founded the first asylums for children (Sebaste anno 335 and Caesarea anno 362).

b)   The Theodosian Code, as well as the Visigothic Laws forbade the sale of children.

c)   The Archpriest Dateus created a children's hospice in Milan in 815, and two centuries later Pope Innocent III founded the first organised "Casa Cuna" in Rome.

d)   In Spain, under the Arab influence, laws and manuscripts on the care of the mother and child were also developed from a legislative and scientific point of view. Already in the 10th century, one of the first treatises on obstetrics and paediatrics was published in Cordoba, called *"The book of the generation of the foetus, the treatment of pregnant women and newborns"*, whose author was Arib Ibn Sa'id.

The art of the Middle Ages transcribes this sympathy for childhood, showing scenes with the child and his mother as the protagonist, often religious (Virgin and Child) or of everyday life. Of great interest for our study is the content of the Regulations of the Hospital de la Santa Cruz in Barcelona, promulgated in 1417, in which the activity of nurses is reflected, within a hospital organisation and specifically, within the activities of the female staff, we find: *"...they also ordered that in the hospital there should be a woman of honest reputation and good manners, to take special care of the children, that is to say, to look after them and keep them clean"*.

We can affirm that in the 14th century we have a figure within the hospital institution, a faithful precursor of the current one. Throughout the 16th century, paediatrics was definitively identified as specialised medical knowledge, with many works already devoted to the study of children's illnesses. A concern for children and for the mission of women as mothers was evident, as can be seen in the work of the great humanist Juan Luis Vives (1492-1540). De subventione pauperum" by Fray Diego de Calahorra, among others, reveals a new social conscience: it is not enough to take care of helpless children in terms of physical care, they must also be educated.

In the second half of the 16th century, Santo Tomas de Villanueva converted part of the Epicopal Palace of Valencia into a hospice, and in 1567 the Inclusa of Madrid was founded, with the others appearing later. Somewhat later, around 1607, it can be seen in some minutes of the Plenary Session of the Cabildo de los Regidores de Sevilla, in which D. Andres Herrera remarks:

"Parents have been seen to have taken their poor little children of both sexes and left them at the gates of Seville, as well as those of Granada and Malaga. The same thing is done by some parents who live in these cities who, forgetting their natural and paternal love, abandon their children, leaving them in the contingency of never seeing them again, naked in the hands of the insult and rigour of the weather, hungry and begging for alms and obliged to collect themselves at night in the doors, plots or the entrance hall of the houses if they are allowed to do so".

The child care institutions in the 17th century had scarce means because they lived on charity; this, together with the lack of knowledge of hygienic practices and the correct preparation of milk mixtures for artificial lactation, were the factors causing high mortality (quoted by De Toni in his History of Child Care). In one maternity hospital in DubKn, out of 10,000 infants admitted between 1775 and 1796, 45 survived (99.6% mortality).

We must mention St. Vincent de Paul (1576-1660) as a champion of the time in favour of abandoned children. St Vincent de Paul recruited a large number of women for this cause and created an asylum, which in June 1670 was recognised by Louis XIV, giving birth to the "Hospice des enfants Trove".

The real development of medicine came, as with other areas of knowledge, with the Enlightenment, centred on the human intellect as a gwa, and man's self-knowledge, developing it in such a way that observation and experience became the basis of progress, benefiting all areas of it, with health attaining unusual social importance. In this period, greater interest was shown in the most neglected social strata and in illness as a social consequence. The first paediatric care institutions were established during this period, the first of which was the "Dispensary for Poor Children", founded in 1769 by G. Armstrong in London. Numerous works on paediatrics appeared in Europe, the culmination of which was the "Textbook on Paediatrics" by the Swede Nils Rosen von Rosenstein, published in 1765, who was the first to introduce the teaching of paediatrics, and who laid the foundations of paediatrics as a speciality, and consequently emphasised the specialisation of all professionals dedicated to the care of the child.

An important milestone in the history of paediatrics was the establishment of the Necker Hospital in Paris in 1778, which marked the birth of the French School of Paediatrics. This example soon spread throughout Europe, and new children's hospitals appeared, and new schools sprang up around them:

- Paediatric Clinic of the "Berliner Charite" (1830) in Germany.
- Hospital for Sick Children" in England.
- St Petersburg Paediatric Hospital" (1834), Russia.
- Hospital del Nino Jesus", (1876), in Madrid.

In spite of this scientific development, there are still children's institutions, mainly aimed at the illegitimate child, famous especially for their high mortality rate, which have been modernised and modern concepts of hygiene and prevention have been introduced into their structures, and the public authorities themselves have taken care of this by means of legislation:

- Rousell Law" (1874), in France.

- Rundwerfungung" (1880), in Germany.
- Infant Life Protection Act" (1872), in England.
- "Ley de Proteccion a la Infancia" (1904), in Spain.

The existence of paediatrics as an autonomous speciality within medical education did not appear in Spain until almost the end of the 19th century. In 1887, Dr. Criado Aguilar occupied the first chair of paediatrics founded at the University of Madrid. A few years earlier, in 1876, the first hospital dedicated exclusively to paediatric care had been founded in Madrid: the Hospital del Nino Jesus. The concern for infant mortality, whose main causes, apart from infectious diseases, were to be found in poor attendance at birth and nutritional deficiencies in the first days or weeks of a child's life, led to the creation, from the end of the 19th century, of institutions aimed at remedying these defects.

The origins of the "Clinics for babies with breasts and drops of milk" date back to the 19th century in France, and there are several people and key moments in their development. The first known maternity clinic is that of the Hospital de la Charité de Pans, opened in 1892 by the Frenchman Pierre Budin. In Spain, the arrival of the first maternity clinic was not long in coming. La Gota de Leche de San Sebastian opened to the public on 15 August 1902 and was officially inaugurated on 28 September 1903.

To speak of 20th century paediatrics is to speak of the great achievements that have occurred in this century in the field of preventive medicine. The development of vaccination programmes has even made it possible to eradicate diseases which, as in the case of smallpox, were responsible for a high morbidity and mortality rate. Advances in nutrition have evolved along with social and technological development; however, *"just when paediatricians in developed countries thought they had traditional diseases under control, migratory movements have brought back the old problems. In the meantime, the major ills of the Third World continue to exist and the richer children suffer from new ones, especially of a psychological nature"*.

Other facts such as the development of bloodless diagnostic techniques, the development of surgery and the advances in the field of obstetrics and neonatology have allowed a notable decrease in infant mortality. In this field it is worth mentioning the work developed by Dr. Virginia Apgar, the first connection of this doctor with the paediatrics was after the study that ended with the concretion of the Apgar score, it could be demonstrated that the children with a low score in the incipient Apgar scale were hypoxic and acidotic. The Apgar score was first investigated in 1949 and formally presented at a congress in 1952. This effective and easy method of assessing a newborn, at one minute (as initially proposed by Dr. Apgar) and at five minutes, is based on scores ranging from 0 to 2 for each of the parameters of heart rate, respirations, muscle tone, skin colour and reflexes.

The word *Paediatrics,* made up of the Greek words *Paidos* (child) and *latreia* (cure), is etymologically the *"Science that deals with the cure of the child"*. Modern paediatrics is a science that deals with the health of the child, but in its broadest sense, not only in the curative sense, which constitutes clinical or welfare paediatrics, and deals with the study and treatment of children's illnesses, but also in the preventive sense, child care, which takes care of the prevention of diseases and general hygiene of the healthy child, and Social Paediatrics as a part that takes care of the child, healthy or sick, but not as an isolated being, but included in his family environment and society, Rehabilitative Paediatrics, which is considered to simplify as a part of the last one. Nowadays, developmental paediatrics has been incorporated, which, as Cruz Hernandez says, is a new approach to children's medicine which is becoming more widespread, especially in developed countries, but which is of equal interest to all. Its aim is to promote an optimal state of physical and mental health and to ensure the early diagnosis and treatment of possible anomaKas.

Since the establishment of paediatrics as an independent branch of medicine, it has been a constant in the thinking of all the great masters to establish the concept of such a unique speciality, which breaks with the classical schemes, being a branch of medicine, but which is concerned with the human being as a whole, during a period of his or her life. Czerny, one of the great pioneers of European paediatrics, opened the academic year each year at the turn of the century with the following words addressed to his students: "*Paediatrics is internal medicine limited to the human being from the day of birth to puberty*". With these words he made clear, even in his early days, the concepts of an independent and total speciality in the care of the child. Jacobi, the proponent of American paediatrics, defined it at the end of the 19th century as follows: "*Paediatrics does not deal with miniature men and women, with reduced doses and with the same diseases in smaller bodies, but has its own rank and horizon, and gives to General Medicine as much as it receives from it*", thus perfectly establishing that paediatrics does not constitute a speciality according to the classical model, but represents a new concept, a chronological speciality, but with the category and doctrinal content of total medicine. The American Blackfan conceives it as: "*Paediatrics is not a speciality in the common sense of the term, because it does not deal with a single organ, but with the whole body. The diseases of childhood and their treatment do not constitute the whole of modern paediatrics, because, although their study is important, the problems of growth and development which have a direct relation to the preservation of health, both physical and mental, and the prevention of disease, are emphasised. Paediatrics aims not only to maintain health, but to actively promote the physical and mental aptitudes and well-being of the child*". This advanced and current conception brings together the three aspects of paediatrics: oncological, preventive and social, to which we must add developmental paediatrics.

In our country, prominent paediatricians have also explored the concept of paediatrics from the point of view of a singular speciality, as follows: Collado points out that: "*paediatric medicine studies the child in its aspects of care, teaching and research, with the ultimate aim of monitoring, maintaining and, when necessary, recovering his or her health*". Sanchez Villares, expresses this conceptual notion as follows: "*From its beginnings, paediatrics has acquired the conceptual characterisation of a different sign to that of the classical specialities. Its main objective is not the attention to an organ, apparatus, system or illness, nor even to the illnesses of the child. Its true personality is provided by the biological attributes of the period of existence from birth to the end of adolescence, during which the phenomena of growth and evolutionary maturation take place. It is these attributes which confer peculiarities, both in terms of the preservation of health and in terms of illness situations, as well as in terms of the problems posed by their treatment or care".*

More recently, the same Sanchez Villares says: *"Among its objectives are included all those relating to the care of the healthy child in the first years of life, those of prevention in the rest of the infant period (Preventive Paediatrics), those aimed at the total and continuous care of the child in a state of illness (Clinical Paediatrics), and those relating to the healthy and sick child in its correlation with the physical and human environment in which it develops in an uninterrupted manner and with its own rhythm (Social Paediatrics)".*

For Cruz Hernandez: *"Paediatrics is the science of the child and its diseases. If in terms of its scientific content it is the total medicine of the infant age, in terms of its chronological limits it is medicine applied to a period of life that begins at birth and ends with adolescence".* But perhaps the most complete conceptual definition of Paediatrics, which we believe faithfully expresses its current notion, was given in 1979 by the Commission of Paediatrics and its medical specialities of the A.E.P., constituted by experts who define Paediatrics as: *"The integral medicine of the evolutionary period of human existence, which runs from conception to the end of adolescence"*; paediatrics is concerned with the care of the healthy child (preventive paediatrics), with the integral, total and continuous medical care in the state of illness (clinical paediatrics) and with its individual and community interrelations, with the physical and human environment in which it develops in an uninterrupted manner, and with its own characteristics (social paediatrics). From this definition we can deduce the need to include the prenatal period, since with the progress made with the development of new diagnostic techniques and even intra-uterine treatment, in which the paediatrician can collaborate.

According to the Committee of Experts of the Pan American Health Organisation (PAHO) in 1969, "the child is a dependent, growing being, with peculiar biological characteristics, vulnerable to multiple pathological processes, which is influenced in intrauterine life and projected into adulthood.

The basic peculiarities that condition the separation between adult and child medicine, as independent sciences, obey to different orders, and constitute the biological, medical, social and psychological foundations of paediatrics.

Many anatomical and functional characteristics of the infant organism are markedly different from those of the adult:

a)   *Growth.* It is the main characteristic of infancy, and common to all of it. It is more pronounced the closer one is to birth. This causes a continuous evolution, that the child organism of today is not the same as it was yesterday or will be tomorrow, justifying different reactions to the same cause. Paediatrics is responsible for the study of growth and development in its physical, psychological and social aspects.

b)   *Morphological evolution.* The child not only grows, but its morphology changes, a clear example being the proportion between the head and the total length of the body, which in the newborn is 1/4 and in the adult 1/8, and there are many other examples at other levels of the organism.

c) *Organic immaturity*. The human being presents at birth certain still immature functions, which will be perfected until reaching adulthood.

d) *Importance of nutrition and metabolism*. The fact that it is precisely in the paediatric age when growth and development are most active means that correct and adequate nutrition is of transcendental importance, as it is the mainstay of growth and development.

e) *Immune peculiarities*. The infant is born with a passive immunity, transmitted from its mother, but its specific and unspecific immunity is immature, however, it is capable of forming antibodies in its early stages, if subjected to sufficiently potent stimuli. In addition, the limiting barriers are often insufficient, and often a gateway for infections. Throughout childhood, the child builds up its immunity at the expense of repeated infectious processes (clinical or subcKnical), and the lymphatic system plays an important role in this.

f) *Functional solidarity*. It is rare for a pathological process in one organ or system of the child not to have repercussions on others, with immune insufficiency, and neurovegetative and metabolic lability being conditioning factors in these responses.

Bibliograffa

1. Bartsocas S. *La puericulture dans l'Antiquite grecque*. Arch Fr Pediatr. 1955; 12: 71-83.

2. Arib Ibn Sa'id. *The book of the generation of the foetus, the treatment of pregnant women and newborns. Treatise of the 10th century.* Arjona Castro, Ed. 1991.

3. Granjel LS. *History of Spanish Paediatrics*. Barcelona. XVI International Congress of Paediatrics, 1980.

4. Crespo M. *A new paediatrics*. Pediatr Integral 1998;3(2):193-207.

5. Cruz M. *Paediatrics: basic concepts*. In Tratado de Pediatna. 7^ Edition. Barcelona, Ed. Spaxs, 1993.

6. Galdo Munoz G. *Bases historicas de la Pediatna*. Actualidad Medica. 1983; 69: 39-52.

7. Hernandez, M.: *Physiology of Growth and Somatic Development*. In: Sanchez Villares: Pediatna basica. Ed. Idepsa. Madrid. 1980.

8. Stickler, GB: *Clinical guidelines for the paediatrician*. Pediatrics (ed.esp), 1987, 24:57-58.

9. Kofman, I et al.: *Curso General de Pediatna*. Volume I, part one. Ed. Ergon. 1.981

10. Gartfa C.: *Pediatna social*. Ed. D^az de Santos S.A., Madrid, 1994.

11. W.H.O. *Research in Paediatrics*. Technical Report Series, n S 440. 1980.

2.Term and preterm newborn. Initial care of the newborn.

Dr. Jose Uberos Fernandez

Dr. Elisabeth Fernandez Marin

The WHO defines a premature newborn as a baby born before 37 weeks gestational age.

Although "maturity" "prematurity" and "gestational age" "preterm" may be considered synonymous, in reality they are not, with "prematurity" referring to those born at less than 2500 g or those born below gestational age and "preterm" to all newborns born before 37 weeks gestational age. Term newborns are those born between 37 and 42 weeks postmenstrual age and post-term newborns are those born at more than 42 weeks postmenstrual age.

Newborn at term

The status of the newborn is defined by gestational age, weight and presence of pathology.

Gestational age. This is the time elapsed from the first day of the last menstrual period (LMP) until birth. It is established that term gestation is 40 weeks. For clinical purposes, a full term NB is between 37 and 42 weeks gestation. If it is 36 weeks or less, it is preterm, and if it is 42 weeks or more, it is post-term or postmature.

Table 2.1. Birth classification by gestational age.

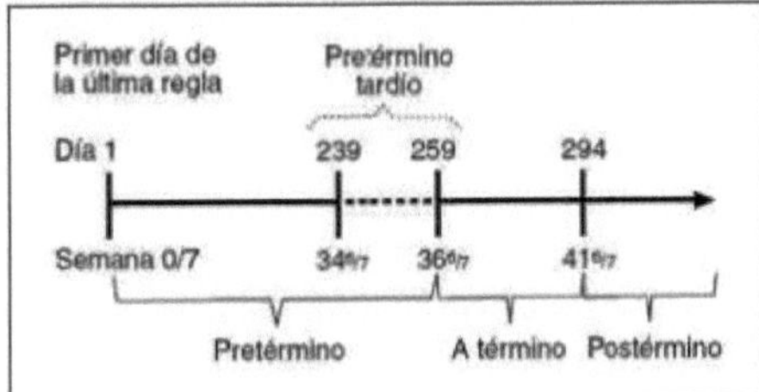

Prematuro	< 37 semanas
Prematuro extremo	< 28⁰ semanas
Gran prematuro	28⁶ a 31⁶ semanas
Prematuro moderado	32 a 33⁶ semanas
Prematuro tardío	34⁰ a 36⁶ semanas
A término	37⁰ a 41⁶ semanas
A término precoz	37⁰ a 38⁶ semanas
A término tardío	39⁰ a 41⁶ semanas
Postérmino	42⁰ o más semanas

Weight. It should be assessed in relation to gestational age and is appropriate when it is between the 10th and 90th percentile. These values represent approximately 2,500 to 4,000 g for a full term baby. When the weight is below the 10th percentile, it refers to a low birth weight for gestational age; on the other hand, a weight above the 90th percentile refers to a high birth weight for gestational age. Generally, a baby weighing less than 2,500 g is referred to as underweight and a baby weighing more than 4,000 g is referred to as macrosomic.

Assessment of neonatal status. It should be carried out through:

a)   Anamnesis with maternal, obstetric and perinatal data

b)   Complete clinical examination of the newborn, as well as scores on various scales (Apgar, Silverman).

c)   Gestational age determination

d)   Weight assessment.

The normal neonatal state is that of a full-term infant, of adequate weight and without pathological disorders.

Apgar test

The Apgar test is a rapid test performed at the first and fifth minute after birth, established by Virginia Apgar in 1952. The score at minute 1 determines how well the newborn tolerated the birth process and is related to the pH in umbilical arterial blood. The score at minute 5 is related to the response to resuscitation measures, therefore, in cases of perinatal asphyxia it is an indicator of the duration of asphyxia and is related to the neurological prognosis of asphyxia. It is sometimes assessed at 10 and 15 minutes as a prognostic indicator.

The Apgar test takes into consideration the following parameters. Each of these categories is given a score of 0, 1 or 2 according to the condition observed.

- Respiratory effort: If the newborn is not breathing, the score is 0. If the breaths are slow or irregular, the baby's respiratory effort score is 1. If the newborn cries well, the respiratory score is 2.
- Heart rate: The heart rate is assessed with the stethoscope. This is the most important assessment. If there is no heartbeat, the infant scores 0 in heart rate. If the heart rate is less than 100 beats per minute, the newborn's score is 1 in heart rate. If the heart rate is greater than 100 beats per minute, the newborn's score is 2 in heart rate.
- Muscle tone: This is assessed by passive flexion tone, normal in the newborn. If there is no flexion of all four limbs a score of 0 is given, if there is only flexion of the lower limbs a score of 1 is given, if there is flexion of all four limbs a score of 2 is given.
- Reflexes: If there is no reaction, the newborn scores 0 for reflex irritability. If there is grimacing or grimacing, the newborn scores 1 for reflex irritability. If there is grimacing and a cough, sneeze or vigorous cry, the newborn scores 2 for increased irritability reflex.
- Skin colour: If the skin colour is pale blue on the finger pads and lips, the newborn scores 0 for colour. If the colour is pink on the lips and blue on the fingers, the score is 1, if the colour is pink on both, the score is 2.

The Silverman and Anderson test is a test that assesses the respiratory distress of a newborn, based on five criteria. Each parameter is quantifiable and the sum total is interpreted in terms of difficulty. A score of 1 to 4 indicates mild respiratory distress, 5 to 7 is moderate and above 7 is severe.

- Thoracic or abdominal elevation: synchronised (0), little elevation on inspiration (1), thoracoabdominal wobble (2).
- Ribbing: none (0), barely visible (1), marked (2).
- Xiphoid retraction: none (0), barely visible (1), marked (2).
- Nasal flaring: absent (0), minimal (1), marked (2).
- Whining: absent (0), audible with stethoscope (1), audible without stethoscope (2).

Growth and development

Weight. The birth weight is subject to variations depending on sex (higher weight in boys), parental constitution, social situation of the parents (malnourished mothers or with toxic habits due to tobacco, alcohol or other drugs), race, maternal or gestational disease and other factors such as maternal work or altitude above sea level. The weight in the first days after birth undergoes a so-called "physiological loss", which reaches approximately 10% and starts to recover from the 5th day onwards, to be the same as at birth on the 9th or 10th day. This physiological weight loss has been linked to an increased fluid loss related to the low neonatal urine concentration capacity.

Length. The average length at birth is 50 cm, with differences related to the same factors that condition weight. The normal lower Kmite is 46 cm.

Periods. The average cephalic circumference of the healthy term newborn is 34 cm. The thoracic penis measured at the level of the nipples should be 2 cm less than the cephalic penis. In the absence of pathology, the sitting height should be equal to the maximum cranial penmetre. Cranial penmetre is the parameter that best relates to gestational age. Brachial penmetre and tricipital fold, which are less commonly used, relate well to nutritional status.

Bone maturation. Although there are differences with gestational age, at birth, most term infants have *six secondary ossification points*: the inferior epiphysis of the femur, the superior epiphysis of the tibia, the proximal epiphysis of the humerus and three of the tarsus (calcaneus, astragalus and cuboid).

Nutritional status. During the neonatal period it is assessed with the weight in relation to gestational age, when it is below the 10th percentile it indicates a situation of malnutrition. In the newborn, the relationship between weight and height is assessed by the Rohrer index (weight in grams/height in cm).[3]

Newborn care

The care of the normal newborn aims to monitor the normal adaptation process of the newborn and to help the mother to understand the characteristics of the newborn and physiological phenomena that do not occur at any other age. The care of every newborn includes at least one special assessment at three points in time during the first days of life: immediate care at birth, during the transition period (first hours of life), at about 6 to 24 hours prior to discharge with the mother from the hospital.

1. ***Immediate evaluation.*** The first assessment and examination of the newborn includes the following aspects:

• Assessment of respiration, heart rate and colour. If these are altered, follow the newborn resuscitation algorithms described in subsequent chapters of this book.

• Apgar test. At one minute and at 5 minutes. More than 70 years after its description, this test is still fully valid as an expression of the good vital adaptation of the newborn to the extra-uterine stage.

• Rule out major malformations. Some are life-threatening emergencies that may present immediately or within the first hours and days of life: choanal atresia, diaphragmatic hernia, oesophageal atresia, pulmonary hypoplasia, renal malformations, spinal dysraphism, ambiguous genitalia, and anal imperforation. Clinical semiology and guided physical examination together with certain procedures (e.g. passage of nasogastric tube) allow to rule out the main malformations that carry a higher life-threatening risk, if not detected in a timely manner.

• Anthropometry and first gestational age assessment. Gestational age and weight will allow the classification of the newborn. For the parents it is very important to provide quick information on sex, weight, height, absence of malformations in a preliminary report.

2. ***Transitional care.*** The first hours of a newborn's life require special monitoring of temperature, vital signs and general clinical status. This should be done together with the mother if the child has no problems, taking care that good temperature control is maintained.

During the first hours of life the most important changes in the adaptation of the newborn to the extra-uterine environment take place. There are variations in respiratory rate, heart rate, alertness and motor activity. During the first 15 to 30 minutes of life, a tachycardia of up to 180 beats/minute (first 3 minutes), breathing of 60 to 80 beats/minute, sometimes somewhat irregular, and some rib retraction and nasal flaring may be common.

Secretions in the mouth are frequent. The body temperature and especially the skin temperature always drops. This first stage has been called the first period of reactivity. In the following hours, the heart rate decreases to 120-140 beats/minute and the respiratory rate to less than 60 breaths/minute. The child appears calmer and tends to fall asleep. This period lasts about 2 to 6 hours, followed by a second period of reactivity. The child is more active and very responsive to stimuli.

Passage of urine and meconium. The first urine output and meconium expulsion (first bowel movements of the newborn) are recorded. 92% of newborns pass their first urine within the first 24 hours of life, a high percentage of them in the delivery room. All should have done so by 48 hours of life. Otherwise a renal or urinary tract abnormality should be suspected. As for meconium expulsion, about 69% do so in the first 12 hours of life, 94% in the first 24 hours and 99% within 48 hours of life.

3.   *The puerperal period.* This period is of great importance from an educational and preventive point of view. The mother is in a unique position to take an interest in and acquire knowledge and educational content that will facilitate the subsequent care of her child.

• Breastfeeding. This is one of the moments to provide the mother with information regarding breastfeeding and its advantages, to receive support for its initiation and technique and to be reassured regarding common breastfeeding problems. The support of all health care staff during her stay in the hospital is decisive for good breastfeeding.

• Appearance of meconium and transitional stools. The stools of the first few days change in colour, consistency and frequency. The meconium, which at the beginning is very dark greenish brown, almost black, changes to a lighter brown colour. Between the 3rd[er] and 4th day, the stools take on the typical golden yellow colour of breastfeeding. From the 2nd and 3rd[er] days onwards, it is common for the baby to pass a stool every time he is put to the breast with a lot of noise, expelling semi-fluid and foamy stools. It is important to explain to the mother that this is normal. The primigest mother requires special attention in this respect.

• Colour and skin. In the first 24 hours and after the first 2 hours of life it is normal for babies to have a pinkish or reddish colour. It is common for the hands and feet to be pale and somewhat bluish in colour. On the second or third day, erythematous-papular spots often appear, known as erythema toxicum neonatorum. This is variable in intensity with an irregular distribution, preferably on the trunk and extremities. Occasionally, some of the papules have a small pustule in the centre. Washing with a neutral soap reduces the intensity of this erythema. It is easily differentiated from other skin lesions of pathological character.

• Jaundice. The mother should be aware that this is a phenomenon that occurs to varying degrees in most newborns during the first days of life. It is not a disease and only in exceptional cases is it pathological. However, it is also important to know that exceptionally jaundice can be severe and that bilirubin levels can reach potentially dangerous levels.

- Behaviour and reflexes. The position and tone of the newborn as well as the reflex movements are unfamiliar to the expectant mother. She is particularly struck by the Moro reflex, which is produced with a wide variety of stimuli. All these facts seem very abnormal in an adult or older child.
- Hormonal effects. Maternal hormones related to gestation remain circulating in the newborn during the first days and often cause an increase in mammary size. This occurs in both sexes around the 5th day when lacteal secretion appears, which can be observed by compressing the mammary nodule. Occasionally in girls a pseudo menstruation may appear. These are normal phenomena which disappear spontaneously.
- Evolution of weight. In the first few days, it is physiological that weight loss occurs. This is a physiological fact within a certain range. A drop of 7 to 10% of the birth weight is accepted as normal. This is regained around the 7th day. When this has not been achieved by the tenth day, special reinforcement of breastfeeding is required and the need for supplementation with a starter formula should be evaluated. Children under 3 kg generally drop less, and those over 4 kg may drop more and take longer to regain their birth weight.
- Care of the umbilical cord. The umbilical cord suffers from dry gangrene, which is more rapid the more contact it has with the air. After 5 to 10 days it falls off. Humidity prolongs this process, so bathing should be postponed until two days after it has fallen off. The umbilicus is a potential entry point for infection, so care should be taken to clean it with alcohol or other local antiseptic at each change of comb. It is normal for the base of the umbilicus to have some moisture and yellow-fibrinous discharge. It is not normal to have purulent discharge or redness around the umbilicus, which should raise suspicion of infection. An umbilical hernia is often present and becomes more noticeable after the cord has fallen off. In the vast majority of cases this does not require treatment and disappears spontaneously before the age of 4 years.

General appearance

In the first hours of life, the **face** is usually puffy, with palpebral oedema that makes it difficult to open the eyes. After one or two days, these signs disappear and the constitutional or pathological facial features become more evident. Subconjunctival haemorrhages are sometimes seen in the eyes, but these will disappear spontaneously. The nose should be checked for patency and symmetry of the nostrils to rule out traumatic dislocation of the nasal septum, which is common in facial deliveries. In the neck, special attention should be paid to the sternocleidomastoid, due to the frequency of a nodule or haematoma, and to rule out fistulas.

Thorax. It is bell-shaped, the ribs being horizontal and not oblique as is the case at later ages. Muscle tissue is scarce and, when present, agenesis of the pectoralis major can be detected, as in Poland's syndrome, which also presents hypomastia or unilateral amastia. The clavicles should be explored to rule out the presence of a fracture: pain, swelling, crepitus, asymmetrical Moro reflex.

Abdomen. Slightly bulging, above the level of the thorax. There is physiological hepatomegaly which may extend beyond the costal margin. The spleen is palpable in some children. The kidneys are usually not palpable.

Limbs. They are short, with the lower limbs showing a curvature of the tibiae, a physiological deformity which may persist until the end of the second year of life, as it is usually accentuated at the age of the first steps. Both hips should be carefully explored with the Ortolani and Barlow manoeuvres to rule out congenital dislocation or coxofemoral dysplasia. Femoral pulses should also be palpated.

Attitude or posture. The term newborn adopts flexion of arms and legs with a discrete degree of physiological hypertension (comfort attitude). Preterm babies between 35 and 37 weeks usually adopt the "frog" attitude: hypotonic lower limbs, open book. In breech delivery the lower extremities usually have different anomaKas of position.

Head. It is moulded during delivery and is usually oval or "apexed" in shape. It is common to find a discrete soft tissue tumefaction, which constitutes the so-called *"caput sucedaneum"* or birth tumour: it should be distinguished from cephalohaematoma or subperiosteal haemorrhage. It should be distinguished from cephalohaematoma or subperiosteal haemorrhage. There may also be a parietal endometrium, with a consequent reduction in the size of the fontanelles, which may even be inappreciable on palpation. A few hours after delivery, the diameter of the anterior fontanel is 3-4 cm.

Digestive system

Mouth. With thick lips and sometimes with a central prominence on the upper lip, called a *suction callus*. Enaas are toothless, although congenital teeth may sometimes be present (one per 2,000 live births), which can cause ulcers at the base of the tongue and the theoretical risk of aspiration if they become dislodged. *Inclusion cysts* are small, hard, whitish nodules in the enaa that disappear spontaneously and can be mistaken for congenital teeth. On the soft palate there is often a fine, whitish stippling called *palatine millium, Bohn's nodules* or *Epstein's epithelial pearls.*

The stomach has a capacity of approximately 30 ml, from 28 weeks gestational age the secretory function is normal, with sufficient lactase for normal lactase digestion and with an underdeveloped autonomic nervous system which explains the hypervagotonia involved in the development of infant colic and gastro-oesophageal reflux. Gastric emptying begins immediately after ingestion and is completed within 2-4 hours.

The LMP presents a relative functional insufficiency with enzymatic immaturity represented by the defect of the enzyme glucuronyltransferase, responsible for the physiological jaundice of the newborn. Fat absorption is impaired in the premature infant and polyunsaturated fats and medium chain triglycerides (MCT) are better absorbed.

Respiratory system

After birth, the newborn undergoes major physiological changes, mainly due to pulmonary expansion and decreased pulmonary vascular resistance. The newborn has a physiological tachypnoea of 40-60 breaths/minute. The intensity, rhythm and type of respiratory movements, as well as the possible presence of thoracic retraction and superimposed noises, should also be taken into account in the examination. The *Silverman and Andersen score*, based on clinical parameters, measures neonatal respiratory distress.

Circulatory system

At birth, placental circulation is interrupted and pulmonary circulation is established, with a decrease in pulmonary vascular resistance and a consequent decrease in pulmonary pressure, which will be lower than the systemic pressure. During the first week of life, the increase in PaO2 leads to maturation of the pulmonary arterioles towards vessels of low resistance. In situations of sustained hypoxaemia this transition does not occur and high pulmonary resistances persist, leading to pulmonary hypertension, also known as persistence of foetal circulation.

There are three physiological arteriovenous shunts in the foetus which are abolished under normal conditions after birth. The foramen ovale and the ductus arteriosus close functionally progressively and transient murmurs may be heard. The ductus venosus connects the umbilical vein to the inferior vena cava. The ductus arteriosus connects the pulmonary artery to the aorta. In the newborn there is physiological tachycardia of 120-150 beats/minute.

Genitourinary system

The most significant feature of the newborn's urinary system is its inability to concentrate urine. Among the factors that may contribute to the low renal concentrating ability of the neonate the most interesting are: reduced glomerular filtration rate, short loop of Henle in the cortical and juxtamedullary glomerulus, low nitrogen metabolism with low serum nitrogen concentrations and low renal medullary osmolality. Both glomerular filtration rate and tubular function is about 1/3 of that observed at later ages. In the first 24 hours, diuresis is scarce and a brick-red sediment can be seen in the first urine samples, which is due to urate deposition. After 48-72 hours, diuresis is normal, 1.5-2 ml/kg/hour.

In relation to the male genitalia, phimosis (rarely complete) is frequent, as well as balanopreputial adhesion and uni- or bilateral hydrocele. In girls, the labia majora are underdeveloped and may leave the hymen, labia minora and the opening of the urethra visible. There is often a vaginal discharge with desquamative cells (physiological desquamative vulvovaginitis) and even a haemorrhagic discharge related to breast intumescence and facial acne, related to maternal hormone levels. Synechia of the labia minora may be seen in the neonatal period or, rather, later.

Haematological and immunological characteristics

The haemoglobin count is 5.5 to 6 x 10^6 /mm3 on average increased compared to the adult. Foetal haemoglobin constitutes 70% of the haemoglobin of the child at birth and gradually disappears and is replaced by adult haemoglobin. The normal haematocrit value ranges from 45 to 60%. Leukocytes are normally elevated, from 10,000 to 25,000 in the first 48 hours.

Nervous system - Assessment of motor development

The autonomic nervous system is well developed, there is a situation of hypervagotome already mentioned. The newborn behaves to a large extent as a subcortical and medullary "mesencephalic" being, with a tendency to irritability, hypertonia and spontaneous reflex movements (archaic reflexes). These aspects are developed in later chapters of this book.

Post-mature newborn

Post-preterm or post-term newborn is a newborn whose pregnancy has lasted 42 weeks or more. These infants may be of adequate, low or high birth weight for their gestational age. Between 4.5 and 9.5 per cent of all deliveries are post-term pregnancies, in which perinatal mortality is increased.

Factors influencing post-maturity can be grouped into maternal, foetal and idiopathic.

• Maternal factors: Uterine malformations, malnutrition, primiparity, genital infantileism, pelvic narrowness, decreased progesterone production, prolonged bed rest, comfortable standard of living.

• Fetal: Trisom^as 13 and 18

• Idiopathic

The most frequent characteristics are: apparent weight loss, unusual alert appearance, lively gaze, absence of vernix caseosa, dry and parchment-like skin, wrinkled "washerwoman's" hands, with early and intense desquamation, elongated and brittle hands, absent lanugo, and usually a greenish colouring of the umbilical cord and skin. She will often have required resuscitation manoeuvres in the delivery room, and will have had both meconium and amniotic fluid aspiration and secondary pulmonary hypertension. Hypoglycaemia is common, as is hyponatraemia; haemoglobin values are high, with albuminuria and glycosuria in a large number of infants.

Preterm newborn

Approximately 8% of live newborns are preterm, of which approximately 1% are ELBW infants (Figure 1). Gestational age largely determines survival, so we distinguish between "moderate preterm", between 32-36 weeks, with low mortality in our environment, and "late preterm", those born between 34 and 36 weeks of gestational age. Extreme preterm", less than 32 weeks (generally weighing less than 1,500 g), also called "very low birth weight infants" (VLBW infants); within this group, "very extreme preterm" or "very low birth weight infants" (VLBW infants), with gestational age less than 28 weeks and generally weighing less than 1,000 g.

Prematurity is responsible for more than half of all neonatal deaths. ELBW infants account for 1.5% of all live births in our setting, but contribute 50% of total neonatal mortality. In spite of all the efforts made in the medical and research fields, the frequency of prematurity in developed countries is increasing. In the United States, the number of preterm births has risen from 9.5% in 1981 to 12.7% in 2005. In Denmark, with universal health coverage and optimal prenatal care standards, it has also been shown that the increase and proportion of preterm births has risen by 22% from 1995 to 2004. Risk factors for prematurity include maternal age and ethnicity. In our setting, the age of mothers of very low birth weight preterm infants has progressively increased from an average of 30.3 (SD 5.6) years in 2008 to 34.4 (SD 3.9) years in 2014.

In relation to ethnicity, the prevalence of prematurity in the black population (16%) is twice that in the white population (8.4%). Other factors implicated in prematurity such as multiple gestations account for 12-27% of all preterm births. Other possible predisposing factors considered include infection, stress, poor nutrition, drug use, metabolic imbalance and inherited factors. Looking at each of the risk factors individually, the most significant predictor of preterm birth is a previous preterm birth. In fact, studies on twins and recurrences in families confirm that the recurrence of prematurity in subsequent gestations is 3 - 7 times higher in medically induced preterm births and in extreme preterm births; in addition, there is a higher risk of recurrence of preterm birth at the same gestational age in the next gestation. Therefore, in the opinion of some authors, genetics may explain about 40% of the risk of prematurity.

There are three primary categories of prematurity: 1) Medically indicated preterm birth, resulting from specific conditions such as pre-eclampsia or intrauterine growth restriction and affecting both mother and foetus; this category accounts for 30-35% of all preterm deliveries. 2) 25-30% of preterm deliveries are caused by premature rupture of membranes and are closely related to infection, placental abruption or anatomical defects. 3) in 35-45% of cases preterm labour is spontaneous, with no clear aetiology.

Clinical manifestations and complications

The alterations that a preterm newborn presents depend fundamentally on the gestational age. *Early* life-threatening *disorders in* preterm infants in the first week of life are:

1. Poor control of thermoregulation with frequent tendency to hypothermia.
2. Respiratory disorders: hyaline membrane disease, apnoea crises.
3. Cardiocirculatory disorders: early arterial hypotension and persistent ductus arteriosus.
4. Encephalic lesions, related to anoxia and intraventricular haemorrhage.
5. Feeding difficulties, leading to malnutrition; paralphtic liver, meconium plug and necrotic enterocolitis.
6. Tendency to metabolic disorders: hypo/hyperglycaemia, hypocalcaemia, hyperbilirubinaemia, hypo/hypernatraemia, hypo/hyperkalaemia, hypophosphataemia.

Among the *disorders* or *complications are* retinopathy of prematurity, anaemia, osteopenia of prematurity, late respiratory disorders (bronchopulmonary dysplasia, aspiration) and central nervous system disorders (post-hemorrhagic hydrocephalus, periventricular leukomalacia).

Morphological characteristics of the preterm new-born baby

Growth. Weight is less than 2,500 g. Physiological weight loss is intense (up to 15% of birth weight) and recovery is slow. Length is proportional to immaturity and always less than 47 cm at birth. As a gwa, apart from the tables, it should be remembered that from the 5th month, when the foetus measures 25 cm, the foetus grows 5 cm every 4 weeks. The cranial penmetre is always less than 33 cm at birth.

General morphology. The large size of the head and the poor development of the lower limbs, which are slender, with little muscular development, no fatty muscle and covered with thin skin, are striking. The nails are soft and short. The transverse folds on the soles of the feet are limited to the one on the front side.

Skull and face. The sutures are open and the fontanel is wide. The cranial bones are soft (craniotabes of prematurity). The hair is short and underdeveloped. Palpebral aperture occurs at 25-26 weeks of gestation. The pinnae are small, soft and poorly developed. The face is sharp and wrinkled.

Skin. Reddish at first, soon turns pale. Jaundice is early, intense and prolonged. The absence of adipose muscle makes the vessels easily visible through the skin and the bony reliefs stand out. Distal cyanosis is frequent, as well as oedema. There is a large amount of lanugo.

Genitalia. From the 28th week of gestation, the testis at the entrance of the inguinal canal is guided by the *gubernaculum testis* into the scrotum, which it reaches by the 35th week. In girls the labia majora do not cover the labia minora. The mammary glands are underdeveloped and the mammary intumescence common in the term newborn does not usually appear. Bilateral inguinal and umbilical hernias are common.

Functional characteristics

Respiratory system. Breathing movements are rapid, shallow and irregular. Periodic breathing is characterised by apnoeic episodes lasting 5 to 10 seconds with no change in heart rate or colour, as opposed to apnoeic crises lasting more than 20 seconds, with bradycardia and cyanosis. Respiratory disorders are due to: surfactant deficiency (hyaline membrane disease), immaturity of the respiratory centres (physiological respiratory acidosis) and respiratory complications (infectious pneumonias, aspiration syndrome).

Digestive system. The sucking and swallowing reflexes are weakened and coordination between the two does not appear until 32-34 weeks. The musculature of the mouth has little strength. At 28-30 weeks of gestation, the preterm baby has the same digestive capacity as a normal newborn, although insufficient fat absorption leads to steatorrhoea. The aforementioned alterations easily lead to two opposite situations: if feeding is scarce, intense weight loss, hypoglycaemia, acidosis, hypoproteinaemia and malnutrition appear; if it is excessive, vomiting, gastric dilatation or necrotic enterocolitis may appear.

Thermoregulation. The absence of brown fat in the premature newborn means that a constant feature is hypothermia, although there is also a tendency to hyperthermia caused by environmental factors, due to poor management of the thermoregulatory mechanisms.

Nervous system. The premature infant is drowsy. It has hypotoma and the reflexes of the newborn are diminished or absent. The central nervous system is very sensitive to aggressions such as perinatal asphyxia or acidosis, which can favour the appearance of intraventricular haemorrhage and periventricular leukomalacia.

Sensory disturbances. The most affected is the eye. The iris is poorly pigmented, eye movements are very uncoordinated. Retinal vascularisation is complete after premature birth. Uncontrolled vascular proliferation is the cause of *retinopathy of prematurity, the* cause of amaurosis.

Circulatory system. Variable tachycardia. Extreme preterm babies have a tendency to arterial hypotension in the first hours of life. Functional and transient murmurs are frequent. Persistent ductus arteriosus may be seen in extreme preterm infants and is related to increased intravenous fluid intake.

Urinary system. As a consequence of renal immaturity, albuminuria, glycosuria and discrete haematuria are frequent.

Haematopoietic organs. In the red series, a higher number of erythroblasts is initially observed (20%). The physiological polyglobulia disappears quickly, so hyperbilirubinaemia will also become more frequent. Anaemia of prematurity soon sets in. During the first 10-15 days it is mainly iatrogenic, due to repeated extractions for laboratory tests.

The secretion of erythropoietin, which starts in the foetal midgut, moves progressively along the gestational period to the kidney at the end of gestation, thus moving from a secretion of low sensitivity to stigmata to a high sensitivity to stigmata, mainly to hypoxic stigmata. Some authors (5), have proposed a *fetal type* of O_2-independent erythropoietin secretion, which takes place in the liver, and an *adult type* of O_2-dependent erythropoietin secretion, which takes place in the kidney.

In the white series, there is a tendency to leukopenia and after 2-3 weeks and coinciding with weight recovery, eosinophilia is usually observed. In the platelet series, normal platelet counts are observed, but there are alterations in aggregation. From 6 months of life onwards, thrombocytosis may be found. Hypoprothrombinaemia and increased clotting time are also observed.

Immunity. Neutropenia, low maternal IgG and lack of IgA and IgM are common. Phagocytosis and bactericidal capacity of leukocytes and inflammatory response are decreased.

Prognosis of prematurity

Prematurity is responsible for more than half of all neonatal deaths. ELBW infants account for 1.5% of all live births in our setting, but contribute 50% to total neonatal mortality.

Retinopathy of prematurity. ROP is defined as a fibro- and vasculoproliferative vitreoretinopathy that occurs as a consequence of abnormal retinal vascularisation in preterm infants (< 1500 grams birth weight or < 32 weeks gestational age) and may result in loss of visual acuity or blindness.

Bronchopulmonary dysplasia. Bronchopulmonary dysplasia (BPD) is a chronic lung disease of multifactorial origin characterised by an early lesion that affects mainly the most immature newborns. Its incidence is related to gestational age, coexisting infections, nutrition and genetic factors. The average prevalence for very low birth weight infants is about 40%.

Necrotic enterocolitis. Necrotic enterocolitis (NEC) is defined as coagulative necrosis and inflammation of the infant's intestine. It is another comorbidity present in our environment in 15% of very low birth weight infants.

Preterm newborn care

Assistance during delivery. Whenever the birth of a premature infant is expected, a specialised team, a prepared portable incubator and resuscitation devices should be present in the delivery room. The baby should be received gently, wrapped in a dry, warm, sterile cloth. Late clamping of the umbilical cord is recommended (wait until 30-60 seconds of life). Respiratory resuscitation should be performed if necessary, according to the resuscitation protocol (see Neonatal Resuscitation Seminar).

Feeding. Preference is given to breastfeeding, however, the energy requirements of the preterm infant may be greater than those provided by breast milk, and fortifiers are often used.

Control of thermoregulation. Place these infants in a thermal cot or incubator, at a neutral temperature in relation to weight and age. A humid atmosphere proportional to the degree of immaturity should be maintained.

Infection prevention. Systematic administration of antibiotics should be avoided, unless there are coexisting infectious risk factors. An important aspect is to surround the preterm infant in an aseptic environment, including confinement to the incubator, use of gowns, proper cleaning of hands and forearms with the handling of each infant, use of gloves and sterilisation of the main equipment.

Control of respiratory disorders. Oxygen should be administered only if the blood gases indicate it, maintaining a transcutaneous PaO2 between 50 and 80 mmHg and Hb saturation between 90 and 93%. Apnoea crises should be treated with diffuse skin stimulation, and if breathing does not start, bag and mask ventilation should be used after suctioning of mucus.

Other treatments. Preterm newborns, especially the most extreme and in the first hours of life, should be handled with great care and disturbed as little as possible. As soon as their condition permits, visits and contact with the parents should be facilitated in order to develop the necessary stimuli and emotional bonds. In order to prevent osteopenia in premature infants, in addition to vitamin $_{D3}$, formulas with a high calcium and phosphorus content should be prescribed, or breast milk should be fortified. Regarding anaemia of prematurity, blood transfusions are useful in its treatment, but the administration of recombinant human erythropoietin associated with iron reduces transfusion needs. To prevent iron deficiency anaemia, iron administration is also useful.

Hospital discharge. This will be given when the baby feeds properly every 3 hours and gains adequate weight. It generally assumes a gestational age of 34-35 weeks and a body weight of 2,000-2,100g.

Low birth weight newborn

A low birth weight infant is defined as a full term infant weighing less than 2500g. Low birth weight is sometimes equated with intrauterine growth restriction (IUGR) also known as low birth weight for gestational age (LBWGA). We speak of SIR or SGABW when the birth weight at any time during gestation is below the 10th percentile or 2 SD on the fetal growth curves and there is a known cause for its development. Small for gestational age newborns are those with birth weights below the 10th percentile and where there is no demonstrable cause for the low birth weight. The fetal growth curves used in our environment are the Fenton curves.

The main clinical types of newborns with RIC are:

Symmetric or harmonic RIC. It results in small-for-gestational-age newborns with global delay in weight, length and head circumference, but with normal weight index (they cannot be considered malnourished). Between 5-15% of intrauterine growth restricted foetuses have malformations, including dysmorphic smdromes. It is usually categorised as intrauterine growth restriction (IUGR).

Asymmetric or disharmonic RIC. The newborn has a low amount of subcutaneous fat and a lower than average weight index, therefore, with signs of malnutrition. It is usually an extended RIC due to uteroplacental insufficiency, maternal malnutrition or conditions that acted in the last stage of development.

Intrauterine growth is subject to fetal control by genetic and hormonal determinants, but is also dependent on the supply and transfer of energy and nutrients across the placenta. Low birth weight for gestational age infants form a heterogeneous group with respect to the nature, onset and duration of the mechanism by which fetal growth and development is retarded.

The foetus depends on maternal nutrient intake, the supply of substrates for the synthesis of new tissues and the ene^a necessary for foetal oxidative metabolism. Insulin is considered to be the "fetal growth hormone"; it is mostly fetally produced as it crosses the placenta with difficulty; its actions are to promote adipose tissue and glycogen deposition, stimulating protein synthesis.

Maternal nutritional factors have a great influence on foetal growth, especially in the last trimester of gestation. Maternal protein intake in the first trimester of gestation has been shown to have little influence on fetal growth. It has been shown that acute nutritional problems during the first trimester do not seem to influence the weight of the newborn. On the other hand, situations leading to decreased intake during the last trimester may be responsible for low fetal weight. Two variables have a decisive influence on newborn weight: pregestational maternal weight and gestational weight gain.

The maternal medical causes associated with RIC are the best known and of these the most important is maternal AHT, it is considered that this factor alone can be responsible for a 10% reduction in birth weight. Of the environmental causes, the most frequent cause of RIB is tobacco consumption during gestation; the percentage of low birth weight triples in pregnant women who smoke more than 20 cigarettes a day.

The LBW usually has a thin, lean appearance with little adipose muscle; dry, parchment-like skin with intense scaling; sparse hair; alert sensorium. The umbilical cord is yellowish and thin, and dries early. Frequent absence of urination during the first hours of life. The pathological processes of particular importance in these infants are:

Neonatal asphyxia and meconium aspiration syndrome. After strict application of resuscitation measures, some of these infants will show signs of perinatal asphyxia and hypoxic-ischemic encephalopathy.

Hypothermia. Occurs easily, especially during resuscitation.

Hypocalcaemia. More frequent in low birth weight for gestational age infants.

Hypermetabolism. The needs for ketones and calories per kilogram of body weight are increased.

Behavioural changes. Low birth weight infants often have impaired reflex activity, poor muscle activity and are irritable. The EEG shows patterns of immaturity. In the study of behaviour by means of the Brazelton scale (NBAS) it is possible to demonstrate some temperamental traits characterised by less activity, tendency to hypotomia, less responsiveness to environmental demands and different organisation of behaviour, which makes them unrewarding for close adults by making interaction difficult, which modifies the behaviour of the child and the adult.

Hypoglycaemia. It is the most common problem. In addition to low birth weight and prematurity, there are many other causes of neonatal hypoglycaemia.

Hypoglycaemic crises accompanied by symptoms such as convulsions and tremor can damage the brain, leading to mental retardation and cerebral paralysis. To prevent hypo-glycaemia, feeding should be early (within two hours after delivery), with systematic blood glucose monitoring during the first 72 hours.

In the presence of acidosis, an increase in lactate and ketone bodies will point to a defect in gluconeogenesis, ketosis hypoglycaemia, glycogenosis, growth hormone deficiency or cortisol deficiency.

In the absence of acidosis and decreased ketone bodies, decreased free fatty acids will point to genetic hyperinsulinism, transient neonatal hypoglycaemia, hypopituitarism or stress hyperinsulinism. An increase in free fatty acids points to a defect in fatty acid oxidation.

The symptoms of hypoglycaemia are not specific and their expressiveness and severity is highly variable:

- Changes in level of consciousness: Irritability; abnormal crying; lethargy; stupor.
- Apatfa, slight hypotoma.
- Tremor.
- Poor sucking and feeding, vomiting.
- Irregular breathing. Tachypnoea. Apnoea.
- Cyanosis.
- Convulsions, coma.

In infants who, despite adequate oral feeding, do not maintain normal glucose levels and have clinical symptomatology, rapid correction of blood glucose levels is necessary. The use of peripheral lines for glucose infusion is preferable to the umbilical line; umbilical arterial glucose administration has been associated with hyperinsulinism due to direct pancreatic stimulation.

Despite adequate nutrition in the neonatal period, most NBs will have growth arrest after birth. Rapid recovery of growth catch-up (in green) will lead to better future neurodevelopment in both high birth weight and small newborns. However, extrauterine and intrauterine growth delays will lead to delays in future mental and motor development.

In terms of growth, slow prenatal development shows, when nutritional intake is adequate, a later growth spurt or *catch-up*. Weight regain occurs between 9-12 months of life, so that by the year 56% have a weight in the normal range for their age. In 22% of adults with short stature there is a history of RIC.

Symmetrical RIC, with some decrease in growth potential, have a poor neurological prognosis, while asymmetrical RIC with preserved brain growth usually have a good prognosis. These children, in general, are less active and respond less well to social stimuli, and may have alterations in sleep and eating patterns and lower school performance with learning difficulties.

Treatment should, as far as possible, be aetiological. In the case of RIC of the endouterine type, action in the intrauterine fetus includes, apart from the treatment of the maternal condition, absolute rest, a hypercaloric diet with vitamin supplements, avoidance of smoking. The indication of the type of delivery corresponds to the obstetrician, with correct information to the paediatrician who has to take care of this newborn. The monitoring of these deliveries is essential, as RICs present a higher frequency of foetal distress, requiring neonatal resuscitation.

The neonatal pathology detailed above will require the appropriate prophylactic approach (early feeding; preferential use of breast milk; monitoring of possible hypothermia or hypoglycaemia) and the appropriate treatment according to the disorders presented by the newborn (infection, malnutrition, etc.). Care should be completed with proper postnatal monitoring in the maturational consultation, and "early stimulation" techniques should be implemented if necessary.

Bibliograffa

1.   Slattery MM, Morrison JJ. Preterm delivery. Lancet. 2002;360(9344):1489-97.

2.   Ananth CV, Vintzileos AM. Epidemiology of preterm birth and its clinical subtypes. J Matern Fetal Neonatal Med. 2006;19(12):773-82.

3.   Uberos J. The significance of genetics in pathophysiologic models of premature birth. Minerva Pediatr. 2018;70(4):383-90.

4.   Parets SE, Knight AK, Smith AK. Insights into genetic susceptibility in the etiology of spontaneous preterm birth. Appl Clin Genet. 2015;8:283-90.

5.   Uberos Fernandez J, Munoz Hoyos A, Molina Carballo A, Bonillo Perales A, Gartfa del Rfo C, Ruiz Cosano C, et al. Evaluation of erythropoietin in umbilical cord: importance of gestational age and blood rheology. An Esp Pediatr. 1995;43(5):355-60.

6.   Jimenez-Gonzalez R, Figueras-Aloy J, Thio-Lluch M. Prematurity. In: Cruz-Hernandez M, editor. Tratado de Pediatna. 10 ed. Madrid: Ergon; 2006. p. 97-105.

7.   Fenton TR, Kim JH. A systematic review and meta-analysis to revise the Fenton growth chart for preterm infants. BMC Pediatr. 2013;13:59.

8.   Cruz Hernandez M, Botet Masons F. Characteristics of the normal newborn. In: Cruz-Hernandez M, editor. Tratado de Pediatna. 10 ed. Madrid: Ergon; 2006. p. 47-55.

9.   Walker AM. Circulatory transitions at birth and the control of the neonatal circulation. In: Hanson MA, Spencer JAD, Rodeck CH, editors. Fetus and Neonate. Physiology and clinical applications. 1 ed. Cambridge: Cambridge University Press; 1993. p. 160-96.

3.Neonatal resuscitation

Dr. Elisabeth Fernandez Marin

The success of the transition from intrauterine to extrauterine life will depend on the physiological changes that occur at the time of birth. Most newborns will make this transition successfully without assistance, but there is a small group that will require resuscitation in the delivery room. For this reason, it is necessary to have standardised algorithms of action with the best scientific evidence, with the aim of unifying the assistance of any professional involved in the birth of newborns.

Periodically, the main international resuscitation societies, such as the International Liaison Committee on Resuscitation (ILCOR), the European Resuscitation Council (ERC), the American Heart Association (AHA) or the Australian-New Zealand Committee on Resuscitation (ANZCOR), draw up a universal gwa from which each group or local committee can adapt it to its own reality and draw up its own gwa or recommendations.

In the case of Spain, the Neonatal Resuscitation Group of the Spanish Society of Neonatology (GRN-SENeo) is in charge of updating and adapting these international recommendations.

Neonatal resuscitation algorithm (Figure 3.1)

The main parts of the neonatal resuscitation algorithm consist of the following sections:

1) Communication, anticipation and preparation (human and material resources)
2) Initial assessment
3) First steps in stabilisation
4) Initial assessment
5) Ventilation-oxygenation
6) Thoracic compressions
7) Fluid and drug administration

1) Communication, anticipation and preparation (human and material resources)

Preparation is the first and most important step to achieve success during neonatal resuscitation. Communication between the obstetric and neonatal team allows the preparation of a safe environment: knowing the situation and risk factors (anticipation), preparing the necessary material (check-list), the human team (distributing roles: coordinator and assistants) and the

overall assessment of our performance in order to optimise teamwork.

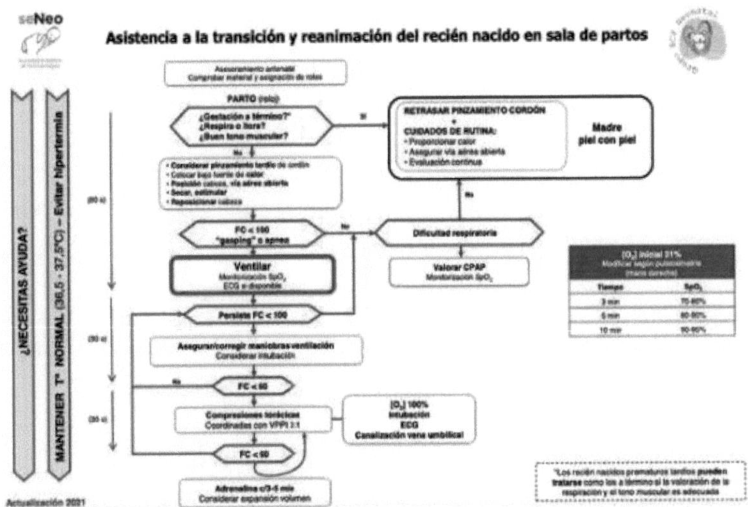

Figure 3.1. Generic neonatal resuscitation algorithm, GRN-SENeo.

Few newborns require resuscitation in the delivery room. Of those who require assistance, most only need respiratory support and a minority may need intubation or chest compressions for a short period of time.

Those babies who are more likely to need resuscitation may be identified by the presence of one or more risk factors: maternal, fetal, prenatal or delivery complications. In this group of patients, if time permits, the team should meet with the parents prior to delivery and discuss anticipated problems and plan the baby's care, addressing the parents' questions and concerns.

Regarding the number of rescuers and the role of each of them, the GRN-SENeo proposes (figure 3.7):

• At every birth, a person capable of performing the initial steps must be present in the delivery room and easily reachable, a person who is able to carry out all the resuscitation manoeuvres.

• In high-risk deliveries there should always be one person trained in full neonatal resuscitation and in high-risk or special situations there should be at least 2 resuscitators and an assistant (e.g. extreme preterm).

• In multiple births there should be one resuscitation team for each NB.

Resuscitation should be performed in the delivery room, in a warm, well-lit, draught-free environment on a soft, pre-warmed surface under a source of radiant heat. It is recommended that the delivery room and resuscitation equipment (table 1) be prepared prior to delivery. All equipment should be easily accessible and should be checked and replaced after each delivery.

Table 3.1. Neonatal resuscitation equipment.

Heat and transport

- Heat source
- Warm gauze, cap
- Plastic bag or wrap (preemies <32 weeks)

- Transport incubator

Suction equipment
- Hoover with pressure gauge
- Suction probes (12 and 14 Fr)

Monitoring equipment
- Stethoscope for auscultation
- Saturation and heart rate monitor
- ECG monitor

Oxygenation and ventilation
- Oxygen/air source and oxygen blender
- Positive pressure device (preferably T-piece resuscitator vs. self-inflating bag)
- Masks of different sizes

Intubation equipment
- Laryngoscope (size 00, 0 and 1)
- Endotracheal tubes (size 2.5, 3, 3.5 and 4 with/without double lumen)
- Devices for endotracheal tube fixation
- Lung mask (different sizes)
- Capnograph

Vascular access
- Umbilical venous catheter and material for cannulation
- Peripheral intravenous catheter
- Needles and syringes

Medication
- Adrenaline (1mg/ml vial or preloaded diluted 0.1mg/ml)
- Physiological saline solution
- 10% glucose serum
- Naloxone (0.4mg/ml vial)

Adapted from Neonatal Resuscitation in the delivery room, Uptodate, 2022

2) Initial assessment

The initial assessment is carried out in the seconds immediately after birth by answering three questions:
- eGestation at term?
- Breathe or cry?
- Good muscle tone?

When all questions are answered in the affirmative, the mother is placed skin-to-skin, late cord clamping and routine care is provided, with continuous assessment of the newborn during the first few minutes of life by assessing respiration, activity and colour.

In case the answer to any of the questions is negative, initial stabilisation steps should be initiated. Delayed cord clamping (at least one minute) should be the strategy of choice in term and preterm infants of any gestational age, born vaginally or by caesarean section, who do not require immediate resuscitation. In neonates requiring resuscitation, priority should be given to initiation of positive pressure ventilation (PPV). Umbilical cord clamping is not currently recommended and is expressly discouraged below 28 weeks.

The temperature of the newborn without asphyxia after birth should be maintained between 36.5 and 37.5°C, with particular importance the lower the gestational age. To achieve this goal it is proposed:
- Keep the delivery room at 26°C and avoid draughts.
- If resuscitation is not required, place the newborn in skin-to-skin contact with

continuous assessment, in preference to any other heat source, as this avoids 50-90% heat loss and promotes maternal bonding. Cover the head and body with a warm cloth to prevent further heat loss.

- If resuscitation is required, place the newborn on a warm surface and under a source of radiant heat, avoiding hyperthermia.
- In preterm infants less than 28 weeks, use polyethylene wraps or plastic bags under the source of radiant heat, without pre-drying them.

In asphyxial patients who may be candidates for active hypothermia (gestational age greater than 35 weeks with asphyxial sentinel event), the temperature of the thermal cradle should be switched off once the patient is stabilised, in order to initiate passive hypothermia pending further assessment.

3) First steps in stabilisation

The first steps of stabilisation comprise:

- Prevent colour loss by placing the newborn on a warm surface under a radiant heat source.
- Optimise airway patency. The correct position for this is in the supine decubitus position with the head in the sniffing position. Aspiration of orophanegeal secretions is only indicated when there is airway obstruction and not systematically (suction tube 8-10 French, pressure <100 mmHg, 5 s maximum, mouth first, then nose.
- Drying and gentle tactile stimulation, both manoeuvres being sufficient in most cases for the child to initiate breathing and/or crying.

4) Initial evaluation

After stabilisation manoeuvres, the NB is reassessed using two parameters:

- Heart rate (HR): preferably determined by auscultation of the precordium, or alternatively by palpation of the base of the cord (requires HR < 100 bpm to be detected). A HR greater than 100 bpm, or an increase in HR, is the most reliable and quickest indicator of adequate ventilation. Colour is not a good parameter to assess oxygenation.
- Breathing: apnoea or ineffective breathing (gasping/ gasping)

These two parameters are assessed every 30 seconds throughout resuscitation. If both parameters are positively assessed (HR > 100 bpm and effective respiration), the newborn may be transferred to the mother and routine care continued under continuous assessment. If one or both parameters are altered, it is necessary to initiate intermittent positive pressure ventilation (IPPV) and neonatal resuscitation manoeuvres are initiated. At this time it is recommended to place a preductal pulse oximeter (right upper extremity) to obtain information on HR and haemoglobin oxygen saturation (sat_{O2}). To get a faster reading, it is advisable to place the sensor first and then connect it to the monitor when it is turned on. If available, HR monitoring can also be initiated via ECG.

In the case where the assessment is positive but the newborn shows signs of respiratory distress, continuous positive airway pressure support (CPAP - with initial PEEP settings at 5-7 cmH_2O and flow rate 6-8 bpm) should be initiated. It is considered that in 60 seconds the most important steps of resuscitation (initial steps and IPPV) can be performed and this is known as the "golden minute".

5) Ventilation-oxygenation

In a newborn infant with apnoea and/or bradycardia, the establishment of adequate pulmonary ventilation is a priority. Although PIP is involved in initial aeration, maintaining this aeration to avoid alveolar collapse, improve gas exchange, distensibility and achieve adequate functional residual capacity (FRC) is more dependent on optimising positive end-expiratory pressure (PEEP).

IPPV should ideally be delivered via a T-piece resuscitation system; this is a device that maintains constant positive inspiratory pressure (PIP) and PEEP. It is connected via tubing to a mask to provide IPPV to the newborn.

If this resuscitation system is not available, a self-inflating bag can be used, which has clear disadvantages compared to the T-piece resuscitation system: the PIP provided is not stable as it depends on the pressure exerted by the resuscitator, it has a pressure release valve (pop-off valve) which when open provides 30-40 cm H_2O increasing when closed, the FiO2 cannot be regulated exactly (variable from 40-100% depending on pressure valve opening or use of reservoir) and respiratory rate regulated by the rate of insufflation of the resuscitator. For this reason it should only be used as a backup device in the event of failure of controlled resuscitation systems.

An appropriately sized face mask should be selected to achieve an airtight seal between the rim of the mask and the infant's face, which is essential to achieve the desired positive pressure. The mask should cover the chin, mouth and nose, leaving the eyes free. It is held to the face by positioning the hand so that the little, ring and middle fingers extend over the jaw like the letter "E" and the thumb and index finger form the shape of the letter "C" on the mask. The ring and little fingers lift the chin forward to keep the airway permeable. The airtight seal is achieved by exerting slight downward pressure on the edge of the mask and gently pressing the jaw towards the mask.

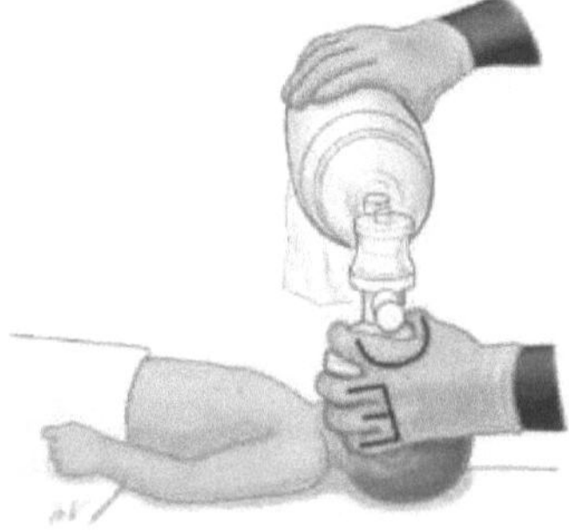

Figure 3.2. *Face mask seal (Neonatal Resuscitation in the delivery room, Uptodate, 2022).*
We recommend a rate of 40-60 rpm, a PEEP of 5-7 cmH_2O and a PIP of 2025 cmH_2O in preterm infants (PTNB) and 25-30cmH_2O in term infants (TGA), adjusting these parameters as soon as possible according to heart rate (HR) response.

There is currently no evidence to justify sustained insufflation (IS-use of inspiratory time > 1 second during the first few breaths), so it is recommended to avoid this clinical practice and focus aeration and lung recruitment on optimising PIP and PEEP.

If after 30 seconds of ventilation a HR < 100 bpm persists, it is necessary to ensure/correct the ventilation manoeuvres (positioning, opening of the airway, interface) by considering endotracheal intubation at this point. Endotracheal intubation is a technique that must be performed by expert personnel, requiring two resuscitators, one performing the procedure and the other monitoring the condition of the newborn. The time required for intubation should be limited to 30 seconds in order to minimise hypoxaemia.

It is indicated when face mask ventilation is ineffective or prolonged, accompanying chest compressions, in special situations (extremely low birth weight newborn, congenital diaphragmatic hernia), if there is an undetectable HR and if it is decided to perform direct endotracheal suctioning due to airway obstruction. The size of the endotracheal tube (ETT) should be selected and the centimetres to be inserted should be known according to the gestational age and/or weight of the newborn.

Table 3.2. Endotracheal tube size by gestational age and birth weight.

Tube size, mm, inside diameter	Gestational age weeks	Weight in grams
2.5	<28	<1000
3	28 to 34	1000 to 2000
3.5	34 to 38	2000 to 3000
3.5 to 4	>38	>3000

Table 3.3. Initial depth of endotracheal tube insertion ("tip to lip") for orotracheal intubation.

Gestational age weeks	TET centimetres to the lip	Weight in grams
23 a 24	5.5	500 a 600
25 a 26	6	700 a 800
27 a 29	6.5	900 a 1000
30 a 32	7	1100 a 1400
33 a 34	7.5	1500 a 1800
35 a 37	8	1900 a 2400
38 a 40	8.5	2500 a 3100
41 a 43	9	3200 a 4200

Intubation procedure: the laryngoscope is held in the left hand using the right hand to stabilise the newborn's head. It is introduced through the right side of the tongue and pushed to the left and advanced to the vallecula (behind the base of the tongue). The laryngoscope is lifted in the direction of the handle to allow visualisation of the vocal cords, avoiding levering. Once visualised, a TET is passed through the vocal cords until the thick black knea at the tip of the tube is level with the vocal cords, ensuring correct location of the TET above the carina. A gwa can be used to provide rigidity and curvature to the TET, avoiding protrusion from the tip of the tube and taking care that the tube does not come out when it is removed.

Successful endotracheal intubation is confirmed by: immediate increase in heart rate (if low), adequate oxygenation on pulse oximetry, auscultation of ventilation in both lung fields, symmetrical chest movement, positive capnography and vapour condensation within the TET during exhalation.

The use of supraglottic airway devices (nasal mask) may be considered in neonates > 34 weeks (>1500-2000 grams) when face mask ventilation is ineffective or intubation is not possible or considered unsafe due to congenital anomaKa, lack of equipment or lack of training. Learning to use them should be encouraged primarily in personnel who are not accustomed to advanced neonatal resuscitation and intubation practice.

As far as oxygenation is concerned, it is recommended to start resuscitation:

-    In NB > 35   weeks with   FiO2 0.21.
-    In newborns <   35 weeks with   FiO2 0.21 in newborns > 30 weeks   and < 30   weeks without   distres.
-    In NB < 30   weeks with   distress with FiO2 of 0.30
-    In NB < 28 weeks consider FiO2 of 0.30 irrespective   of   presence of stress
-    If chest compressions are given, increase FiO2 to 1 and decrease it later once spontaneous circulation is restored.

Oxygen supply is then adjusted according to pulse oximetry$_{con}$ with the goal of achieving SpO2 > p25, from Dawson's graphs avoiding SpO2 > 90%. Target saturation values according to minutes of life are included in the resuscitation algorithm.

IPPV will be maintained until a positive assessment is achieved (HR > 100 bpm and effective breathing). If the HR is less than 60 bpm, initiation of chest compressions is required.

6) Thoracic Compressions (TC)

Initiation of external chest massage is indicated when after 30 s of adequate ventilation with intermittent positive pressure ventilation (IPPV), the HR is less than 60 bpm. The technique of choice for TC is the two-thumbs technique (figure 6). The chest of the NB is embraced with both hands, which act as a hard plane under the back, and the two thumbs are used to perform CT scans in the lower third of the sternum, below the imaginary Knea that joins the two nipples. The appropriate depth is one third of the anterior-posterior diameter of the thorax.

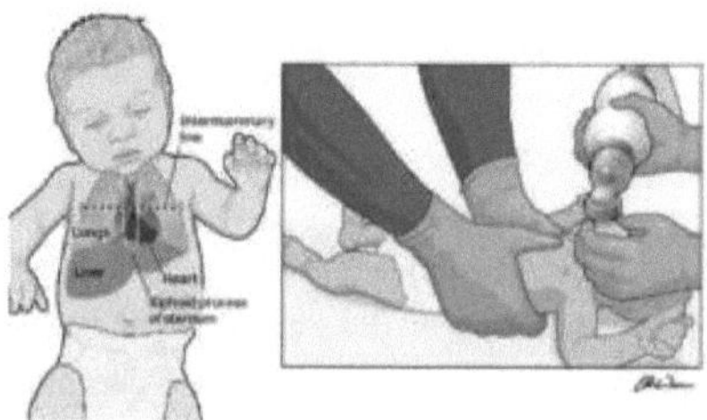

Figura 3.   *. Two thumbs technique (Neonatal Resuscitation in the delivery room, Uptodate, 2022).*

As an alternative technique, 2-finger CT scans can be performed (figure 7). Compression is performed at the same location, with a second hand placed on the back to serve as a hard plane, using the index and middle or middle and ring fingers which should be placed perpendicular to the sternum, avoiding pressure on the ribs.

The compression/ventilation ratio should be 3 compressions for each ventilation (3/1), coordinated with IPPV. With this ratio, 90 compressions and 30 breaths can be reproduced in one minute, thus prioritising ventilation (due to the frequent respiratory origin of bradycardia). At the start of TC, FiO2 should be increased to 1.

Every 30 seconds, assessment should be performed and cardiac massage should be stopped when the heart rate is greater than 60 bpm. If it persists below 60 bpm, CT should be continued and adrenaline administered.

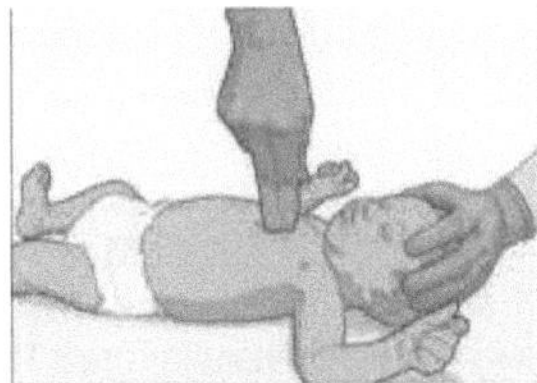

Figura 4.   *. Two-finger technique (Neonatal Resuscitation in the delivery room, Uptodate, 2022).*

7)   Fluid and drug administration

The use of adrenaline, volume expanders or both should be considered in the presence of persistent bradycardia (HR<60lpm) despite effective ventilation and properly performed chest compressions. The use of other drugs such as bicarbonate and naloxone has no place in neonatal resuscitation.

The preferred route for drug administration is the intravenous route (preferably umbilical venous route, but peripheral and intra-osseous routes are also possible); if this is not possible, endotracheal route can be used, only valid for the use of adrenaline.

Adrenaline

Administration is recommended if the HR remains below 60 bpm after effective ventilation has been ensured and CT has been performed correctly for 30 seconds, therefore no sooner than 90 seconds after the start of resuscitation manoeuvres. The preferred route of administration is intravenous, as it is more effective. However, the endotracheal route can be used while intravenous access is being obtained or if intravenous access is not possible. Whatever the route of administration, the recommended dilution is 1:10,000 (0.1mg/ml), which may come in a ready-to-use form or be obtained by diluting one ampoule of adrenaline 1mg/ml in 9 ml of saline or water for dilution.

-   Intravenous administration: doses of 0.01 to 0.03 mg/kg (0.1 to 0.3 of 1:10,000 dilution).

-   Endotracheal administration: 0.05 to 0.1 mg/kg (0.5 to 1ml/kg of 1:10,000 dilution).

The dose may be repeated every 3-5 minutes if the HR remains < 60 bpm. If the initial dose was administered by endotracheal route, subsequent doses may be administered intravenously once access is obtained.

Bicarbonate

Although theoretically sodium bicarbonate should be beneficial in correcting acidosis, there is also evidence that it negatively affects myocardial and brain function.

Given this uncertainty of risk/benefit, the routine use of sodium bicarbonate as part of neonatal resuscitation is not recommended.

On rare occasions, the newborn will not respond to initial resuscitation efforts. In this case, first check that all resuscitation steps have been performed correctly and completely. If there is no response despite correctly executed resuscitation, the following findings may help to identify the cause:

- Lack of response to IPPV ventilation: airway obstruction (meconium, mucus, choanal atresia, malformation) or impaired lung function (pneumothorax, pleural effusion, diaphragmatic hernia, pulmonary hypoplasia, congenital pneumonia or hyaline membrane disease).
- Central cyanosis: congenital cardioparesis
- Persistent bradycardia: heart block
- Apnoea: brain injury, congenital neuromuscular disorder or respiratory depression due to maternal medication.

Resuscitation in special situations

1) Amniotic fluid had

Currently, recommendations on resuscitation of the newborn with amniotic fluid indicate that the same general algorithm should be followed with no delay in resuscitation measures, with special emphasis on initiating ventilation within the first minute of life.

Aspiration of upper airway secretions should not be performed systematically and is only indicated if obstruction is suspected. Visualisation and orotracheal suctioning may be considered if there are signs of meconium airway obstruction despite initiation of ventilation, and provided the resuscitator is skilled in intubation. Repeated intubations are not indicated.

In this group of patients, it is advisable to carefully assess the onset of respiratory distress after delivery and during routine skin-to-skin care with the mother.

2) Prematurity

Preterm infants present a greater challenge, as they are more likely to require resuscitation and develop complications, particularly newborns under 1000 grams.

Resuscitation in this group of patients includes a number of specific recommendations, some of them already described in previous chapters. The algorithm refers to preterm infants less than 32 weeks. Late preterm infants may be managed as term infants if assessment of breathing and muscle tone is adequate.

a) Antenatal counselling

If possible, delivery should take place in a facility with personnel fully trained in the care of preterm infants. The obstetric and neonatal team should meet with the parents prior to delivery to establish a joint plan of action, this being essential in cases with a gestational age in the limits of viability.

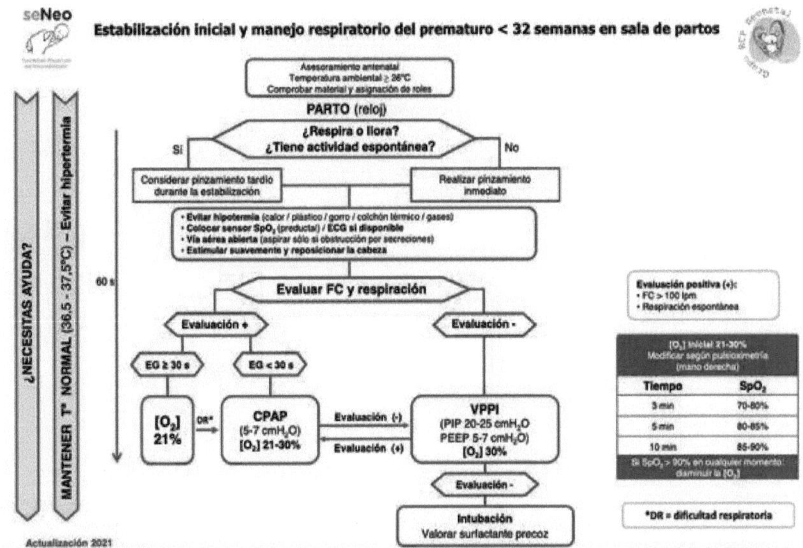

Figure 3.5. *Algorithm for initial stabilisation and respiratory management of preterm infants < 32 weeks in the delivery room, GRN-SENeo.*

b)   Ambient temperature

Thermal stabilisation is essential and should be maintained between 36.5 and 37.5°C. For this purpose, an ambient temperature higher than 26°C should be achieved and polyethylene wrapping or plastic bags and beanie should be used under a source of radiant heat, without drying them beforehand.

c)   Check material and assign roles.

As for the number of resuscitators, there should be at least 2 resuscitators and an assistant. Resuscitation should be performed in the same delivery room, with all the necessary equipment to perform a complete neonatal resuscitation.

After delivery and within the first 60 seconds, measures for initial stabilisation and respiratory support of the preterm infant are initiated.

In the first assessment of the newborn we will consider:

-   Breathing or crying?
-   Does it have spontaneous activity?

If the answer to both questions is yes, late cord clamping may be considered during stabilisation. If one or both is negative, immediate clamping will be performed.

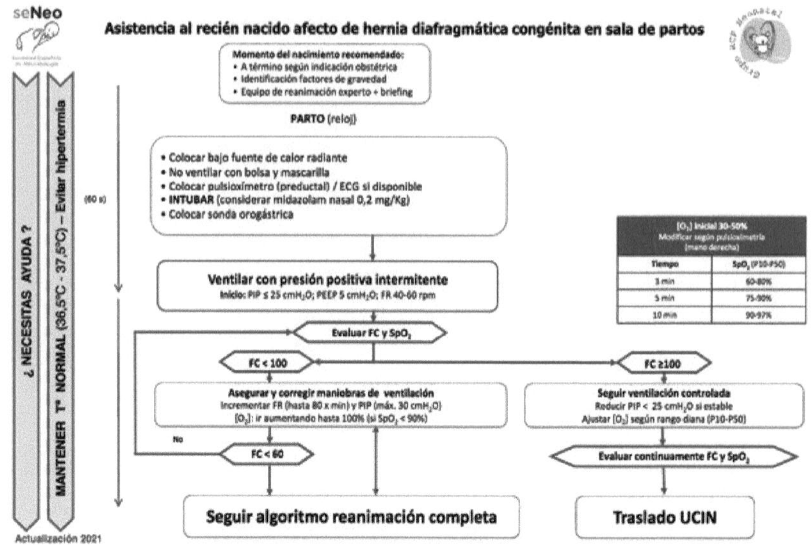

Figure 3.6. *Algorithm of care for the newborn affected by congenital diaphragmatic hernia in the delivery room, GRN-SENeo.*

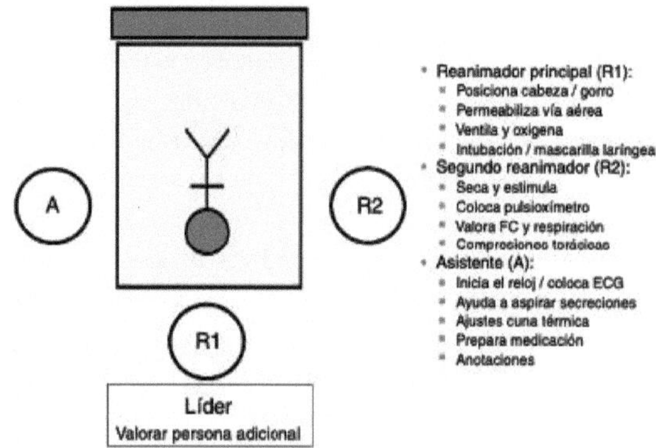

Figure 3.7. *Distribution of roles in neonatal resuscitation, GRN-SENeo.*

After clamping, the newborn shall be placed under a source of radiant heat with the implementation of measures to prevent hypothermia:

- Attach preductal SpO2 sensor and ECG if available.
- Opening of the airway, aspirating only if there is obstruction by secretions
- Gently stimulate and reposition the head

After initial stabilisation, HR and respiration are assessed, with HR<100 bpm and spontaneous breathing being considered a positive assessment. Accordingly, the following scenarios may be encountered:

- Evaluation (+)
* If GA > 30 weeks with no signs of respiratory distress, no respiratory support is required.

*   If GA >30 weeks with signs of respiratory distress or presenting with GA < 30 weeks, respiratory support with CPAP will be initiated.

(PEEP 5-7 cmH2o and FiO2 21-30%)

The evaluation will be carried out every 30 seconds, changing the support according to the result.

- Assessment (-): start IPPV (PIP 20-25 cmH2O, PEEP 5-7 cmH2o and FiO2 30%). If after 30 seconds the evaluation is positive, switch to CPAP, if negative, assess intubation and administration of surfactant.

If after 30 seconds of adequate ventilation a HR<60 bpm persists, chest compressions coordinated with IPPV at a 3:1 ratio should be initiated. If after 30 seconds, adrenaline is administered (similar to the general algorithm).

3) Diaphragmatic hernia

The birth of newborns with diaphragmatic hernia should take place in a hospital with the necessary resources to care for these patients, with multidisciplinary teams.

Post-reanimation care

1) Glucose

Experimental studies indicate that glucose is, along with hypothermia, one of the most effective protectors of the central nervous system in situations of asphyxia.

Hypoglycaemia has been associated with adverse neurological outcome and reduced survival and hyperglycaemia is also associated with neurodevelopmental damage.

Given these findings, current recommendations advise that in the asphyxiated NB, perfused glucose administration should be initiated during stabilisation to maintain the blood glucose range between 47 and 150 mg/dL.

2) Temperature

In non-asphyxiated infants it is a strong predictor of morbidity and mortality and an indicator of quality at all gestational ages, especially in preterm infants. There is evidence of a dose-related effect on mortality, with an increased risk of at least 28% for each °C below 36.5°C on admission.

The new algorithm reflects maintaining the axillary temperature on admission at 36.5 to 37.5°C, avoiding hyperthermia and hypothermia.

In the asphyxial newborn >35 weeks, passive hypothermia should be initiated at 33-34°C central in a susceptible patient, once stabilisation has been achieved during resuscitation. Its neuroprotective benefit is time-dependent, so active hypothermia should be initiated before 6 hours of life.

Ethical aspects

The presence of the parents is recommended during resuscitation in the delivery room, whenever possible. In those patients who will later be admitted to the neonatal unit, early skin-to-skin contact or at least visual or tactile contact should be encouraged, always under the supervision of healthcare staff. In cases with uncertain prognosis or survival in the Kmite, with high morbidity and sequelae, it is recommended to individualise the action and conduct an interview with the parents to make a consensual decision and thus assess whether to initiate resuscitation or therapeutic abstention with welfare care.

If it is decided to suspend resuscitation or not to initiate it (under 23 weeks, lethal chromosomopathies or severe congenital malformations), care should focus on the comfort of the neonate and the well-being of the parents, allowing them to be with their child, if they so wish. It is necessary for each centre to have a protocol for perinatal palliative care which should include the following basic measures: warmth, analgesia, sedation, accompaniment and continuous information for the parents, allowing them to be with their child for as long as they need and as they wish (tucked in, family accompaniment, spiritual or religious counselling), favouring an appropriate place with privacy.

It is difficult to set a specific time to stop resuscitation. If after approximately 20 minutes, having completed all steps of resuscitation, the HR remains undetectable, it is reasonable to discuss with the clinical team and inform the family to discontinue resuscitation manoeuvres. This decision should be individualised taking into account other factors: previous fetal pathology, perinatal circumstances, gestational age and availability of therapeutic hypothermia.

Regarding the Kmite of viability, this should be established in each centre based on a joint decision and action plan of the obstetrics and neonatology teams, taking into account the centre's own results and the opinion of the family. The current recommendations of the Neonatal Reanimation Group of the Spanish Society of Neonatology (GRN- SENeo) are as follows:

- Active resuscitation from $24^{0/7}$ weeks post-menstrual.

- Between $23^{0/7}$ and $23^{6/7}$ weeks, considered the grey zone, consensus should be reached with the family (information on morbidity and mortality risks, assessment of perinatal risks), considering that in those cases with favourable conditions a proactive approach can be taken.

- At gestational age < $22^{6/7}$ weeks, a palliative approach, although between $22^{0/7}$ and 226/7 weeks, an active approach may be considered if the parents wish and favourable conditions exist.

In the event of any threat of labour in pregnancies > $22^{0/7}$ weeks, corticoids should be administered and the mother should be transferred to a 3er level centre, in order to have the possibility of an adequate prenatal assessment and counselling by multidisciplinary perinatal teams.

Bibliograffa

1. Fernandes, C.J. (2022). Neonatal Resuscitation in the delivery room. In L. E Weisman, L. Wilkie (Ed). *Uptodate.* Accessed November 2022, from www.uptodate.com/contents/neonatal-resuscitation-in-the-delivery-room.

2. Zeballos Sarrato G, Avila-Alvarez A, Escrig Fernandez R, Izquierdo Renau M, Ruiz Campillo CW, Gomez Robles C, Iriondo Sanz M; on behalf of the Neonatal Resuscitation Group of the Spanish Society of Neonatology (GRN-SENeo). Guia espanola de estabilizacion y reanimacion neonatal 2021. Analysis, adaptation and consensus on international recommendations. An Pediatr (Engl Ed). 2021 Jul 23:S1695-4033(21)00213-7. Spanish. doi: 10.1016/j.anpedi.2021.06.003. Epub ahead of print. PMID: 34304987.

3.   Zeballos Sarrato G, Salguero Garda E, Aguayo Maldonado J, Gomez Robles C, Thio Lluch M, Iriondo Sanz M; Grupo de Reanimacion Neonatal de la Sociedad Espanola de Neonatolog^a (GRN-SENeo). Adaptacion de las recomendaciones internacionales en estabilizacion y reanimacion neonatal 2015. An Pediatr (Barc). 2017 Jan;86(1):51.e1-51.e9. Spanish. doi: 10.1016/j.anpedi.2016.08.007. Epub 2016 Oct 13. PMID: 27746074.

4.   Iriondo M, Szyld E, Vento M, Buron E, Salguero E, Aguayo J, Ruiz C, Elorza D, Thio M; Grupo de reanimacion neonatal de la Sociedad Espanola de Neonatolog^a. Adaptation of the international recommendations on neonatal resuscitation 2010: comments. An Pediatr (Barc). 2011 Sep;75(3):203.e1-14. Spanish. doi: 10.1016/j.anpedi.2011.04.005. Epub 2011 Jun 16. PMID: 21683665.

5.   Perkins GD, Graesner JT, Semeraro F, Olasveengen T, Soar J, Lott C, Van de Voorde P, Madar J, Zideman D, Mentzelopoulos S, Bossaert L, Greif R, Monsieurs K, Svavarsdottir H, Nolan JP; European Resuscitation Council Guideline Collaborators. European Resuscitation Council Guidelines 2021: Executive summary. Resuscitation. 2021Apr ;161:1-60. doi: 10.1016/j.resuscitation.2021.02.003. Epub 2021 Mar 24. Erratum in: Resuscitation. 2021 May 4;163:97-98. PMID: 33773824.

6.   Highlights of the 2020 American Heart Association Gwas for CPR and CEA

4. Operation of a neonatal unit

Dr. Jose Uberos Fernandez

Dr. Ana Campos Martinez

Neonatology was born as a branch of Obstetrics, in this respect it is important to highlight the figure of Pierre Budin, who in the 19th century made his first contributions to the care of the premature newborn in the 19th century, through his book The Nursling (1888). It should be noted that in the 1950s only 30% of newborns weighing less than 1300 g survived. Improvements in neonatal survival go hand in hand with improvements in hygiene and nutrition, mainly with the development of new formulations of parenteral nutrition for very low birth weight preterm infants, development of enteral nutrition supplements and management of breast milk fortifiers, better obstetric monitoring, incorporation of fetal lung maturation with corticosteroids in the pregnant woman with threatened preterm delivery and exogenous surfactant therapy in the preterm infant with respiratory distress. In the 1970s, positive pressure ventilation using the Gregory chamber was introduced, improved ventilatory means and volume-guaranteed ventilation have contributed to the reduction of long-term comorbidities in preterm infants, especially retinopathy of prematurity and bronchopulmonary dysplasia.

Neonatology was recognised as a medical speciality in 1960. In 1967, Prof. Angel Ballabriga created a Section of Prenatal Biology and Neonatology within the Spanish Association of Paediatrics (A.E.P.), which was gradually joined by various members.

The work between obstetricians and neonatologists is the basis of perinatal medicine and has clear benefits for parents and their children. The aims of perinatal medicine include:

•   To provide families with the best care and advice during the prenatal stage, during childbirth and after birth.

- Prevent or treat causes of maternal, foetal and neonatal morbidity and mortality.
- To achieve these goals in a way that is most acceptable to the parents and their child,

respecting ethical principles.

A neonatology unit is defined as the paediatric clinical unit that guarantees the care coverage of healthy newborns and neonatal patients, as well as birth assistance and resuscitation in the delivery room and operating theatre. A newborn baby is accepted as a newborn baby up to the 46th week of post-menstrual age. Depending on the number of deliveries, the area of reference and the services offered, the neonatal units are classified into levels I, II and III.

Among the care processes included in a neonatal unit are the following:

- Prenatal and perinatal care in collaboration with other specialists, especially obstetricians.
- Assistance to the newborn during childbirth.
- The care of the newborn baby who stays with its mother in the maternity ward.
- Care for newborns in intensive care, intermediate care, special care, observation or short-stay wards.
- Home care in home hospitalisation.
- Follow-up care for newborns at risk.
- Breastfeeding support consultation care in difficult situations.

Level I neonatal unit

Its functions include:

- Assistance to low-risk gestations, healthy term newborns and those newborns of 35-37 weeks gestational age who are physiologically stable.
- Resuscitation in the delivery room and operating theatres.
- Identification of patients who may require transfer to a higher level of care.
- Stabilisation of unexpected neonatal problems.
- Attendance, examination and identification of neonatal disease in healthy newborns.
- Primary care follow-up system for discharged newborns.

The **Level I Neonatal Unit** requires the following support services:

- Pharmacy service with a pharmacist available for consultation 24 hours a day.
- Support staff for breastfeeding promotion.
- Basic radiology (portable X-ray equipment, ultrasound) available 24 hours a day, 7 days a week.
- Laboratory performing haematology, biochemistry and other urgent techniques 24 hours a day, 7 days a week, with the ability to report results immediately.
- Staff with the ability to perform blood typing, crossmatching and availability of blood products.
- Detection of newborns at high social risk and provision of social services.

It requires a **resuscitation and stabilisation** room located in the delivery room/surgery room with a minimum surface area of 4 m^2 and a **basic care room** with a thermal cot, an oxygen socket for every 5 beds, an electrical socket per bed and a washbasin for every 5 beds, with a surface area of 2 m /bed.^{2}

Level II neonatal unit

The **level IIa neonatal unit** is located in a hospital with at least 1000 deliveries/year. It is conceived as a level of care for:

- Assistance to selected complicated pregnancies and newborns > 32 weeks gestation and > 1,500 g.
- Care of neonates with mild illness and problems that can be resolved quickly and without the need for assisted ventilation or arterial cannulation (the availability of nasal CPAP for short-term processes is an asset).
- Assistance to neonates coming from the referral centre who have passed the gravity stage (return transport).
- Developmental monitoring programmes for high-risk newborns.

It must offer the following features:

- Designated space for the care of sick/convalescent neonates.
- Cardiorespiratory monitoring for continuous observation.
- Peripheral intravenous insertion for administration of fluids, glucose and antibiotics.
- Basic radiological and ultrasound diagnosis for newborns at risk of traumatic and/or malformative lesions.

The **level IIb neonatal unit** is located in a hospital with at least 1500 deliveries/year.

- Care of moderately ill neonates including those who may require conventional mechanical ventilation of short duration (< 24 h) or non-invasive respiratory support.

It offers the following features:

- Peripheral or central administration of total parenteral nutrition and/or medications.
- Insertion of umbilical or peripheral arterial catheter for monitoring.
- Conventional mechanical ventilation of short duration (< 24 h) or non-invasive ventilation.

2 neonatal specialists and 5-7 nursery stations are needed for every 1000 deliveries (70% incubators).

Level III neonatal unit

Level III neonatal units must be integrated in a referral hospital with its own or a contracted maternity ward and a paediatric department where all or most of the paediatric specialised areas are performed. In addition, there must be more than 2,000 deliveries/year in their reference area.

Level IIIA. In addition to Level IIB functions, it will include:

- Assistance to selected complicated pregnancies and newborns > 28 weeks gestation and > 1,000 g.
- Care of the critically ill neonate including those requiring conventional mechanical ventilation.
- Minor surgical procedures.

Level IIIB. In addition to Level IIIA functions, it will include:

- Care of all complicated pregnancies and newborns of any gestational age.
- Possibility of advanced respiratory support (high frequency oscillatory ventilation and administration of inhaled nitric oxide (iNO).

*   Paediatric surgery for major surgical intervention with immediate availability.

Level IIIC. In addition to Level IIIB functions, it will include:

*   Neonates requiring a full spectrum of subspecialised paediatric medical and surgical care.

Bibliograffa

*   . M. Ceriani. Neonatolog^a practica 3^ Ed. Panamericana. Buenos Aires 1999.
*   . Ministerio de Sanidad, S.S.e.I. Unidades de Neonatolog^a: Estandares y recomendaciones de calidad. Madrid, 2014.

5.Newborn at risk. Early intervention and care programmes

Dr. Irene Machado Casas

General aspects of Neurodevelopment and Neuroplasticity

It is not possible to understand the concept of early care and its importance without first having some basic notions of neurodevelopment and neural plasticity.

Neurodevelopment is the process of growth, development and training of the nervous system. In the human species it is a long and complex path that begins at conception and lasts throughout childhood and adolescence to reach "brain maturity", although it reaches its peak in the first years of life in which the child:

*   Builds knowledge about the surrounding environment.
*   Learn the motor skills necessary for survival.
*   Acquires language skills, which enable him/her to communicate and develop his/her own inner reasoning.
*   He becomes aware of himself, learns to self-regulate his emotions and acquires the necessary behaviour to integrate into society.

It is a dynamic process, in continuous change, aimed at the progressive acquisition of the person's skills in order to achieve independence and adaptation to the environment.

It begins with the formation of neurons, or neurogenesis, which occurs in the first half of pregnancy and gives rise to the 100 billion neurons that the human brain possesses. All neurons must move to their final location in the cortex during a process called migration, which occurs from the deepest part of the brain where they are formed to the cortex. All this happens in the second trimester of pregnancy.

After 25 weeks of gestation, the formation of new neurons is exceptional. However, the weight of the brain triples from birth to the first three years of life and this is due to the appearance of millions of synaptic connections between neurons and dendritic arborisation (synaptogenesis). It is estimated that each neuron can have between 7,000 and 10,000 synapses, and these will appear and be modelled according to exposure to external and internal factors and experiences (learning) that permanently modify their conformation.

This process of modification of brain structure to change according to learning is called neural plasticity, which is maximal in the first four years of development coinciding with the learning of innate skills (eating, walking, talking....etc).

The last process to begin is myelination, in which the axons of neurons are coated with myelin to improve the speed of transmission of nerve impulses. It begins at 8 months gestation and is virtually complete by 2 years of age.

These are not consecutive stages, they overlap in a complex process in which there are critical periods for normal brain development, during which brain structures are mature and optimally prepared to acquire a new function, and if a particular skill is not acquired at the optimal time it will be much more difficult, and sometimes impossible to learn it.

The child at risk

The concept of the at-risk child began to emerge thanks to scientific advances in relation to perinatology. From the 1980s onwards, an improvement in health care during pregnancy and childbirth began, which together with the apogee of intensive care in Neonatal Intensive Care Units, especially with premature infants, has been responsible for the decrease in the mortality of these infants. But this increase in survival has been accompanied by an increase in morbidity, i.e. an increase in the number of patients with chronic disabling disorders, including "infantile cerebral palsy", which has led to the need to improve the care of children with problems and to promote their health and all-round development.

Table 5.1. BIOLOGICAL risk factors in the newborn *(Modified from Libro Blanco de la Atencion Temprana y del Procesos Asistencial Integrado de del Servicio de Salud Publico de Andaluaa SSPA).*

- Newborn with birth weight <-2ds for gestational age.
- **Weight less than 1,500 gr.**
- Prematurity, especially gestational age (GA) < 32 weeks.
- APGAR < 3 at 1 minute, or < 7 at 5 minutes, or loss of fetal wellbeing.
- **Severe asphyxia.**
- Newborn on mechanical ventilation for more than 24 hours.
- Hyperbilirubinaemia requiring exchange transfusion.
- Neonatal seizures.
- **Infections of the central nervous system (meningitis, encephalitis or ventriculitis).**
- Neonatal sepsis.
- **Persistent neurological dysfunction (more than seven days).**
- **Brain damage as evidenced by neuroimaging.**
- **Malformations of the central nervous system.**
- Malformational syndromes with hearing compromise.
- Malformative syndrome with visual compromise.
- **Neurometabolopathies.**
- **Chromosomopathies y other dysmorphic syndromes.**
- Polycythemia-hyperviscosity syndrome (especially if symptomatic).
- Child of a mother with mental pathology and/or infections and/or drugs that may affect the foetus.
- Newborn with a haemoptysis with unclear neurological pathology o at risk of recurrence.

- Twin, if the sibling is at neurological risk.
- Use of ototoxic drugs, mainly aminoglycosides over a prolonged period o with elevated plasma levels.

Table 5.2. Specific risk factors VISUAL SENSORY

• Prolonged mechanical ventilation
• Weight less than 1,500 gr.
• Prematurity, especially gestational age (GA) < 32 weeks.
• Hydrocephalus.
• Infections of the central nervous system (meningitis, encephalitis or ventriculitis).
• Intracranial pathology in neuroimaging.
• Malformational syndrome with visual compromise.
• Postnatal infections.
• Severe asphyxia.

Table 5.3. Specific risk factors SENSORY AUDITORY SENSORIAL

- Hyperbilirubinaemia requiring exchange transfusion.
- Weight less than 1,500 gr.
- Prematurity, especially gestational age (GA) < 32 weeks.
- Infections of the central nervous system (meningitis, encephalitis or ventriculitis).
- Use of ototoxic drugs, mainly aminoglycosides over a prolonged period or with elevated plasma levels.
- Polymalformative syndrome with hearing impairment.
- Family history of hearing loss.
- Postnatal infections.
- Severe asphyxia.

Table 5.4. BIOLOGICAL risk factors in the newborn (Modified from Libro Blanco de la Atencion Temprana y del Procesos Asistencial Integrado de del Servicio de Salud Publico de Andalutfa SSPA).

• Mental illness or intellectual disability in parents or carers.
• Toxic habits in parents or caregivers.
• History of mistreatment or abuse.
• Low socio-economic status.
• Situation of isolation or marginalisation.
• Family disruption.
• Institutionalised children.

A newborn is considered to be at risk if, as a consequence of his or her personal history (pregnancy, birth, perinatal period), he or she is more likely to present, in the first years of life, problems in his or her neurological development (motor, sensory, cognitive or behavioural) in a transitory or definitive manner. The factors that lead to this situation are classified as biological, neurosensorial, psychological, social or an association of these, the association of risks being an aggravating factor for the possible neurological deficit of the child.

Early Childhood Care

As we have seen, this situation of maturation in the early years conditions a greater vulnerability to certain adverse conditions (prematurity, genetic disorders, sensory or affective deprivation, etc.) that may jeopardise optimal development; but it also endows the nervous system with greater plasticity that allows a greater capacity for recovery and organic and functional reorganisation, and it has already been demonstrated that early and appropriate intervention will condition a better prognosis of the overall development of the child.

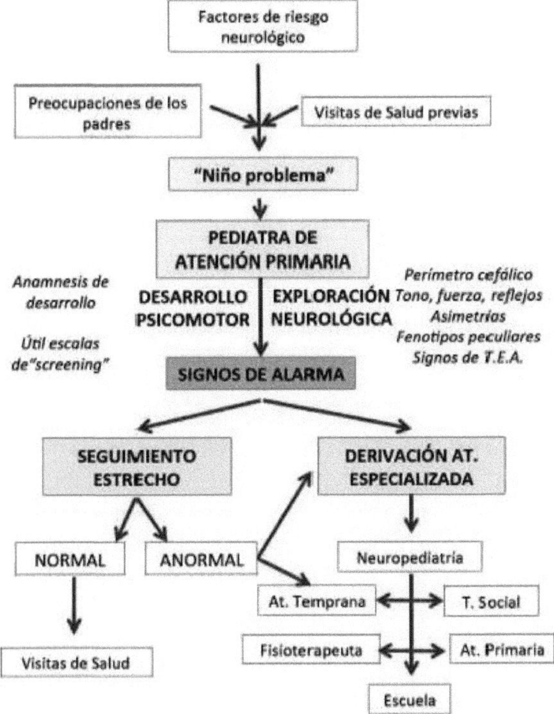

Figure 5.1. Identification of the at-risk child in primary care and referral.

From this arises the concept of Early Intervention (ECI), defined in the white book on ECI, published by the Ministry of Labour and Social Affairs and the Royal Board on Disability in 2000, as *"...the set of actions, aimed at the child population aged 0-6 years, the family and the environment, whose objective is to respond as soon as possible to the transitory or permanent needs of children with development disorders or who are at risk of suffering from them. These interventions, which must take into account the globality of the child, must be planned by a team of professionals with an interdisciplinary and transdisciplinary orientation".*

In other words, the main objective of ECI is to strengthen the child's capacities so that he/she can achieve the fullest possible personal autonomy and integration into the family, school and social environment.

Early Childhood Care Programmes

The early care programmes applied to the child must therefore be individualised, flexible and accessible in order to respond to the real needs of the child and his or her family, allowing an adequate follow-up and periodic evaluation of the child at risk detected in the neonatal period; or of those in whom, without presenting risks, warning signs are detected with the aim of confirming normal development or, failing that, to detect early deviations from normal psychomotor development and to establish therapeutic measures at an early stage.

The team is made up of TA specialists from health, social and educational backgrounds (psychologists, speech therapists, occupational therapists, physiotherapists, etc.) who must have special training in neurodevelopment in order to treat each child's problems in a comprehensive way, including creative approaches, and normalisation strategies to ensure that the child's full potential is developed, with or without established injuries.

Intervention is therefore provided to all children between 0 and 6 years of age who have a diagnosis according to the "Organisational Diagnostic Manual for Early Childhood Care (ODAT)" (presence of one or more risk factors) or warning signs throughout their development.

This manual attempts to compile a list of causes and factors that influence child development, grouping them in axes that allow a common language among the different professionals who work with children with developmental disorders or at risk of suffering them, and is based on three levels:

• Level 1: describes the risk factors for developmental disorders and is further divided into Axis I (biological risk factors), Axis II (family risk factors) and Axis III (environmental risk factors).

• Level 2: describes the type of disorder that can be diagnosed in the patient, family or environment (axis IV, V and VI) e.g. motor development disorders, visual disorders, emotional disorders etc.

• Level 3: includes resources also divided into three axes referring to the child, the family and the environment.

At present, it is estimated that approximately 10% of the Spanish child population between 0-6 years of age present problems or their families have developmental concerns at some point in their development. Hence, ECI has been promoted and recognised in the different Autonomous Regions of Spain, thus establishing a network of Early Attention and Intervention Centres (CAIT), which try to support all these needs, although insufficiently, as in recent years, we are experiencing a boom in new morbidities in child development. The CAITs are becoming an observatory, where the new factors that influence child development are analysed, called the "new morbidities of the millennium" which are linked to the profound change of upbringing, family and social life style that occur today in childhood and adolescence.

It is curious to observe how the problems linked to the classic concept of disability (blindness, deafness, cerebral palsy, syndromic conditions) are decreasing in these centres, coinciding with an improvement in health care, and at the same time there is a significant increase in disorders of affectivity, communication and the regulation of behaviour (bonding, adaptive, autistic spectrum, behaviour and attention), as well as problems in the area of language acquisition, habits or personal autonomy. These problems have also been observed in other countries, which has concerned international organisations such as UNICEF and WHO, which after several studies have drawn up manuals to try to develop environments for a child to reach his or her greatest developmental potential.

Bibliograffa

1. Pons Tubio A et al. Proceso Seguimiento recien nacido de riesgo: proceso asistencial integrado. Seville: Junta de Andalutfa - Consejena de Salud; 2009. [accessed 25-10-2022]. Available in   :
https://www.juntadeandalucia.es/export/drupaljda/salud_5af1956dcfafc_0_riesgo.pdf

2. ODAT Organizacion Diagnostica Atencion Temprana. GAT (Federacion de profesionales de la Atencion Temprana) 2004. Ed. Real Patronato Discapacidad. https://gat- atenciontemprana.org/

3. White Paper on Early Intervention. GAT and Real Patronato. 2000. http://gat-atenciontemprana.org/recursos/

4. Poch Olive ML , Ramos Sanchez I . Early childhood screening programmes. In: Retos de Futuro en el desarrollo infantil. PP 45 - 54. Ed. GAT (Federacion de profesionales de la Atencion Temprana) February 2022.

5. Ares Segura, C. D^az Gonzalez Follow-up of the premature newborn and high biological risk infant. Pediatr Integral 2014; XVIII(6): 344-355. 6-WHO 2020 Improving early childhooddevelopment :   WHOguideline.
https://www.who.int/publications/i/item/97892400020986

6. Perinatal asphyxia and hypoxic-ischemic encephalopathy

Dr. Jose Uberos Fernandez
Dr. Aida Ruiz Lopez

Perinatal asphyxia (PA) is the condition in which there is a severe disturbance in the gas exchange of the foetus or newborn as a consequence of different noxae acting before or during labour, or in the first minutes after birth. Perinatal asphyxia causes severe hypoxaemia with significant disruption of acid-base balance. In survivors of moderate and severe asphyxia, the main sequelae are early onset hypoxic-ischemic encephalopathy (HIE), which, together with prematurity, is the main cause of infantile cerebral palsy. From a general point of view, we can define perinatal asphyxia as a group of smdromes that condition a tissue oxygenation defect that arises around birth. It is a highly prevalent pathology affecting 1-3% of term newborns and 7% of preterm infants in industrialised countries.

It is a fact that most foetuses with alterations in the foetal cardiotocographic record (FCR) or with pH < 7.20 are born well and do not show signs of encephalopathy or organ repercussion, hence the term foetal distress, used in past decades by obstetricians and paediatricians, has been replaced by the term "non-reassuring foetal state" or "loss of foetal wellbeing".

Pathophysiology of asphyxia

Both maternal, placental and foetal factors are involved in the oxygenation of the foetus and newborn. Animal experimental studies have established that after an anoxic insult there is a symptom-free period of 1 minute after which an increase in blood pressure and a sudden decrease in foetal heart rate can be observed. A redistribution of blood flow occurs, so that it increases in "noble" areas such as the adrenal glands, myocardium or brain and decreases in other areas of the economy. As a consequence of the increased vascularisation in the adrenal glands, an adrenergic and catecholamine response is produced to try to compensate for the decrease in oxygenation.

The uterine blood flow is about 500 ml/min and the umbilical blood flow fluctuates around 250 ml/min. The difference in flow rates favours diffusion from the mother to the foetus. The higher oxygen pressure of the maternal blood favours its diffusion to the foetus. The difference of CO_2 pressures in foetal blood is 4 to 26 mmHg higher than in maternal blood, which also favours its diffusion.

Although the placenta has been referred to as the foetal lung, the structures separating the maternal and foetal circulation are thicker than the pulmonary structures, which hinders gas diffusion due to the increased interstitial space. This situation is partly compensated by the higher content of foetal Hb with a high affinity for oxygen and a haemoglobin dissociation curve shifted to the left.

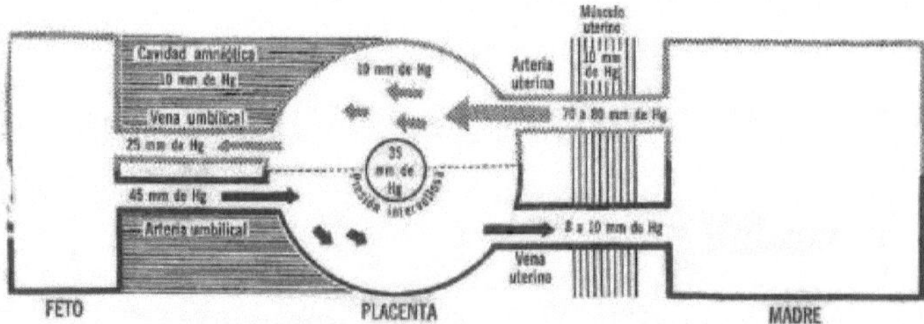

Figure 6.1. Placental flow during uterine quiescence.

During labour, the flow from the umbilical vein to the foetus and back through the umbilical arteries generates a placental pressure gradient which corresponds to a higher pressure in the uterine arteries than in the uterine veins. It should be noted that during the uterine resting situation the intervillous pressure is 35 mmHg. This situation of net gas exchange is altered during uterine contractions, as the intervillous pressure increases to 75 mmHg, which decreases arterial blood flow through the uterine arteries and interrupts blood flow in the uterine veins. Although it must be accepted that all newborns after delivery are hypoxaemic to a variable degree and by virtue of their HbF percentage tolerate oxygen deprivation better than the adult. It should be remembered that the higher HbF content in the foetus and neonate condition a shift of the dissociation curve to the left so that with lower pO2 higher O_2 saturation is achieved.

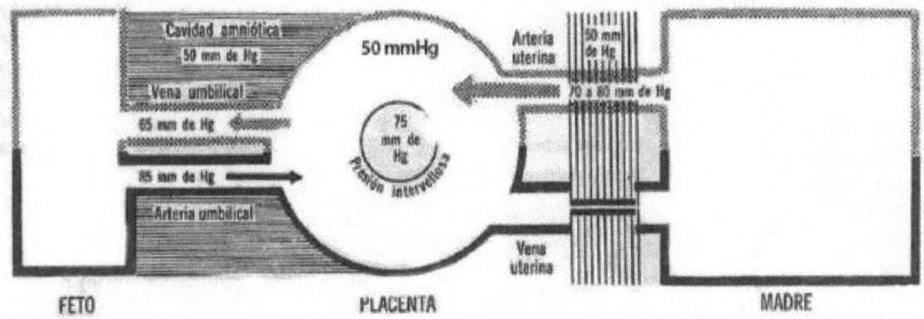

Figure 6.2. *Placental flow during uterine contraction.*

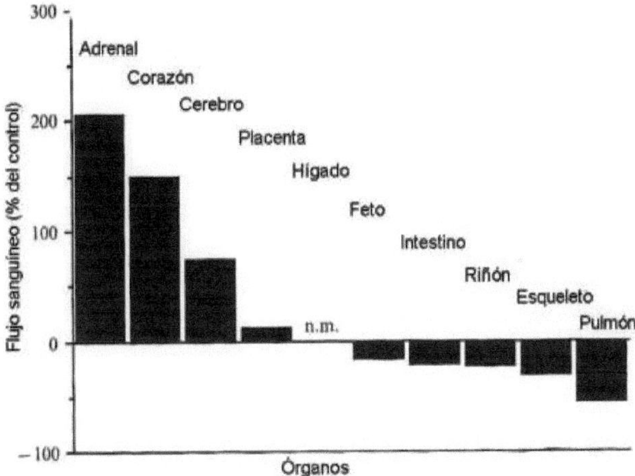

Figure 6.3. *Redistribution of blood flow in the foetus after sustained maternal hypoxaemia (Taken from Jensen & Berger, with permission).*

The blood that reaches the foetus through the umbilical vein is the best oxygenated with a SO2 of 80%. The passage through the ductus venosus of Arancio allows the left lobule of the liver to be the best oxygenated organ. The oxygenated blood that reaches the inferior vena cava mixes in very low proportion with the blood that reaches this vessel so that its passage to the left cavities through the foramen ovale ensures that the blood that reaches the foetal brain has a high proportion of oxygen.

Risk factors for perinatal asphyxia

These include prenatal risk factors dependent on maternal and obstetric pathology, intrapartum risk factors and postnatal risk factors.

Prenatal risk factors include:
*   Hypertension
*   Kidney disease
*   Diabetes
*   Cancer
*   Thyroid pathology
*   E. cardiovascular
*   Rh sensitisation
*   Tuberculosis
*   Lupus erythematosus
*   Alcohol and/or narcotics addiction
*   Psychosis
*   Neuropathic disease
*   Severe anaemia

Among the obstetric history should be considered:
*   Great multiparity
*   Surgical delivery
*   Prolonged labour (>24 h)
*   Foetal loss
*   Prematurity or low   birth weight
*   Neonatal death
*   Previous child after traumatic birth, cerebral palsy, respiratory distress.

Of the obstetric pathology should be taken into account the presence of:
*   Arterial hypertension
*   Bleeding after the 12th week
*   Current multiple gestation
*   Anomalous fetal presentation or position
*   Hydramnios
*   General anaesthesia
*   Intake of some drugs during pregnancy
*   Anaemia (Hb <8 g/dl)
*   Absence of pregnancy monitoring
*   Failure to follow medical indications

Intrapartum risk factors:
*   Alteration of uterine dynamics
*   Foetal malposition, disproportion
*   AnomaKas of the umbilical cord, prolapse
*   amniotic meconium fluid, fetid
*   Intrapartum fever

Postnatal risk factors include the existence of:
*   Respiratory diseases
*   Congenital malformations
*   Congenital heart disease

*   Sepsis

Pathogenesis of perinatal asphyxia

The anoxic situation implies the use of anaerobic metabolic pathways over aerobic pathways which are much more efficient in the production of ene^a. Anaerobic glycolysis generates only 2 molecules of adenosine triphosphate (ATP), whereas aerobic glycolysis generates 38 molecules of ATP. The decrease in energy reserves can lead to failure of the Na^+ -K /H^{+++} pump responsible for an increase in intraneuronal Na concentration$^+$ with cellular oedema. In addition, the increased secretion of catecholamines that always occurs in a stress situation is responsible for increased lipolysis and increased lactic acid production, metabolic acidosis leading to pulmonary vasoconstriction.

In the foetus, tissue oxygenation failure may be due to *anoxic anoxia*, when there is an oxygenation defect; *anaemic anoxia* if there is a defect in oxygen distribution; *circulatory anoxia* if there is a circulatory defect in oxygen transport; and *cytotoxic anoxia,* if there is a cellular defect in oxygen uptake.

The mechanisms by which anoxia causes brain damage are primarily twofold: ischaemia and excitotoxicity due to increased glutamate and intracellular Ca .$^{++}$

The pathophysiological mechanisms of perinatal asphyxia can be broken down as follows:

*   Circulatory

*   Metabolic

*   Bioqwmics

*   excitatory amino acids (excitotoxicity)

*   Oxygen free radicals

*   Proto-oncogene activators

After one minute of asphyxia, a primary apnoea occurs, which can be reversed after correction of the oxygen deficiency and application of sensory stimuli. When a primary apnoea persists in the first few minutes, a secondary apnoea situation develops in which recovery is only possible if cardiopulmonary resuscitation (CPR) manoeuvres are performed. The duration of asphyxia is proportional to the intensity of the CPR manoeuvres required to reverse the situation. The changes caused by asphyxia in the newborn were documented by G. Dawes (1968); however, the newborn is more resistant to hypoxia/acidosis than later in life:

*   Increased red cell mass (polyglobulia).

*   High fetal haemoglobin ratio

*   Elevated heart rate and increased systemic flow.

*   Low tissue metabolic rate.

*   Use of lactic acid/ketoacids with ene^a generators (anaerobiosis).

Clinical manifestations of perinatal asphyxia

Perinatal asphyxia affects the respiratory, cardiocirculatory, central nervous, renal, gastrointestinal and haematological systems. The involvement of the respiratory system can be summarised by the possibility of occurrence of:

*   Respiratory depression

*   Respiratory Distress Syndrome

*   meconium aspiration syndrome

*   Persistent pulmonary hypertension syndrome

Cardiovascular system involvement can be summarised by the presence of:

*   Myocardial depression

*   Tricuspid regurgitation (TPPH)

*   Arterial hypotension

It should be remembered that hypoxaemia will lead to increased angiotensin and vasopressin secretion responsible for the pallor and bradycardia common in perinatal asphyxia.

The renal system involvement in asphyxia can be summarised by the possibility of presenting:

*   Acute tubular necrosis

*   Renal vein thrombosis

It should be remembered that during an episode of asphyxia there is a drastic decrease in renal flow, which is responsible for these manifestations.

Affection of the gastrointestinal system manifests itself as:

*   Eating disorders

*   Necrotising enterocolitis

The biochemical modifications described include:

*   Biochemical modifications

*   Alteration of membrane permeability

*   Hyperkalemia

*   Increased lactate: responsible for intracellular metabolic acidosis and cerebral oedema.

*   Initial hyperglycaemia followed by hypoglycaemia

*   Hypocalcaemia

*   Hyponatraemia

*   Hypothermia

*   Hyperbilirubinaemia

Central nervous system involvement can manifest itself as:

*   Hypoxic-ischemic encephalopathy

*   Seizures

*   Cerebral haemorrhage and infarction

*   Inappropriate secretion of antidiuretic hormone (ADH)

Diagnosis of perinatal asphyxia

The diagnosis of severe perinatal asphyxia is based on several criteria including evidence of cardio-respiratory depression, severe acidosis (defined as arterial blood pH less than 7 or base excess greater than 12 mmol/L), poor postnatal vitality (Apgar at 5 minutes less than 5).

Thus, we speak of severe asphyxia criteria if they are present:

*   Apgar 1' < 2

* Apgar 5' < 5
* Acidosis in foetal *scalp* pH<7.0

Prognosis of perinatal asphyxia

Several factors will be related to prognosis, on the one hand, the response to neonatal resuscitation, baseline pH, lactate/creatinine levels and urinary ₽2- microglobulin levels. Of particular prognostic importance is the existence of clinical manifestations, especially the degree of IHD.

Complications of perinatal asphyxia

They can be early or late.

Early complications include:

* Bleeding
* Multi-organic parenchymal injury (hypoxia)
* Disseminated intravascular coagulation (DIC)
* Hypoxic-ischemic encephalopathy
* Shock
* Persistent pulmonary hypertension
* Inadequate ADH secretion

The complications ta^as derive from the existence of hypoxic-ischemic encephalopathy and include neurodevelopmental disorders of varying intensity, which will be discussed in the next topic.

Treatment of perinatal asphyxia

The existence of a sentinel event in the obstetric history should motivate us to be alert to the existence of perinatal asphyxia, in these cases we must control hyperoxia and initiate passive hypothermia. Fluid restriction and correction of water and electrolyte disorders are indicated. It should be remembered that the therapeutic objective in severe perinatal asphyxia is neuroprotection, i.e. to prevent neuronal death secondary to ischaemia.

Hypoxic-ischemic encephalopathy

Hypoxic ischaemic encephalopathy (HIE) is a frequent pathology in the neonatal units of our country and is one of the most important causes of mortality and neurological sequelae in the newborn at term. By EHI we mean a constellation of neurological signs that appear immediately after birth following an episode of perinatal asphyxia and are characterised by impaired alertness, impaired wakefulness, altered muscle tone and motor responses, altered reflexes, and sometimes seizures.

Astic brain damage in the foetus and neonate selectively affects vulnerable areas of the brain, which are related to the different metabolic rate of the cells and the degree of maturity of the brain at the time of the noxious event. Assessment of early neurological dysfunction is the most useful clinical indicator that asthmatic encephalopathy has occurred.

The different neurological sequelae observed after a severe asthmatic noxa reflect the location, identity and extent of the affected neuronal population. Injury in term infants is diffuse and multifocal, so that the sequelae may be more global and varied, expressed as an increased risk of cognitive-intellectual compromise and the development of epileptic smdromes.

The main cerebral ischaemic lesion in the term infant is parasagittal ischaemia involving cortical necrosis with involvement of the immediately underlying white matter in a characteristic distribution, most frequently affecting posterior regions (parietal-occipital). Term infants show greater motor and tone involvement as the ischaemic hypoxic damage to the cortex, thalamus, basal ganglia and brain stem is more extensive and selective, which may be expressed clinically as cerebral palsy, constituting a non-progressive, early-onset motor and postural deficit (see spastic theme); the incidence of spastic quadriplegia increases with involvement of the basal ganglia and other diencephalic structures.

The effects of EHI in preterm infants may be more severe due to:

1) Have primitive vascularisation, especially in the white matter and subcortical region.

2) That cerebral blood flow is irregular.

3) Oligodendrocyte precursors are more vulnerable to excitatory amino acids (glutamate) and free radicals.

Severe psychomotor delay (which may correlate with later cognitive deficit) in term NBs is a consequence of injury to several cortical areas due to hypoxia or multifocal ischaemic brain injury. Hearing, visual or language disorders reflect extensive parasagittal lesions that may involve parietal-occipital regions.

Classically, three degrees of increasing intensity are described after an asphyxitic period: Period I of hypervigilance, Period II of lethargy or dullness and Period III of stupor. Newborns who reach period II and this lasts only a few days usually improve without major sequelae. Patterns of involvement also depend on gestational age; in preterm infants older than 36 weeks there is a vascular distribution with infarcts in the cortex and subcortical areas; in preterm infants younger than 36 weeks, more periventricular areas are affected.

Intracranial haemorrhages are an important clinical problem due to their high frequency. Their locations include:

- **Subdural haemorrhage.** Infrequent, usually related to traumatic antecedents in term newborns.

- **Subarachnoid haemorrhage.** Pathogenesis involves obstetric trauma or circulatory events related to prematurity. The earlier ones are more common in term newborns.

- **Cerebellar haemorrhage.** Haemorrhage is most frequent in preterm infants less than 32 weeks gestational age or less than 1,500 g at birth, where it reaches rates of 15-25%. It is multifactorial, but of particular importance are traumatic delivery (breech, forceps, or both), hypoxic events, especially with respiratory distress syndrome, and prematurity. In preterm infants, the pathogenesis is similar to intraventricular haemorrhage, whereas, in the term infant, the pathogenesis is mainly related to traumatic events.

- **Intraventricular haemorrhage.** Most common form of intracranial haemorrhage. neonatal, characteristic of the premature newborn. The subependymal germinal matrix is characteristically the site of origin of intraventricular haemorrhage. Among the factors involved in its pathogenesis, the most frequent are: cerebral blood flow fluctuations influenced or not by elevations in central venous pressure or cerebral vasodilatation associated with acidosis, coagulation disorders and haemostasis. The first classification of HIV was made by Papile et al. in 1978, based on CT findings, nowadays applied to ultrasound findings. Four grades are distinguished according to severity:

- Grade I: Subependymal haemorrhage
- Grade II: Intraventricular haemorrhage (IVH). Intraventricular bleeding and occupies between 10 and 50 % of the ventricle.
- Grade III: HIV with ventricular dilatation. Intraventricular bleeding is greater than 50%.
- Grade IV: HIV with ventricular dilatation and parenchymal extension.

IHD goes through several clinical phases related to pathophysiology. On resuscitation of the asphyxiated newborn, the neurological response is nil, but after resuscitation, within 30 to 60 minutes it improves due to reperfusion. The newborn enters a latency phase, remaining relatively stable for 6 to 15 hours and then deteriorating again. At this stage, secondary seizures occur as a consequence of the damage associated with reperfusion and necrosis. In the following days, apoptosis of the damaged areas occurs, which will later be associated with long-term sequelae.

Table 6.1. Classification of hypoxic-ischemic encephalopathy according to Sarnat criteria.

Signs	Stage 1	Stadium 2	Stage 3
Level of awareness	Hyperalert	Lethargic	Stupor/coma
Muscle tone	Normal	Hypotonic	Flaccid
Posture	Normal	Flexion	Brainless
Tendon reflexes/clonus	Hyperactive	Hyperactive	Absent
Myoclonias	Present	Present	Absent
Reflection of Moro	Strong	Debil	Absent
Pupils	Mydriasis	Myosis	Poor reflex/anisocoria
Seizures	No	Common	Decerebrate
EEG	Normal	Low voltage changing to convulsive activity	Isoelectric suppressions
Duration	Less than 24 hours	1 to 14 days	Days to weeks
Forecast	Good	Variable	Death/significant neurological deficit

Diagnosis of hypoxic-ischemic encephalopathy

After resuscitation of the newborn we speak of mild asphyxia when the minute Apgar test is equal to or less than 5. In severe asphyxia the minute Apgar test is equal to or less than 2 and at 5 minutes, less than or equal to 5. There is a high concordance between minute Apgar and umbilical cord pH and between Apgar at 5 minutes and neurological prognosis (severity of asphyxia). After resuscitation, the infant's condition may appear to be good for the next 8-10 hours, the so-called latency period, after which the symptoms of EHI start to become evident. There are several criteria for assessing the severity of EHI after anoxic insult. These criteria are contained in the Sarnat and Garda-Alix scales.

The diagnosis of severe perinatal asphyxia is based on several criteria including evidence of cardio-respiratory depression, severe acidosis (defined as arterial blood pH less than 7.0 or base excess less than -12 mmol/L), poor postnatal vitality (5-minute Apgar less than 5) and early evidence of hypoxic-ischemic encephalopathy (Sarnat-Garcia Alix score > 6). All of them with a history of events of loss of foetal wellbeing:

* Fetal heart rate anomaKas (<100 L/min or >160 L/min)

* The existence of variable or late DIPs (fetal heart rate drop) in cardiotocographic recording

* Amniotic meconium fluid

In newborns of gestational age greater than or equal to 35 weeks with IHD, it is recommended that clinical grading systems based on the Sarnat scale be applied during the first 6 hours of life to classify the severity of encephalopathy and to identify candidates for therapeutic hypothermia (patients with moderate or severe encephalopathy).

Postnatal criteria for moderate to severe hypoxic-ischemic encephalopathy are considered to be present if any of the following are present:

* Multi-organ failure

* Neurological symptoms of moderate - severe EHI (Sarnat / Garda Alix scale score > 6)

The amplitude-integrated electroencephalogram (EEGa) is an accessible technique for monitoring electrocortical activity in preterm and term infants in neonatal intensive care units. There is a good prognostic correlation in IHD with EEGa recording in the first 6-12 h of life, EEGa has shown its validity in establishing the severity of IHD and helping to establish early neurological prognosis. Children with normal continuous or discontinuous voltage tracing had a favourable neurological development, while those with an abnormal tracing (burst-suppression, low voltage, inactive) progressed to death or severe neurological sequelae.

It should be noted that only 20% of electrical seizures lead to clinical seizures in the newborn. The current approach is to treat electrical seizures as soon as they are detected in the newborn.

Brain involvement in HD is characteristically bilateral and symmetrical, but structures such as the hippocampus, medial layer of the cerebral cortex, striatum, thalamus and Purkinje cells are more severely affected. Certain characteristics of these areas contribute to their selective vulnerability to oxygen deprivation: a higher relative metabolic demand, a greater amount of excitatory neurotransmitters, a more modern phylogenetic origin that justifies that the striatum is affected but not the globus pallidus, and the location at the crossroads of two arterial territories.

Prognosis of hypoxic-ischemic encephalopathy

Several factors will be related to the prognosis, especially the extent of the affected brain areas, which will be determined by nuclear magnetic resonance imaging, it is considered that from one week onwards the lesions are already fully established. Complications of EHI are numerous and include neurodevelopmental disorders of varying intensity.

Treatment of hypoxic-ischemic encephalopathy

Therapeutic measures include:

* Appropriate resuscitation manoeuvres
* Avoiding hyperoxia
* Passive hypothermia
* Normalise blood pressure (Ensure effective brain flow)
* Adequate haematocrit (40-60%)
* Normalise blood glucose
* Water restriction (65 ml/kg^a) up to diuresis > 2 ml/kg/h
* Treating seizures
* Passive and active hypothermia

It should be remembered that the therapeutic goal in severe perinatal asphyxia and IHD is neuroprotection, i.e. avoiding neuronal death secondary to ischaemia.

Bibliograffa

1.   Alfredo Garda-Alix, Miriam Martinez Biarge, Juan Arnaez, Eva Valverde, Jose Quero. Intrapartum asphyxia and hypoxic-ischemic encephalopathy. Protocols Diagnostico-Terapeuticos de la AEP: Neonatolog^a. Pags. 242-252. Accessed 22/9/2015. In: *https://www.aeped.es/sites/default/files/documentos/26.pdf*

2.   A. Jensen and R. Berger. Regional distribution of cardiac output. In: *Fetus and Neonate. Physiology and clinical applications,* edited by M. A. Hanson, J. A. D. Spencer, and C. H. Rodeck, Cambridge:Cambridge University Press, 1993, p. 23-74.

3.   G. S. Dawes, B. V. Lewis, J. E. Milligan, M. R. Roach, and N. S. Talner. Vasomotor responses in the hind limbs of foetal and new-born lambs to asphyxia and aortic chemoreceptor stimulation. *J Physiol. 1968; 195 (1):55-81.*

7.   Anaemias,   haemorrhages   and polyglobulias in newborns

Dr. Jose Uberos Fernandez

Dr. Enrique Blanca Jover

Neonatal anaemia

From birth and during the first two months of life there is a decrease in haemoglobin levels, which, by reaching values below those considered normal for adults, are the basis of what has come to be known as physiological anaemia in infants. However, haemoglobin values at birth can be altered depending on factors such as gestational age, maternal smoking, intrauterine growth retardation or maternal diabetes, situations that can lead to an increase in haemoglobin values in the newborn. While in the 10-week foetus haemoglobin values oscillate around 9 g/dL, in the 22 to 24-week foetus haemoglobin values are close to 14-15 g/dL, and during the third trimester and until the end of gestation the mean haemoglobin values are close to 16.6 g/dL. Among the factors that have been described to explain the decrease in erythrocyte production after birth, the increased availability of oxygen in the extrauterine environment has been implicated, remembering that it is during this period that erythropoietin synthesis changes from being predominantly hepatic to renal.

We consider anaemia in the first 7 days of life of a term newborn as less than 5 million haematfes, a central haematocrit of less than 45% or haemoglobin of less than 14 g/dL.

Aetiopathogenesis of neonatal anaemias

Anaemia in the newborn is usually caused by acute blood loss before, during or after delivery. Losses originating before or during delivery include placental transfusion, which may be responsible for the loss of up to 20% of the newborn's blood volume. Maternal transfusions presuppose a placental lesion that allows the passage of blood from the foetus to the mother, in these cases the diagnosis can be made by the demonstration of foetal haemoglobin in the maternal blood, this easily performed technique is known as the Kleihauer-Betke test. Occasionally, velamentous cord insertion or cord tearing during delivery can cause acute haematic loss in the newborn. Feto-fetal transfusion may be observed during twin pregnancies, this finding presupposes the existence of an anaemic newborn and a polyglobulic newborn; we speak of feto-fetal transfusion when the difference in haemoglobin between the twins is greater than 5 g/dl. Less frequent causes of neonatal anaemia involve iatrogenic attitudes such as puncture of the newborn's calf during birth monitoring or trauma to the newborn during amniocentesis. Another cause of neonatal anaemia, common in neonatal intensive care units, is the frequent analysis necessary for the proper management of the disease, which leads to the need for repeated transfusions, increasing the morbidity of these patients.

Haemorrhagic disease of the newborn is due to a defect of vitamin K-dependent clotting factors. At one time, the non-prophylactic use of vitamin K, together with the low concentration of vitamin K in breast milk, made this pathology common during the neonatal period.

Separate considerations must be made regarding physiological anaemia in infants; various factors have been implicated in the decrease in erythropoiesis that occurs in the first 2 months of life under physiological conditions. Both before and after birth, an adequate supply of nutrients is necessary for normal erythropoiesis. Among the nutrients considered essential are iron, folates, vitamin E, vitamin B_{12} and copper. When iron intake is deficient, iron deficiency anaemia usually develops between 6 months and 3 years of age, but in mothers with severe iron deficiency during pregnancy, iron stores in the foetus are lower and the risk of developing iron deficiency anaemia is higher and the onset of iron deficiency anaemia is earlier. The diagnosis of iron deficiency anaemia is based, in addition to the quantification of circulating iron, on the decrease in haematopoietic size; a decrease in mean corpuscular volume (MCV) occurs after birth, with a decrease up to 6 months of life of up to 67 fl being considered normal. Vitamin E depletion is a cause of haemophthalmic anaemia, especially in premature infants, and the mechanism of action seems to be related to the prevention of lipid peroxidation that this vitamin exerts on the haemarie membrane. The administration of iron to infants may have an inhibitory effect on the absorption of vitamin E, especially when this supplementation is carried out in the first 2 weeks of life. Clinical manifestations of vitamin E deficiency include jaundice, anaemia, reticulocytosis, thrombocytosis and peripheral oedema. Recommendations for vitamin E prevention consist of supplementation with 2-25 IU/d(a) during the first 2-4 weeks of life. Folate is a coenzyme necessary for both amino acid production and DNA synthesis. Folate deficiency is not usually a cause of megaloblastic anaemia during the first 2-4 weeks of life.

the neonatal period, in fact folate concentrations in the umbilical cord are 5 to 7 times higher than those observed in maternal serum; moreover, milk is a food resource usually rich in folates; when the supply of folates is compromised in the first months of life, given that the requirements at this age are also high, folate deficiency anaemia can develop, especially in premature infants, infants with diarrhoea or treated with diphenylhydantoin. Vitamin B_{12} or cobalamin is an essential cofactor for the production of tetrahydrofolic acid from 5-methyltetrahydrofolic acid. Vitamin B_{12} deficiency is a rare occurrence in the first months of life and only in cases of cobalamin deficiency in the pregnant woman have cobalamin deficiencies been described in the newborn.

Haemophthisic anaemias comprise another important chapter of neonatal anaemias; within this group of anaemias we include haemolysis due to infection (in many of them Heinz corpuscles appear, typical but not characteristic, as they can appear in other diseases), haemopoietic anaemias of constitutional cause (hereditary spherocytosis, enzymopenias, haemoglobinopathies) which mostly give clinical manifestations at a later age, but can exceptionally manifest themselves in the neonatal period; neonatal alloimmune anaemias are the most common type of neonatal haemophthalic anaemias and are due to the existence of antibodies to haematophores. The possibility of reducing neonatal alloimmune anaemia by administering anti-D immunoglobulin to Rh-negative mothers with Rh-positive newborns or those who have had an abortion has considerably reduced the frequency of this type of anaemia, although it has not been able to fall below 4 cases/10,000 pregnancies.

Currently, ABO isoimmunisation has become the most frequent cause of alloimmune neonatal anaemia with 16% of cases compared to 2% of anaemias due to Rh alloimmunisation. The Rh blood system consists of a group of antigens, of which the most logical and widely used nomenclature is that proposed by Fisher and Race in 1948, which proposes the existence of 3 antigenic determinants CDE, the presence or absence of the D antigen denotes whether the subject is Rh positive or negative.

Another important group of anaemias in the neonatal period is represented by aplastic anaemias, those of congenital cause being the most frequent. Blackfand-Diamond erythrogenesis imperfecta manifests itself at birth in 30% of cases. Affected newborns usually present with intrauterine growth retardation, without malformations or abnormal skin pigmentation. Anaemia with decreased reticulocytes (<0.1%), increased haemoglobin F, increased adenosine deaminase activity and presence of "i" antigen are found. Bone marrow examination shows absence of myeloid precursors. Other causes of congenital aplastic anaemia are Fanconi anaemia, dyserythropoietic anaemia, Estem-Dameshek anaemia and idiopathic aplastic anaemia. Secondary aplastic anaemias occur in conjunction with other smdromes, where the predominant cause is usually an invasion of the bone marrow by cells that hinder normal erythropoiesis, including Albers-Schomberg syndrome (infantile osteopetrosis + pancytopenia), Benjamm syndrome (idiocy and prematurity), congenital leukaemia (in Down syndrome) and post-transfusion aplastic anaemia.

Clinical manifestations of neonatal anaemias

The usual clinical manifestations will consist of pallor, and in the most severe cases of acute presentation, tachycardia or the development of heart failure. Meanwhile, in the gradual forms of presentation, the development of foci of extramedullary erythropoiesis and cardiac insufficiency lead to the appearance of hepatosplenomegaly. However, when considering neonatal anaemia, the gestational age of the newborn and the site of collection must be taken into account in addition to the absolute haematological count. Blood samples can be obtained by central vessel puncture, umbilical catheter or skin puncture (capillary samples); the latter are less reliable and generally generate higher count figures than venous samples, these differences can be extremely marked in very sick newborns (with poor peripheral perfusion) and in very premature newborns.

Treatment of neonatal anaemias

The treatment of neonatal anaemia will vary according to the aetiology of the anaemia, as a general rule an adequate blood volume should be maintained to develop adequate gas homeostasis; therefore, in special situations such as critically ill newborns, haemoglobin values considered critical will be significantly higher than in situations without concomitant pathology.

If the haemoglobin is greater than 10 g/dL, transfusion is rarely indicated. If the haemoglobin is less than 7 g/dL, transfusion is usually always indicated. If the haemoglobin is greater than 7 g/dL and less than 10 g/dL, clinical status, venous oxygen pressure less than 25 mmHg and an oxygen extraction ratio greater than 50% decide the need for transfusion.

Neonatal polyglobulia

Polyglobulia, due to the presence of hyperviscosity of the blood, represents a potential risk for 1 to 5 % of all newborns in industrialised countries. As blood viscosity increases, a variety of internal organs can be affected and their blood flow can be reduced, resulting in hypoxia and acidosis. Fortunately, few infants with polycythemia or neonatal hyperviscosity develop complications attributable to these causes. The type of symptomatic manifestations, as well as the foreseeable sequelae in these infants, is a matter of great controversy. In most cases infants with hyperviscosity are also likely to have polycythaemia, and vice versa. Polycythaemia refers only to an abnormal increase in red cell mass, whereas hyperviscosity relates to the force required to achieve flow. Blood viscosity is affected by erythrocyte mass, plasma components and the interaction of circulating cellular elements.

The first descriptions of polycythaemia were due to monochorionic twin boys with placental vascular anastomosis. Often there is a sharp contrast between the small, anaemic twin and its much larger, plethoric sibling. The incidence and symptoms in the neonate vary, their severity appears to be considerable and often ranges from myoclonus and refusal of food to episodes of fatal enterocolitis. Severe illness and mortality appear to be almost exclusively confined to infants with other neonatal problems. These include aqw, asphyxia, premature births or polycythemic infants who have developed enterocolitis or seizures.

The defining features of polyglobulia are the existence in the blood of:

- More than 6 million hematfes.
- More than 20 g/dL haemoglobin.
- Central (venous) haematocrit:
- 60-65 %: Physiological polyglobulia.
- 65-70%: Paraphysiological polyglobulia.
- >70%: Pathological polyglobulia.

The haematocrit of the newborn falls gradually from the first day of life until it reaches its minimum value at about 3 months of age. In the first hours and days of life there are rapid exchanges in the intravascular fluid that make the static measurement of a single haematocrit less reliable. Infants who have their cord clamped immediately show no significant increase in haematocrit in the first hours of life. All infants studied demonstrated a decrease in venous haematocrit between 4 and 24 hours after delivery. However, in later-term, growth-competent newborns who had their cord clamped immediately (with a mean of 14 seconds) show an immediate postnatal increase in haematocrit. These changes in haematocrit have been associated with a significant drop in the incidence of polycythaemia from 2 hours to 12-18 hours of age. Therefore, a delay in venous determination until 12-24 hours of age reduces the incidence of polyglobulia and makes its treatment unnecessary. At the same time, this delay may increase the incidence of neonatal problems and sequelae secondary to undiagnosed polyglobulia.

Most polyglobulias are asymptomatic. Symptomatology is secondary to the situation of hyperviscosity, mainly skin symptoms (cyanosis, redness or jaundice due to haemolysis). They may also present anorexia, respiratory distress, heart failure and neurological alterations.

In severe cases we can observe DIC, thrombosis, priapism, convulsions, necrotising enterocolitis, renal failure. Alphabetically we can find thrombopenia, hypoglycaemia, hypocalcaemia, hypomagnesaemia, acidosis. The variability of symptoms attributed to polycythaemia and hyperviscosity has made it difficult to identify a clinical course in the polyglobulic child. Some follow-up studies have reported a low incidence of severe sequelae in the well-grown term infant with polyglobulic polyglobulia.

Polyglobulia and hyperviscosity result in reduced blood flow and oxygen transport in the foetus. The microcirculation of negotiable organs shows a decrease in blood flow and oxygen transport with haematocrits above 45%. It appears that oxygen consumption can be maintained only when oxygen transport is at least 14 mL/kg/min. The decrease in cerebral blood flow seen in cases of polycythaemia and hyperviscosity may depend on the increased oxygen content and haematocrit. In newborns with polyglobulia and hyperviscosity, cerebral vascular resistance is elevated and the clinical manifestations described have been lethargy, refusal of feeding or seizures. In some cases the permanent neurological disturbances described are due to multiple cerebral infarctions. Regarding cardiological manifestations, electrocardiograms of patients with polyglobulia mostly only demonstrate the existence of an ECG that was considered normal; however, ECG alterations have been described including right ventricular hypertrophy, ST-segment changes and less frequently left ventricular hypertrophy. Echocardiographic changes and radiological evidence of cardiomegaly have also been described.

The treatment of neonatal polyglobulia is reserved exclusively for symptomatic cases. In general, if the central haematocrit is 65.1-70%, the newborn must be correctly hydrated. If the haematocrit is over 70%, partial exchange transfusions with plasma protein solution (serum albumin) are performed. This treatment reduces haematological alterations, but is associated with feeding alterations, increased risk of necrotising enterocolitis and thrombosis.

Haemorrhagic disease of the newborn

The term haemorrhagic disease of the newborn is currently reserved for the increasingly rare cases of vitamin K deficiency, since both the exogenous supply (mother's milk is deficient in vitamin K) and the smthesis by the intestinal microbiota, which in the first hours or days of life is still deficient, are normally lacking; This contributes to the appearance of physiological hypoprothrombinemia, more accentuated in premature infants due to their greater degree of hepatic immaturity; this situation is potentially reversible and responds immediately to parenteral vitamin K administration. Before prophylactic administration of vitamin K became widespread, this condition occurred in 0.25-0.5% of breastfed infants.

In haemorrhagic disease of the newborn the haemorrhagic picture develops between the 1st and 5th day of life. It may sometimes be present from birth, and severe haemorrhages have been observed after fetal blood samples have been taken from the scalp to determine the pH. Clmica, which is very polymorphic, is classified according to Willi's classification into two main groups of haemorrhages: external and internal.

External haemorrhages include the following locations:

- Umbilical. Very frequent, poor umbilical cord ligation, and in late cases hereditary factor XIII deficiency (fibrin stabilising factor) or umbilical infection must always be ruled out.

- Gastrointestinal. They usually manifest as haematemesis *and* melena. The existence of maternal blood ingested during delivery must be ruled out, for which the Apt test is useful, which serves to differentiate haemoglobin A, belonging to maternal blood, from the alkaline-resistant haemoglobin F of the child. Exceptionally, the blood may be due to epistaxis, or to intestinal processes such as intussusception, Meckel's diverticulum, volvulus and gastrointestinal ulceration, so an abdominal X-ray should always be performed and, if the clinical picture suggests it, an abdominal ultrasound.

- Respiratory. They do not usually manifest themselves as abundant haemoptysis, but as bloody foam visible during nasopharyngeal suctioning of the newborn. They are accompanied by respiratory distress requiring mechanical ventilation. The prognosis is severe.

- Genitalia. Its frequency has decreased considerably since newborns are not routinely circumcised. Vaginal bleeding observed sporadically in newborns is of no pathological significance and is due to the passage of oestrogen from the mother through the placenta.

- Urinary tract. Microhaematuria is common and has no pathological significance, macrohaematuria may be due to renal infarction or renal venous thrombosis.

- Subconjunctival. They are due to the capillary fragility of the newborn and the increase in pressure at the time of delivery. Their prognosis is good.
- Cutaneous. In the form of petechiae or ecchymosis, they are due to traumatic births, presentation of the buttocks, protrusion of an arm, face, etc. They are frequent in neonatal thrombopenias and DIC.
- Cephalohaematoma. When they are very extensive they can lead to anaemia and/or prolonged jaundice, although as a rule their prognosis is excellent.

Internal bleeding includes the following processes:

- Intracranial haemorrhage. It accounts for up to 16% of all major haemorrhages, and is responsible for 15% of neonatal mortality. They can be intraventricular, due to the increased capillary fragility of the germinal matrix, and subarachnoid or subdural, in which mechanical factors and vessel dyslacerations are more involved.
- Haemorrhage of the adrenal glands. It can be unilateral, usually asymptomatic, or bilateral, which is more serious due to the development of adrenal insufficiency. The finding of unilateral adrenal haemorrhage is sometimes coincidental, following the detection of a calcification image on ultrasound of a newborn baby born with dystocic labour. Palpation of an abdominal mass raises the differential diagnosis with renal venous thrombosis, hydronephrosis and tumours affecting the kidney or adrenal glands.
- Hepatic haemorrhages. Like the previous one, although less frequent, they occur in dystociated births and are located below Glisson's capsule. Its rupture causes haemoperitoneum.
- Peritoneal haemorrhages. They are usually secondary to injury to other abdominal organs (liver, spleen, etc.).
- Retinal haemorrhages. They are a common finding on fundus examination in healthy newborns, are of no clinical significance and usually disappear within 48-72 hours; larger ones may persist for up to 10 days.

For the diagnosis of haemorrhagic disease of the newborn the most significant laboratory finding is a prolonged prothrombin time (Quick's time), higher than normal (25 seconds), which means a prothrombin activity below 50%. The clotting time and cephalin or partial thromboplastin time are also prolonged, while the bleeding time (primary haemostasis), clot retraction and platelet count are normal.

Haemorrhagic disease of the newborn can be prevented by administering vitamin K (1 mg) to all newborns within the first 24 hours, but there is inconclusive evidence that higher doses of vitamin K given to the mother during delivery are equally effective. The use of this treatment is of particular importance in the preterm infant and in infants who have undergone traumatic delivery or hypoxia, given their increased risk of haemorrhage. As a general measure, it is advisable to start feeding as early as possible, even in premature infants, giving preference to breastfeeding.

Bibliograffa

1. Uberos J, Blanca E, Munoz A, Narbona E: Neonatal haematology. In *Neonatologi'a. Volume* 2. 1^ edition. Edited by Munoz Hoyos A, Narbona Lopez E, Valenzuela Ruiz A. Granada: Alhulia S.L.; 2000: 271-289: *Formation continuada en pediatna*].

8. Neonatal jaundice

Dr. Jose Uberos Fernandez

Dr. Ana Campos Martinez

Hyperbilirubinaemia and its clinical expression, jaundice, is the most frequent disorder in the neonatal period. Bilirubin is a final metabolite in heme catabolism. Its clinical significance in the newborn derives from its propensity to be deposited in skin and mucous membranes, producing its yellow colouring or jaundice (from the Greek ikteros). Neonatal hyperbilirubinaemia involves an imbalance between bilirubin production and its elimination, which in turn requires bilirubin uptake by the hepatocyte, its conjugation and excretion of the conjugated products.

Bilirubin metabolism

Haemolysis releases iron protoporphyrin (heme), the oxygen-carrying component of haemoglobin. Heme is catalysed by heme oxygenase in the reticuloendothelial system and converted to biliverdin and then, after action of the enzyme biliverdin reductase, transformed into indirect bilirubin, which is fat-soluble and must be transported to the liver by plasma albumin. Free indirect bilirubin is toxic, as it can cross the blood-brain barrier and bind to tissues. It is therefore important to assess hypoalbuminaemia in newborns, as the binding capacity to albumin may be exceeded and the percentage of free indirect bilirubin increased.

In the liver, indirect bilirubin, taken up by the hepatic sinusoids, enters the hepatocyte by the action of two proteins, ligandins Y and Z, which transport it to the smooth endoplasmic reticulum. Here it binds to glucuronic acid and is transformed into conjugated or direct bilirubin by the enzyme uridin-diphosphate-glucuronyl-transferase. The latter form of bilirubin is water-soluble and can be excreted mainly in the faeces and 2% in the urine. It is estimated that 1 g of haemoglobin gives rise to 34 mg of bilirubin. It has been estimated that, in newborns, during the first day of life, bilirubin production is three times the rate observed in adults. Several factors may explain this increase in bilirubin production in the newborn:

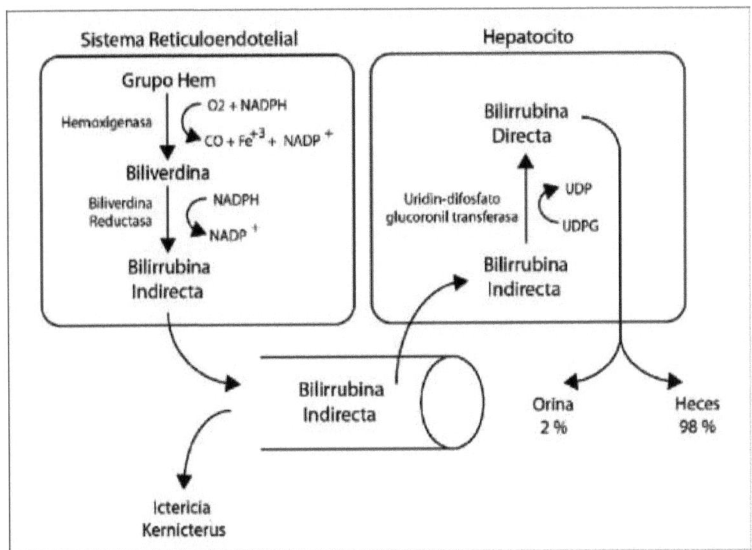

Figure 8.1. Schematic diagram of bilirubin metabolism.

- Shortening of the half-life of haematophores in the newborn to 70-90 days, instead of 120 days in the adult haematophore.
- Higher haematocrit than in adults, essential to maintain adequate oxygenation in the foetus.
- Increased enterohepatic recirculation, as a consequence of deconjugation of conjugated bilirubin in the intestine, which is absorbed and transported back to the intestine.

The bilirubin passes through the bile duct into the gall bladder, where it is stored and concentrated before being excreted into the intestine, where it is reduced by bacterial action to urobilinogen, stercobilinogen and stercobilin. A portion of the direct bilirubin is transformed by P-glucuronidase in the intestinal villi into indirect bilirubin, which is absorbed and passes into the circulation and from there to the intestine (enterohepatic circulation).

Physiological newborn jaundice

In the first days of life there are special internal circumstances that cause the frequent appearance of jaundice, known as physiological jaundice or *fcterus smplex neonatorum*. It is seen in 60% of normal newborns. It is usually seen from the second day onwards, being more evident on the third and fourth days, and then rapidly diminishing, so that in the vast majority of cases it is not noticeable until the eighth day. In some cases it is already visible at the end of 24 hours and exceptionally persists until the 12th day. The icteric tinge of the skin and mucous membranes is considered minimal or moderate, being totally or partially masked by the physiological erythema. The evolution is good, disappearing within the aforementioned period, without the need for therapeutic measures. Hyperbilirubinaemia is predominantly indirect or unconjugated. The most universally accepted Kmite figure in the newborn at term is 13 mg/dL of total bilirubin and, if breast-fed, values below 15.5 mg/dL. The daily increase is less than 5 mg.

Increased bilirubinaemia is detectable in all newborns already in the umbilical cord blood (up to 4 mg/dL), without exerting a pathogenic action; on the contrary, it may have an antioxidant effect. Initially, it was only considered to be related to transient hyperglobulia of the newborn. Other related factors are a deficit of uptake by the proximal pole of the hepatocyte by prothymes Y and Z, with demonstrated insufficiency of the former in this period of life, and increased enterohepatic circulation. However, the major factor in hyperbilirubinaemia in the newborn is the limited ability of the liver to metabolise or modify the bilirubin produced in the first few days, making it suitable for renal elimination. The hepatocyte of most newborns is deficient in the enzyme glucuronyltransferase, which also conditions the occurrence of physiological hyperbilirubinaemia.

Occasionally, episodes of higher incidence of hyperbilirubinaemia are observed in normal term neonates of adequate weight, in which a responsible cause cannot be demonstrated, with the following possible aetiopathogenic factors intervening as possible aetiopathogenic factors: liver dysfunction due to relative immaturity (GA: 37-38 weeks or inductions before the onset of dynamics), drugs administered at delivery that may induce haemolysis (oxytocin) or cause hypoperistalsis with consequent delay in the elimination of meconium, prolonged fasting with increased enterohepatic circulation and other factors that may inhibit the enzymatic activity of hepatic glucuronyltransferase in the newborn (hypothermia, anoxia, cortisone), not to mention the possible role of mono- or oligosymptomatic viral infections and the not uncommon Gilbert's disease. From an evolutionary point of view, it behaves like physiological jaundice, but with higher bilirubin values. Abnormal courses of physiological jaundice may also include breast-fed infants, infants born in populations at high altitude above sea level, newborns subjected to prolonged fasting or who have suffered hypothermia and Lucey's syndrome, since factors similar to those mentioned in physiological jaundice are involved.

Breastfeeding jaundice

Transient and prolonged jaundice in breastfed infants appears around the 4th-7th day, in one out of 200 breastfed infants. It has been attributed to the increased presence of P-glucuronidase, pregnandiol or to an excess of lipase, which leads to an increase in free fatty acids. Pregnandiol, eliminated in the amount of 1 mg daily in the milk of some lactating mothers, acts by inhibiting the glucuronyltransferase system and the cytoplasmic Z-protein of the hepatocyte. Free fatty acids compete with bilirubin in its binding to albumin, leading to indirectly predominant hyperbilirubinaemia. An increase in the frequency of feedings sometimes reduces bilirubinaemia, possibly by increasing the number of bowel movements and thus decreasing the enterohepatic circulation, since in breast milk there is greater activity (3-glucuronidase) which favours the deconjugation of direct bilirubin.

Haemophthalmic jaundice

It is dominated by haemophthalmic disease of the newborn, whether due to maternal-fetal incompatibility of the Rh system, ABO incompatibility or the rarer ones due to other erythrocyte antigens. From being a frequent pathology, it now has an incidence of 1 case per 1000 newborns, following the improvement of the obstetrical controls implemented. Rh immunisation is caused by transplacental passage from the mother to the foetus, the risk depends on the volume of the transplacental transfusion and the ABO group, it is estimated that if the volume transferred is 1 mL the risk of immunisation in an Rh compatible newborn is 3%, for volumes greater than 5 mL the risk is more than 60%. The primary immune response to the D antigen consists of the production of anti-D IgM, which does not cross the placenta and is harmless to the foetus. The secondary immune response is IgG-mediated and is more intense. Unlike the primary immune response, the immunoglobulin crosses the placenta into the foetus, where it binds to susceptible red blood cells that are destroyed extravascularly and in the spleen. The presence of anti-D IgG can be evidenced by a positive Coombs' test or a positive erythrocyte eluate test for anti-D IgG. In the most severe forms of immunisation, severe intrauterine anaemia develops, and increased hepatic erythropoiesis with enlargement of the liver MgD is set in motion. Portal and umbilical venous pressures increase, decreased hepatocellular function and hypoalbuminaemia develop and ascites develops *(hydrops feltalis)*. In less severe forms haemophthalmic anaemia and hyperbilirubinaemia with its complications *(Kernicterus)* dominate the clinical picture.

For the identification of maternal isoimmunisation, at the first prenatal visit, all pregnant women should undergo blood grouping, Rh and antibody screening by means of the indirect Coombs test, and not only Rh negative women, as there are other systems of clinical interest as has already been mentioned. Once the existence of isoimmunisation has been detected, it should be investigated whether it is associated with haemophthalmic disease, for example, the Lewis system is very frequent in producing incompatibility, but as it generates IgM antibodies that do not cross the placenta, it has no clinical significance in the foetus. Practically all maternal isoimmunisations are caused by feto-maternal transfusion, which originates in the course of the third trimester or during delivery.

In any immunised mother (titre > 1:32), the severity of disease in the foetus should be assessed. Fetal surveillance includes serial ultrasound scans to assess the presence of placental oedema (early sign), pleural oedema, ascites. Middle cerebral artery Doppler allows assessment of indirect signs of anaemia. A systolic peak in the middle cerebral artery greater than 1.5 may be indicative of anaemia. Amniocentesis can assess the bilirubin level in amniotic fluid and fetal maturity by quantifying the amount of lecithin. Cordocentesis allows assessment of haemoglobin and haematophilic count in the foetus, as well as transfusion of the foetus if necessary.

The goals of treatment are to prevent death of the foetus or newborn as a result of anaemia and to prevent bilirubin neurotoxicity.

Prevention of maternal anti-D isoimmunisation can be done by administering 300 mg of anti-D Ig at 28 weeks gestation and within 72 hours after any abortion, amniocentesis in non-sensitised pregnant women (negative Coombs test), or after delivery if the newborn is Rh positive.

Resorption of haematomas

The presence of obstetric trauma and cephalohaematomas due to forceps or vacuum extraction, spontaneous, or any extravasation of blood with rupture of blood vessels can lead to an increase in bilirubin, which is often ta^a.

Complications of indirect hyperbilirubinaemia

Free unconjugated bilirubin, because of its lipophilic characteristics, can penetrate the nervous system and damage the mitochondria of neurons.

Kerrn'cterus. The main risk of early hyperbilirubinaemia is the development of "bilirubmic encephalopathy". It is characterised by hypotoma, absence or transient decrease of primitive reflexes, swallowing disorders and decreased motility, which disappear without sequelae. Minor neuropsychological disorders are possible at school age.

Treatment of hyperbilirubinaemia

The most commonly used measures are:

Early feeding and frequent feedings to promote intestinal peristalsis. 2. 2. Plenty of ambient light.

3. Phototherapy, useful for 12-24 hours in non haemophthalmic BPNs, when bilirubinaemia reaches 10 mg/dL.

4. Phenobarbital, administered orally to pregnant women from 36 weeks. It is indicated in populations with a high rate of hyperbilirubinaemia or when there is a presumption of group incompatibility (mother O with father A, B or AB).

5. Hepatitis B prophylaxis.

6. Prevention of haemophthalmic disease.

7. Treatment of sensitised pregnant women with high-dose standard IV gamma globulin.

It is essential to maintain good hydration (normal hepatocyte function, adequate bile permeability).

Phototherapy. A light with a wavelength between 430 and 460 nm (blue light) is used, which causes photoconjugation of the bilirubin found in the skin and dermal capillaries, resulting in conjugated derivatives that are soluble and are eliminated through the kidney and digestive tract. The main disadvantages are: a lamp life of approximately 10,000 hours requires eye protection of the newborn; the light radiation can cause erythema, and the term "tanned baby" has been adopted to refer to the dark greyish skin colouring of some children undergoing phototherapy; this technique should not be used when there is parenchymal liver disease or obstructive jaundice. Hyperthermia-hypothermia and diarrhoea may be observed, due to the passage of photosensitive soluble elements which are irritating to the intestine. Phototherapy rapidly whitens the skin, however, the bilirubin level may remain elevated.

Phenobarbital is a potent, slow-acting enzyme inducer at the level of the hepatocyte smooth endoplasmic reticulum, so it is most useful as a prophylactic. The dose should be around 5 mg/kg^a. Other methods are clofibrate (induces glucuronyltransferase and protein Z transporter synthesis).

Human serum albumin. It is to be used especially before or during exchange transfusion to remove tissue bilirubin, especially in premature infants and intravenously at a dose of 1 g/kg. It is contraindicated in situations with elevated central venous pressure and capillary leak syndrome.

Exchange transfusion. Whenever serum bilirubin exceeds the values indicated for gestational age and chronological age. An increase in the serum indirect bilirubin level at a rate greater than 0.5 mg/dl/hour indicates an intense haemolytic process that will require exchange transfusion within the first 24 hours of life, thus also correcting the anaemia and eliminating a significant proportion of sensitised red blood cells. Its indications are as follows:

- Sepsis of the newborn.
- Umbilical cord bilirubin greater than 5 mg/dl.
- Serum bilirubin in term newborns, greater than 20 mg/dl.
- In newborns weighing less than 1500 g when there is perinatal hypoxia, respiratory distress, acidosis, bilirubin above 15 mg/dl.
- Early anaemia (Hb less than 14 g/dl) associated with jaundice.

Bibliograffa

1. Delgado A: Neonatal indirect hyperbilirubinaemia. (Delgado A ed., vol. 5, 1 edition. pp. 49-64. Bilbao: University of the Basque Country; 1994:49-64.

2. Cruz M, Jimenez R. Jaundice of the newborn (hyperbilirubinaemia). In: Cruz M. *Tratado de Pediatria,* 7^ ed, Ed, Espaxs, Barcelona 1993: 187.

3. Jimenez R, Figueras J, Botet F. Neonatolog^a, 3^ ed, (in press), Jimenez R, Krauel X. Jaundice in the newborn. Pediatr Integral 2000; 5: 491-498.

4. Jimenez R, Krauel X, Jaundice in the newborn (hyperbilirubinemia). In: Cruz M. *Tratado de Pediatna.* 8- ed. Editorial Ergon, Madrid 2001: 165-181.

9. Respiratory distress in the newborn infant

Dr. Jose Uberos Fernandez

Dr. Elisabeth Fernandez Marin

At birth, there is an abrupt transition to foetal respiration. While the first breath causes a sharp and intense drop in pulmonary vascular resistances, the subsequent decrease in these resistances occurs during the first days of life coinciding with the relaxation and maturation of the pulmonary arterioles. Under normal circumstances the pulmonary circulation resembles the adult circulation both in its resistances and histological appearance after a few weeks of life.

The first respiratory movements of the newborn cause the pulmonary alveoli to fill with gas. Alveolar expansion is, above all, what triggers functional pulmonary circulation, through the mechanical effect of a rapid lowering of pulmonary arterial resistance. Endothelial nitric oxide (NO) synthesis, triggered by elevated P_{aO_2}, and the release of prostacyclin, both pulmonary vasodilators, also contribute to the decrease in pulmonary vascular resistance.

Respiratory distress is a common syndrome in the neonatal period that may be due to various pathological entities and is characterised by symptoms such as: tachypnoea, tugging and retractions, expiratory whining, inspiratory stridor or cyanosis. Overall, this pathology constitutes the most frequent cause of neonatal morbimortality and its severity will be related to the aetiological cause and its repercussion on blood gases.

Although the most significant neonatal respiratory distress is hyaline membrane disease (HMD) or respiratory distress due to surfactant deficiency, typical of preterm infants, in this topic we will also focus on respiratory pathologies typical of the term newborn, such as transient tachypnoea or meconium aspiration syndrome.

The causes of respiratory distress in the newborn are summarised in Table 9.1.

Table 9.1. Causes of respiratory distress in the newborn.

Respiratory causes:	**Cardiovascular causes:**
- Hyaline membrane disease.	- Congenital heart disease.
- Mild respiratory distress.	- Cardiac arrhythmia.
-Transient tachypnoea of the NB.	- Myocardiomyopathy.
-Mechanical aspiration.	
- Pneumothorax/Neumomediastinum.	
- Perinatal pneumonia.	
- Persistent pulmonary hypertension.	
- Pulmonary haemorrhage.	
- Pulmonary agenesis-hypoplasia.	
Malformations:	**Infectious causes:**
- Diaphragmatic hernia.	-Sepsis / Neonatal meningitis.
- Oesophageal atresia.	
- Congenital lobar emphysema.	
- Qwstic adenomatoid malformation.	
Upper airway obstruction:	**Metabolic causes:**
- Choanal atresia.	-Metabolic acidosis.
-Sd. de Pierre-Robin.	- Hypoglycaemia.
	- Hypothermia / Hyperthermia.
Haematological causes:	**Neurological causes:**
- Anaemia.	-Suffocation.
- Hyperviscosity.	- Diffuse CNS lesion.
	-Drug withdrawal symptoms.

The Silverman and Anderson test is a test that assesses the respiratory distress of a newborn, based on five criteria. Each parameter is quantifiable and the sum total is interpreted in terms of difficulty. A score of 1 to 4 indicates mild respiratory distress, 5 to 7 is moderate and above 7 is severe.

- Thoracic or abdominal elevation: synchronised (0), little elevation on inspiration (1), thoracoabdominal wobble (2).
- Ribbing: none (0), barely visible (1), marked (2).
- Xiphoid retraction: none (0), barely visible (1), marked (2).

- Nasal flaring: absent (0), minimal (1), marked (2).
- Whining: absent (0), audible with stethoscope (1), audible without stethoscope (2).

Transient tachypnoea of the newborn

It was described in 1966 by Avery, whom he also called "transient tachypnoea of newborn" and more recently "pulmonary maladaptation". It affects 1% of live newborns, most often term newborns, and is responsible for 30% of cases of neonatal respiratory distress. It is a respiratory disease that is present from birth. It is secondary to inadequate mobilisation of the pulmonary fluid in the transition from intrauterine to extrauterine life.

Physiopathology. It is postulated that this entity is produced by the distension of the interstitial spaces by the pulmonary fluid which results in the trapping of alveolar air and a decrease in pulmonary distensibility, which causes tachypnoea, the most characteristic sign of this condition. Other authors consider that it is caused by delayed elimination of pulmonary kyphosis due to lack of thoracic compression (caesarean delivery) or maternal hypersedation. For other authors, there is an immaturity of the surfactant system.

Clinical manifestations. Respiratory distress is present from birth or within 2 hours after birth, with tachypnoea predominating, which may reach 100-120 breaths per minute. The presence of wheezing, cyanosis and retractions are rare, although they may be seen in the more severe forms. The clinical manifestations may worsen in the first 6-8 hours, after 12 hours a slow improvement usually begins and persists for 3-4 days.

Diagnosis. Auscultation usually shows bilateral decreased pulmonary ventilation. Radiological findings range from normal to reinforcement of the hilar bronchovascular tract, presence of pleural fluid, cystic effusion, hyperinflation and even reticulogranular pattern.

Treatment. Although its course is self-limiting, while it lasts, further ventilatory support measures must be instituted to ensure adequate gas exchange.

Hyaline membrane disease

Respiratory distress syndrome (RDS) type 1, also known as hyaline membrane disease, is a clinical picture of early-onset respiratory distress related to prematurity and pulmonary immaturity.

Aetiology. The fundamental cause is a deficit of surfactant, a pulmonary surfactant that can be seen in the fetal lungs from the 20th week of GA onwards.

Pathophysiology. Respiratory distress syndrome type 1 is caused by a transient surfactant deficiency, due to:

- Decreased surfactant synthesis
- Qualitative surfactant alterations
- Inactivation of surfactant.

The loss of the surfactant-mediated surfactant function leads to alveolar collapse, with a decrease in functional residual capacity, with progressive atelectasis leading to alterations in ventilation and the ventilation-perfusion ratio. The lung becomes stiffer and tends to collapse easily and rapidly, increasing the work or respiratory effort. Cyanosis occurs due to hypoxaemia secondary to alterations in ventilation/perfusion, and CO_2 is retained due to hypoventilation. All this leads to mixed acidosis, which increases pulmonary vascular resistance and favours the appearance of right-left shunts at the *ductus* and foramen level, increasing hypoxaemia.

Diffuse microatelectasis, oedema, vascular congestion and damage to the respiratory epithelium appear in the lung. Microscopic examination shows widespread atelectasis, with distal airways occupied by hyaline material composed of fibrin and epithelial cellular debris due to cellular necrosis, the "hyaline membranes", which are the consequence and not the cause of the disease. The surfactant-deficient lung requires high pressures to open the collapsed alveoli, which are higher than 25-30 cm H_2O for smaller radius alveoli. When the patient is on assisted ventilation, overdistension and rupture of larger alveoli can occur, leading to interstitial emphysema and extrapulmonary air accumulation.

Risk factors. These are factors that inhibit surfactant synthesis and can therefore worsen the evolution of a premature infant with HME: asphyxia, hypoxaemia, pulmonary ischaemia, hypovolaemia, hypotension, hypothermia.

Clinical manifestations. At present the clinical picture is not fully established due to early administration of surfactant and respiratory support. The first symptoms appear at birth or in the first hours, progressively worsening, with moderate to severe respiratory distress with polypnoea, rib and xiphoid pull, whining, nasal flaring and cyanosis on room air. Polypnoea, a high Silverman test score and cyanosis are the most frequent clinical signs. The expiratory whine is characteristic and is due to the passage of exhaled air through the half-closed glottis, in an attempt to maintain adequate alveolar volume and avoid alveolar collapse. Auscultation shows marked bilateral symmetrical hypoventilation. The general condition is severely affected, with hypoactivity and poor response to stimuli. Haemodynamic disturbances such as slow capillary refill and arterial hypotension are frequent.

Treatment. Treatment is fundamentally aimed at ensuring good pulmonary function and adequate gas exchange, avoiding complications.

Exogenous surfactant. Tracheal instillation of exogenous surfactant produces a rapid improvement in functional residual capacity and pulmonary distensibility, leading to a decrease in O2 requirements and ventilatory support.

Oxygen therapy. FiO2 should be increased to maintain PaO2 between 50 and 60 mmHg, avoiding higher values to reduce the risk of lung injury and retinopathy of prematurity.

Continuous positive airway pressure (CPAP). It is a common part of the treatment of respiratory distress syndrome. It produces progressive alveolar recruitment, increases FRC, improves oxygenation, promotes surfactant synthesis.

Assisted ventilation. Conventional ventilation synchronised with the patient's respirations is now preferred, ensuring a tidal volume of 4-5 cm H_2O.

Meconium aspiration syndrome

It consists of the inhalation of amniotic fluid containing intrauterine or intrapartum meconium.

Etiology. Occurs in the term or post-term neonate, being exceptional in the preterm. Congenital listeriosis or perinatal asphyxia are the usual triggers of meconium emission by the antepartum foetus. Both meconium emission and the stimulation of respiratory movements in the foetus prior to clamping of the umbilical cord after delivery are considered to be conditioned by foetal hypoxaemia.

Clinical manifestations. They include a wide spectrum of severity, ranging from mild respiratory distress to severe respiratory distress requiring invasive ventilation. These severe forms are often associated with pulmonary hypertension. Increased anteroposterior thoracic diameter due to pulmonary emphysema caused by airway obstruction ("barrel chest") is often seen.

Diagnosis. It should always be suspected in any newborn with meconium amniotic fluid and early onset of respiratory distress. In radiology the most typical finding is the presence of diffuse cottony alveolar condensation.

Prevention and treatment. Airway clearance and establishment of breathing and oxygenation remain essential for resuscitation of all neonates. Treatment should be directed at maintaining adequate ventilation with SaO2 between 85-95% and pH >7.20. Respiratory support can range from ventilation with oxygen therapy and non-invasive positive pressure ventilation to conventional or high frequency invasive ventilation. Administration of antibiotics, corticosteroids and surfactant may be indicated.

Bibliograffa

1.   Lopez de Heredia y Goya J, Valls i Soler A. Respiratory distress syndrome. In: Cruz Hernandez M, editor. Tratado de Pediatna. Madrid: Ergon; 2009. p. 162-5.

PART II

10. Congenital heart disease

Dr. Enrique Blanca Jover

Introduction. General

Congenital cardiopathies (CC) are constituted by different structural anomata of the heart and great vessels. In many cases, their aetiology is not clear, and they may be caused by environmental factors of maternal exposure (diseases such as diabetes or lupus, or exposure to drugs and toxins), genetic factors (chromosomal defects, microdeletions, etc.), or a combination of several of the above factors, which cause the pathology by generating alterations in the embryonic development of cardiovascular structures between the 3rd and 10th week of gestation.

Its incidence is estimated at 8 per 1000 live births, although this figure is currently changing due to the impact of prenatal diagnosis.

It is considered to be the most common malformation. With numerous presentations, its clinical expression ranges from the *absence of symptoms* to the presence of clinical signs of **heart failure**, in varying severity, as well as **cyanosis** - translated as low oxygen saturation.

The greater the complexity and severity of the malformation, the greater the symptomatology and the earlier the manifestations, with the neonatal period being of special interest, as this is when the most serious cases occur. They should be suspected when suggestive symptoms appear (heart failure, cyanosis...) or when characteristic alterations are detected in the physical examination (murmurs, arrhythmias...). The most banal may go unnoticed until adulthood.

The test to diagnose it and assess its severity is *echocardiography*. By performing this test in the foetus (foetal echocardiography), many cardiopathies can be diagnosed before birth, which helps to plan the birth in a tertiary hospital, when it is expected to pose a risk to the newborn, to deal with the clinical picture through knowledge of its possible natural history, or to make decisions about its viability in the face of the only possibility of palliative interventions in the future. However, there are still cardiopathies that are not diagnosed prenatally; this makes it important to assess the various signs and symptoms that may present in the young child as mentioned above in order to detect cardiopathies.

To minimise the risk of possible non-detection of significant CC in apparently healthy neonates, before hospital discharge, the pulse oximetry technique is performed. Oxygen saturation and heart rate are measured in the right upper extremity and one of the two lower extremities. A positive test is defined as a saturation lower than 90% in one of the 2 upper or lower extremities, or between 90-94% in both at the same time, or a difference between both saturations greater than 3%, repeated on 2 or more occasions before the clinical assessment of the newborn. It is an inexpensive, reliable and safe screening test with a low false positive rate.

In the physical examination in this field, the presence of one feature is strongly linked to the possible presence of abnormalities; the existence of a *cardiac murmur*. These are particular sounds, such as whistling or rustling, produced by the accelerated and agitated (turbulent) flow of blood in the heart, which are auscultated with the stethoscope. Their presence does not always imply pathology since in many cases this sound, the murmur may be innocent or functional, appears in normal hearts and has no negative implication. It is a good help in this context.

In relation to diagnostic tests, congenital heart disease usually produces alterations in the electrocardiogram and chest X-ray, but the fundamental diagnostic test, as mentioned above, is **echocardiography**, which allows the diagnosis and assessment of the severity of most of them.

Treatment, when necessary, is usually surgical, and in some cases may require more than one intervention when the heart disease is more complex. Some cases can be solved without intervention by catheterisation, which are closed (percutaneous) procedures, with catheters through the bleeding vessels to dilate stenoses or place closure devices.

Advances in diagnosis and treatment have greatly improved the prognosis, so that today more than 90% of affected children survive to adulthood, and in most congenital heart diseases the average life expectancy is almost comparable to that of the general population.

Classification. Most common congenital heart diseases

There are multiple types of defects which can occur in association in many cases. Systematically, we will divide them according to their predominant pathophysiological effect, with the most frequent congenital cardiopathies, which we will describe in brief.

1.　**CC with left-right shunt**: ventricular septal defect, atrial septal defect, patent ductus arteriosus.

2.　**CHD with obstructed blood flow**: pulmonary stenosis, aortic stenosis, aortic coarctation.

3.　**CC with cyanosis**: Tetralog^a of Fallot. Transposition of the great arteries.

1.　Congenital heart disease with left right shunt.

Ventricular septal defect (VSD).

Concept: The communication is due to a defect in the closure of the interventricular septum. It is the most common CC (15-20%). In most cases (70%) it is located in the membranous part of the septum, a small portion at the subaortic level.

Cytology and pathophysiology: With a small VSD, no symptoms occur. With a moderate or large VSD, growth and developmental delay, decreased exercise tolerance, repeated pulmonary infections and heart failure (HF) are relatively common in early infancy due to left chamber overload.

Diagnosis: On examination, signs of heart failure can be seen, as well as a murmur corresponding to regurgitation in the lower sternal border. The X-ray shows cardiomegaly and the electrocardiogram shows left ventricular enlargement in significant cases. Defect, repercussion and pathophysiology were confirmed by echocardiography.

Treatment: There may be a decrease or closure of the VSD in the first 6 months. After this time, only defects that cause haemodynamic overload need to be closed, and it is not necessary in other cases. It is performed by extracorporeal circulation, and transatrial or transventricular approach, closure with patch or suture with a mortality rate of less than 1%.

Atrial septal defect (ASD)

Concept: Atrial septal defect is a closure defect in the atrial septum. It is also a common cardiopathy, accounting for approximately 8% of cases. The majority of cases (50-70%) are located in the middle part of the septum (ostium secundum type); 30% of cases are located in the lower part (ostium primum type) and are usually associated with failure of the atrioventricular valves and VSD (atrioventricular canal) and 10% in the upper part (sinus venosus type), with special association with alterations in pulmonary vein drainage.

Clinics and pathophysiology: Right atrial shunt overgrowth of the right atrial cavities is usually symptomless.

Diagnosis: In significant cases, auscultatory findings include a hyperflux murmur in the pulmonary focus, in addition to a fixed splitting of the second tone. ECG and radiography reveal cases of right chamber enlargement. Echocardiogram gives the definitive diagnosis.

Treatment: In the case of ostium secundum defects, the defect may shrink or close with time. In large defects that do not close, we usually schedule device closure by catheterisation in ostium secundum cases from the age of 4 years onwards. The other types of ASD (primum, venous sinus), and secundum defects not requiring a device, are closed by patch or suture with extracorporeal surgery with a low mortality rate (less than 1%).

Patent ductus arteriosus (Figure 11.1).

Concept; It is due to persistent patency of a physiological fetal vascular structure between the pulmonary artery and descending aorta slightly distal to the origin of the left subclavian artery. It is a frequent CC (5-10% total).

Clinic and physiopathology: With a physiopathology very similar to that of VSD, in cases of small ductus there are no symptoms. In cases of moderate size and upwards we can find semiology of heart failure.

Diagnosis: Characteristic continuous infraclavicular murmur ("machinery"). Remaining pattern as VSD.

Treatment: In cases with clinical and/or auscultation repercussions, closure is indicated. It can be medical with antiprostaglandmics (ibuprofen, paracetamol, indomethacin) in the case of *premature infants*, but is not effective at other ages. If closure is possible, it will be by means of different devices that are installed by catheterisation. In patients in whom interventional closure is not possible, ligation is performed by surgery, ligation and excision of the duct through a left posterolateral thoracotomy without extracorporeal circulation. Both procedures have virtually no mortality.

2. Congenital heart disease with obstructed blood flow

Pulmonary stenosis (PS)

Concept: Isolated pulmonary stenosis is seen in 10% of all congenital heart diseases (CHD). It is often associated with other CHDs, such as tetralogy of Fallot (TF) and single ventricle situations. It is usually valvular.

Clinic and pathophysiology: Variable, depending on the degree of pulmonary obstruction. In mild and moderate cases it is usually asymptomatic. In the most important cases there is low tolerance to exertion with dyspnoea; in very severe cases, which are usually neonatal, there is tachypnoea and cyanosis.

Diagnosis: Auscultation reveals a crackle and an ejection systolic murmur at the left upper sternal border (pulmonary focus). Electrocardiogram reveals signs of right enlargement when the repercussion is moderate. Radiography does not help the diagnosis with important signs. Echocardiogram confirms and quantifies the diagnosis and is sufficient.

Treatment: Cntic newborns may temporarily improve with prostaglandin E1 infusion to keep the ductus arteriosus open. Balloon valvuloplasty by catheterisation is the procedure of choice for valvular stenosis at any age, generally reserved for severe, moderate-severe in progression or cntic cases. It usually has very good results.

Aortic stenosis

Concept: It affects different levels of the left ventricular outflow tract. Narrowing at the valvular level is the most frequent (71%), followed by subvalvular stenosis (23%). Supravalvular stenosis is very rare (6%). Flow obstruction is caused by a multifactorial congenital malformation of the tricuspid valve, which is either bicuspid or more severely monocuspid.

Clinic and pathophysiology: Variable, depending on the degree of aortic flow obstruction. In mild and moderate cases it is usually asymptomatic. In the most important cases, angina pectoris may occur, with low tolerance to effort, and even syncope; in very severe cases, which are usually neonatal, signs of acute heart failure are present, with low systemic perfusion and pulmonary oedema.

Diagnosis: An opening snap may be auscultated in valvular cases with ejection murmur in the aortic focus. The electrocardiogram reveals progressive changes of left overload in important cases, as well as radiography in which we see inespetffic alterations such as cardiomegaly in important cases. The echocardiogram again localises the level of dysfunction, confirms and quantifies the diagnosis, and is sufficient.

Treatment: In general, treatment is only indicated for severe and/or symptomatic cases. Percutaneous valvuloplasty is usually the procedure of choice, although with less unanimity than in the case of pulmonary valvuloplasty. In many cases restenosis and regurgitation following the procedure leads to surgical repair of the valve (commissurotomy). As an alternative when this is not possible, the Ross operation is increasingly performed, where we replace the diseased aortic valve with the patient's own pulmonary valve with the implantation of a cryopreserved pulmonary homograft. In this way we avoid the anticoagulation to which the patient is subjected for life. In subvalvular and supravalvular cases, only surgical resection of the obstructions with repair of the damaged area is necessary. In the case of cystic newborns, temporary infusion of prostaglandin Ei may be required to keep the ductus arteriosus open until stabilisation.

Aortic coarctation (Figure 10.1).

Concept: It is due to narrowing of the aorta in an area distal to the aortic arch (after giving rise to the left subclavian artery) at its junction with the descending aorta, an area called the aortic isthmus. It has a somewhat lower incidence than stenosis (8% CC). It is particularly common in Turner syndrome (30% of cases). It is also particularly associated with bicuspid aortic valve (present in 85% of cases).

Clinic and pathophysiology: Variable in presentation, it may be asymptomatic in patients who have developed collaterals, with hypertension being detected in routine check-ups. Symptomatic cases in very young children arise from acute heart failure with circulatory failure.

Diagnosis: A systolic murmur may be heard in the lower sternal border, or left interscapular. In severe cases it may be absent. In addition, diminished or absent pulses may be heard in the lower half of the body or diffusely. The presence of hypertension is frequent, especially with arm differences with respect to other lower levels. The electrocardiogram and radiography show similarities with the previous case. The echocardiogram visualises stenosis graphically, associated findings. In some cases, especially in older children, more precise imaging procedures such as magnetic resonance angiography or CT angiography may be necessary.

Treatment: Critical cases in very young children may require temporary medical help with prostaglandin E1 infusion for stabilisation. Surgical repair of the defect by extended resection with end-to-end anastomosis (less frequently patch aortoplasty, subclavian flap) is usually performed in very young children. In older children (above the anus) and recoarctation (can occur in 30% of cases), balloon aortoplasty by catheterisation is the preferred approach; implantation of an expandable stainless steel stent is not uncommon, although it requires larger patient sizes (over 7-8 years of age).

We must not forget to monitor for the presence of hypertension, even after the obstruction has resolved.

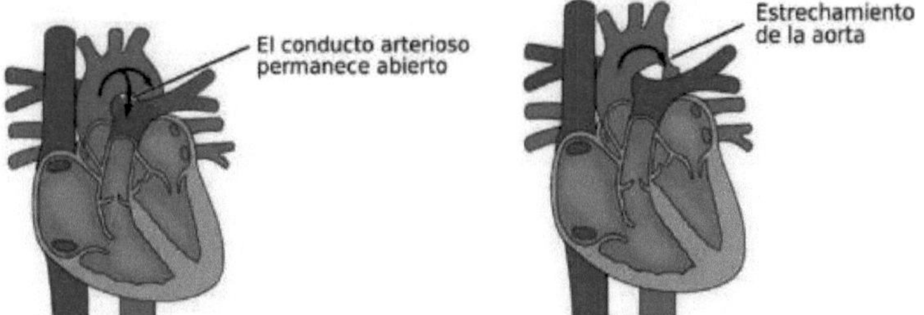

Figure 10.1. Schematic diagram of patent ductus arteriosus (left) and coarctation of the aorta.
(right).

3. Congenital heart disease with cyanosis

Tetralogy of Fallot (Figure 10.2)

Concept: This is the most frequent cyanotic CHD (5%). The defect initially described comprises a large VSD with subpulmonary extension, an obstruction of the right ventricular outflow tract, hypertrophy of the right ventricle reactive to this obstruction and a variable aortic ballooning that moves over the right ventricle. Right aortic arch is present in 25% of cases.

Clinicopathology and pathophysiology: It may be symptomless in its early stages. **Cyanosis** may not be noticeable at its onset or may only be noticed by the somewhat decreased saturation in its measurement. Most patients present with progressive cyanosis, to varying degrees depending on the degree of pulmonary flow obstruction. In some cases they present with hypercyanotic episodes with a sudden increase in obstruction after crying, feeding or defecation, which can be very severe.

Diagnosis: An ejection murmur is heard from birth, usually intense, especially in the upper parasternal border. Monitoring for cyanosis is the cardinal sign of this pathology. The electrocardiogram reveals signs of right ventricular enlargement. Early radiographic findings include a decrease in pulmonary vascularity or right arch. A "boot" or "clog" cardiac image is typical. Two-dimensional echocardiography and Doppler studies usually establish the diagnosis and quantify the severity.

Treatment: Treatment is surgical, with total repair of the defect; it is carried out after 4-6 months in our environment. In a situation of extracorporeal circulation, circulatory arrest and hypothermia, the VSD is closed with a patch, preferably by means of a transauricular and transarterial pulmonary approach, with widening of the right ventricular outflow tract (by sectioning or resection of the infundibular tissue, and pulmonary valvulotomy, avoiding the placement of a tissue patch whenever possible). Surgical mortality is less than 5%.

There are very small patients or patients with a more complicated anatomy (unfavourable coronary anatomy, very marked stenosis in the pulmonary vascular tree), in these cases intermediate procedures may be necessary to increase the flow of the pulmonary artery (modified Blalock-Taussig fistula, a shunt is established between the subclavian artery and the ipsilateral pulmonary artery by means of a Gore-Tex conduit). This would allow a repair surgery at a later stage with adequate guarantees, beyond the usual dates.

In hypoxic episodes, the child should be placed in the genupectoral position, with oxygen therapy, and even subcutaneous morphine.

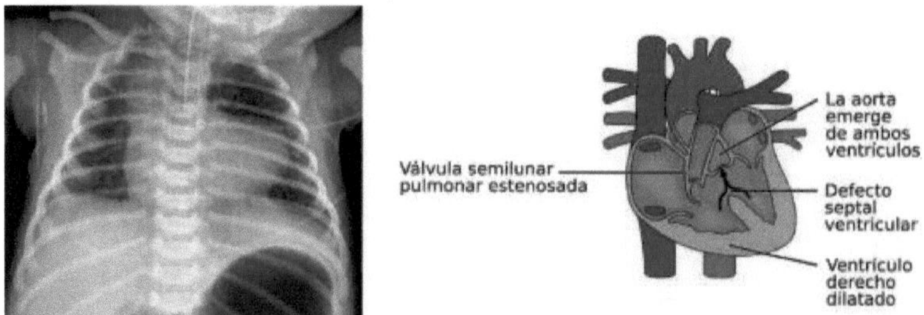

Figure 10.2: Left: Clogged heart. Right: Graphic diagram of tetralogy of Fallot.

Transposition of the great arteries (TGA) (Figure 10.3).

Concept: The aorta originates in the anterior area of the right ventricle, carrying desaturated blood to the body, and the pulmonary artery originates behind it in the left ventricle, carrying oxygenated blood back to the lungs. It accounts for 5% of the CC.

Clinic and physiopathology: There are two parallel circuits, one with hypoxaemic blood throughout the body, the other with hyperoxaemic pulmonary blood. This would not be compatible with life, if there were not different sites in the cardiocirculatory system where both circulations mix (ductus, foramen ovale, ventricular septal defect where present - 30% -).

Cyanosis, which is usually severe, is present from birth, as well as heart failure with pulmonary oedema.

Diagnosis: Auscultation and ECG reveal no remarkable findings. Radiography shows images of pulmonary oedema and a relatively typical "egg-shaped" silhouette. Echocardiography again provides all the information necessary to typify the defect and its possible associated alterations.

Treatment: This is one of the pathologies that has benefited most from prenatal diagnosis, since with this advance warning the birth must take place in a hospital with sufficient resources for the actions that may be necessary after this moment; the ductus arteriosus must be kept open medically by means of PGE1. In many cases a greater opening of the foramen ovale will be required at this time by means of balloon catheterisation (Rashkind technique) to improve the mixing of blood at the atrial level. This is a bridge to surgery, which should generally be performed in the first 2-3 weeks of life. Jatene surgery is the procedure of choice. It consists of an arterial exchange; the coronary arteries are transplanted to the base of the non-transplanted pulmonary artery, and the proximal end of the great arteries is connected to the distal end of the other great artery, which achieves anatomical correction. Mortality is approximately 5%, with relatively few long-term complications.

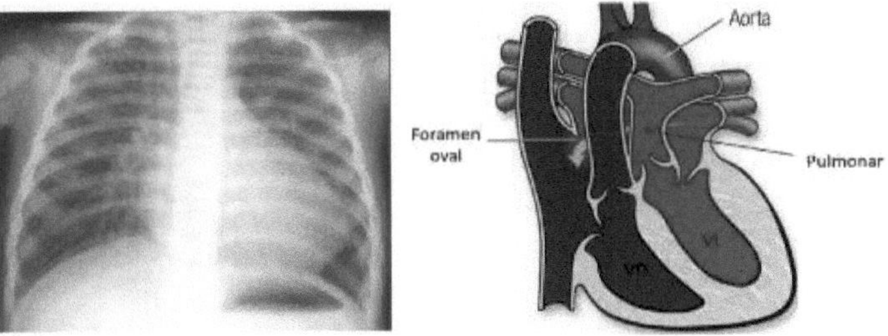

Figure 10.3. TGA: Left. Radiograph with "egg heart" image. Right: graphic diagram of the defect.

Bibliografía

1. Albert Brotoms DC. Cardiología pediatrica y cardiopatias congenitas del nino y del adolescente.1 Ed. Madrid. Grupo CTO 2015.

2. Krishna K. Anderson's Pediatric Cardiology.4Ed. Netherlands. Elsevier. 2019.

3. Park MK, Salamat M. Park's Pediatric Cardiology for Practitioners: Expert Consult. 7Ed.Netherlands. Elsevier. 2021.

4. Sanchez Luna M, Perez Munuzuri A, Sanz Lopez E, Leante Castellanos JL, Benavente Fernandez I, Ruiz Campillo CW, Sanchez Redondo MD, Vento Torres M, Rite

Gracia S; representing the Standards Committee of the Spanish Society of Neonatology. Critical congenital heart disease screening in the neonatal period. Pulse oximetry screening of critical congenital heart defects in the neonatal period. The Spanish National Neonatal Society recommendation]. An Pediatr (Engl Ed). 2018 Feb;88(2):112.e1-112.e6. Spanish. doi: 10.1016/j.anpedi.2017.06.011. Epub 2017 Sep 29.
5. Vijayalakshmi B, Syamasundar P, Chugh RR. A Comprehensive Approach to Congenital Heart Diseases. 2nd edition. New Delhi. Jaypee Brothers Medical Pub; (August 30, 2019).

11. Newborn nutrition. Breastfeeding

Dr. Jose Uberos Fernandez

Dr. Ana Campos Martmez

Breast milk is the first choice of nutrition for newborns and infants, including premature infants. It is a nutritionally, immunologically and microbiologically complete food, being a source of prebiotics and commensal or probiotic bacteria in the infant gut. The composition of breast milk in terms of its macronutrient content and other immunomodulatory components, such as lactoferrin, is adapted to the gestational age and chronological age of the newborn, with greater activity of the proteolytic system of human milk being observed when it is produced in mothers of more premature newborns. In this way, an immature and enzymatically deficient gastrointestinal system is adapted to a milk supply with partially digested proteins and a higher supply of amino acids than that observed in milk from full-term infants.

The World Health Organization and UNICEF recommend that all children be exclusively breastfed from birth for the first 6 months of life, and that breastfeeding continue with appropriate complementary foods for up to 2 years of age and beyond. An estimated one million children die each year from diarrhoea, respiratory and other infections, which breastfeeding could have helped prevent.

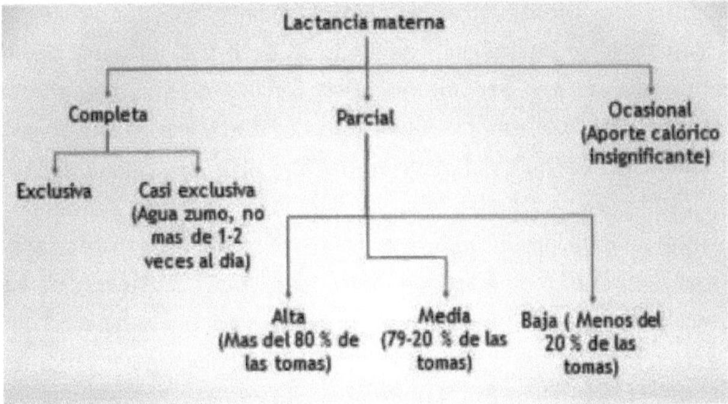

Figure 11.1. Outline of definitions of breastfeeding.

The WHO, in 1981, published an "International Code on Breast-milk Substitutes" which is based on limiting commercial advertising of infant formula and prohibiting the giving of milk samples to mothers.

In 1988 the Interagency Group for Action on Breastfeeding developed a set of definitions to unify terminology for the collection of information on breastfeeding, as shown in figure 11.1.

Physiology of lactation

The histology of the mammary gland is similar in all species: a glandular parenchyma, composed of alveoli and ducts and a supporting stroma. Each alveolar cell behaves as a secretion unit, producing complete milk, synthesising and transporting from the blood plasma proteins, fats, carbohydrates, salts, immunoglobulins and water. The process of cellular synthesis and secretion is similar in all mammalian species. The chemical composition of the milk and the anatomical arrangement of the milk storage and evacuation system varies in the various species.

The ability of the breast to synthesise the components of milk is termed lactogenesis I. Prolactin plays a role in cell differentiation and the formation of galactocytes or secretory cells in breast development during gestation. Breast enlargement and areola growth are related to increased plasma placental lactogen. Nipple growth is related to the level of prolactin. Until the time of delivery, the production of large volumes of milk, or lactogenesis II, is inhibited by antagonism of placental sex steroids, particularly progesterone. The inhibitory effect of oestrogens on lactogenesis is not fully elucidated, but they are known to decrease the amount of prolactin incorporated into the mammary alveolar cells, preventing the increase in prolactin receptors that normally occurs during lactation. Prolactin within the alveolar cell stimulates lactoalbumin synthesis and thus lactose synthesis and secretion.

The lactation period begins after childbirth. During lactation, progesterone receptors disappear from the mammary gland, while the level of progesterone gradually decreases and the inhibitory action of this hormone on milk synthesis is suppressed, and milk secretion begins 30-40 hours after delivery. The breasts fill with colostrum and the volume of milk increases from 50 to 500 ml from the first to the fourth day postpartum.

Galactopoiesis is the process that maintains milk production once lactation is established. This stage of lactogenesis depends on both the hormonal environment of the maternal plasma and the periodic removal of milk secretion from the breast after suckling. Milk does not flow spontaneously into the ducts and is therefore not initially available to the infant. For milk to flow from the alveoli, it is necessary for the alveoli to be squeezed by the myoepithelial cells surrounding them. The contraction of these fibres, or ejection reflex, is produced by the release of oxytocin by the posterior pituitary. The myoepithelial fibres of the breast and uterus have spetffic receptors for oxytocin and these receptors increase during the third trimester of pregnancy, especially in the first 5 days after delivery. Oxytocin is the most important galactopoietic hormone and is indispensable for the emptying of milk during breastfeeding.

Lactational secretion from the breast depends on endocrine control, regulated by prolactin and oxytocin, and autocrine control regulated by breast emptying and the feedback inhibitor of lactation (FIL).

The prolactin-releasing reflex is controlled by dopaminergic neurons in the hypothalamus. The nipple and areola stimulus produces, via a neurohormonal reflex, the inhibition of dopamine secretion (PIF). The amount of dopamine reaching the lactotrope cells of the anterior pituitary determines the amount of prolactin secreted by them. The nipple-areola stimulus inhibits dopamine secretion and thus allows prolactin release by the anterior pituitary.

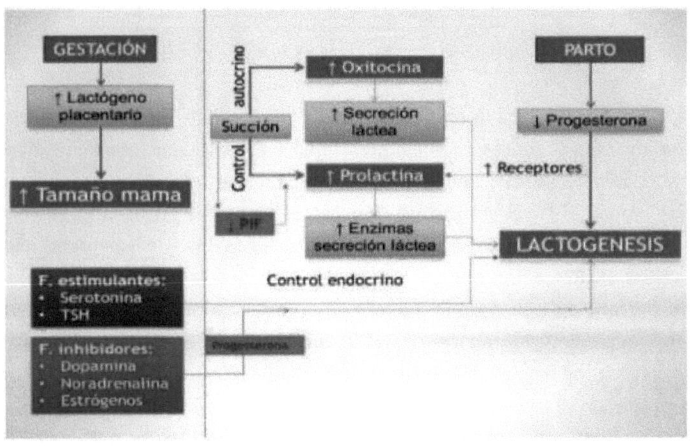

Figure 11.2. Scheme of the process of lactogenesis - galatopoiesis.

The internal control of milk secretion in the alveolus is regulated by the emptying of the milk. It has been clearly established that milk production is related to the requirements of the infant, i.e. it is the infant who establishes a free-demand lactation, who determines the volume of milk produced by the mother. It has also been shown that the degree of emptying of the breast at the end of a feeding determines the rate of milk production in the following hours and that the rate of milk production can be increased by expressing milk after the feeding. All this information supports the clinically tested hypothesis that the breast can regulate the rate of milk production in response to the degree of milk emptying, thus allowing accommodation of requirements.

Composition of breast milk

The composition of breast milk varies over the course of a single feeding. At the beginning it is rich in carbohydrates and watery in appearance. At the end of the feeding, the milk contains more fats and is creamy in appearance.

We have to distinguish the different aspects concerning the colostral milk in the first 5 days of life and the production of mature milk after a period of 15 days.

Table 11.1. Composition of milk of various animal species (mg/dL).

ANALISIS COMPARATIVO: TIPOS LECHE [1]					
	Mujer	Yegua	Vaca	Oveja	Cabra
Hidratos de carbono	6,9	6,3	4,6	4,2	4,4
Grasa	4	1,3	3,4	6,2	4,1
Proteinas	1,5	2,1	3,5	5,2	3,8
Inmunoglobulina A	18,2	19,8	11,7	-	-
Lisozima	1,7	6,6			

Colostrum has 2 g/100 ml fat, 4 g/100 ml lactose and 2 g/100 ml protein. It yields 67 Kcal/100 ml. It contains lower amounts of lactose, fat and water-soluble vitamins than mature milk, while it contains higher amounts of proteins, fat-soluble vitamins (E, A, K), carotenes and some minerals such as sodium and zinc. Beta-carotene gives it its yellowish colour and sodium gives it a slightly salty taste.

Lactose

It is the main carbohydrate in breast milk. It is a disaccharide composed of glucose and galactose. Its average concentration in breast milk is 6-7 g/dL. Lactose values have been inversely related to sodium and chloride values. Lactose levels increase progressively with the duration of lactation. Lactose is an accessible source of galactose, essential for the production of galactoKpids, including cerebrosides, indispensable for the development of the central nervous system. Interesting relationships have been made between the amount of lactose in the milk of a species as opposed to its fat content as an energy source and the relative size of its brain. Lactose levels are fairly constant in milk throughout the day, even in malnourished mothers lactose levels remain constant. The concentration of lactose in breast milk is not related to the nutritional status of the mother. There are other carbohydrates in breast milk besides lactose, classified into monosaccharides, acidic and neutral oligosaccharides, and peptide- and protide-linked carbohydrates.

Proteins

Its concentration ranges between 1.4-1.8 g/dL. As with lactose, the protein content of breast milk must be differentiated between the colostral period and the protein content in mature milk. Colostrum induces enteric mucosal growth, contributing to intestinal development. Studies in various animal species show that the growth rate is directly related to the protein content of breast milk. The free amino acid profile contained in breast milk is also adapted to the different periods of lactation and probably also to the needs of the preterm or term newborn.

The protein content of breast milk decreases over time as the fat content increases and the caloric content of the milk increases. The higher concentration of proteins observed in colostrum is due to non-digestible proteins such as Igs and lactoferrin which have an immunomodulatory role. In addition, the content of prothymes in preterm milk is higher than in the milk of mothers of term infants, with an increase of up to 0.8 g/dL, being proportionally higher in those of younger gestational age.

The acidification of breast milk makes it possible to distinguish two protein fractions: a soluble fraction consisting of whey proteins and a precipitable fraction corresponding to chasema. The proportion of caseme increases progressively with lactation until a caseme:seroprotein ratio of 40:60 is reached in mature milk. The composition of the chasema in milk varies widely according to the animal species. Caseme is a phosphoproteome produced by four genes coding for caseme a s1, a s2, P and κ, which are organised in the form of micelles or soluble units. Some authors report the existence of y-caseme which are actually fragments of p-caseme. a s1, a s2-caseme precipitate with calcium and are not present in human milk.

Casein-beta is degraded to casein-phosphopeptides which keep calcium in soluble form and facilitate its uptake by intestinal cells. Casein-beta from breast milk contains less phosphorus than casein-beta from cow's milk, which explains its better bioavailability of calcium than that obtained from cow's milk.

The casema-kappa serves as a substrate for the intestinal development of the bifidogenic flora. The main function of casema is to provide the infant with amino acids, calcium and phosphorus. Among the proteins identified as whey soluble, alpha-lactoalbumin constitutes 10-12% of the total number of proteins and is a constituent of the enzyme lactose synthetase, which is necessary for the synthesis of lactose. The proportion of whey proteins decreases in the course of lactation, initially the ratio of casema:whey in colostrum is 10:90 and then 40:60 in mature milk.

The digestion of proteins begins in the mammary gland itself. Proteases are found in greater quantities at the beginning of lactation and decrease as lactation progresses. A higher concentration of proteases is found in the milk of premature infants, which supports the idea that breast milk is adapted to the digestive needs of the newborn.

Compared to adults, there is a lower digestive capacity for milk proteins in infants and newborns. Factors responsible include:

- Lower gastric acidification capacity in the newborn, with pH ranging from 6-6.5.
- Pepsin concentration 5 times lower than that observed in adults.
- Reduced trypsin activity.
- Chymotrypsin concentration 10-60% of that observed in adults.
- Enterokinase concentration 20% of that observed in adults.
- Carboxypeptidase 10-20% of adult carboxypeptidase.

Fats

Milk fats constitute 3-5 g/dL. Triglycerides make up 99% of all fats in breast milk, which are covered by a hydrophilic membrane containing phosphoKpids, cholesterol and glycoproteins that are stabilised by emulsion. The fats that are incorporated into breast milk come mostly from circulating maternal fats, which in turn come mostly from the diet. Fat makes up 40-55% of the total energy content of milk. Saturated fatty acids comprise 40% of the fatty acids in breast milk. The predominant fatty acids (FA) in human milk are oleic (38%), palmitic (20%) and linoleic (15%). Approximately 70% of the palm fatty acid is esterified in position 2 of the triglyceride molecule.

The polyunsaturated fatty acids n_3 and n_6 vary considerably with maternal diet. Docosahexanoic acid (DHA) (22:6n3) is strongly influenced by maternal fish intake; whereas the arachidonic acid content of breast milk is less influenced by maternal intake of its precursor linoleic acid. The DHA content of preterm milk is higher than that observed in the milk of term infants.

Vitamin K

The basic requirement of vitamin K in the first 6 months of life is 5 mcg^a, since in the first days of life infants consume small amounts of milk and the vitamin K concentrations in colostrum or mature milk are 0.5mcg/dL and 0.23 mcg/dL respectively, the possibility of vitamin K deficiency is more frequent in the neonatal period than in other periods of life. The haemorrhagic syndrome resulting from this deficiency can occur in the first day, 1-7 days (classical form) or late (2-12 weeks).

Vitamin D

In the exclusively breastfed infant, vitamin D levels are dependent on vitamin D stores, which in turn are dependent on the vitamin D status of the mother. The vitamin D intake in breast milk is low (4-40 IU/L) concentrations which are far below those recommended to prevent rickets and regulate bone mineralisation (300-400 IU/d(a), therefore, the total intake will depend on sun exposure in different cultural environments. Universal supplementation is not necessary, but it should be necessary in spedific geographic latitudes and during the winter months.

Iron

In healthy breastfeeding mothers, additional iron supplementation is not recommended. The normal breastfed infant usually has sufficient iron in its iron stores to cover its requirements for at least 3 months. The iron concentration in breast milk in the first months is 0.1-1.6 mcg/mL, this concentration decreases progressively throughout lactation.

Immunology and breastfeeding

Breast milk is composed on the one hand of the nutritional elements already mentioned, and on the other hand of elements that characterise the defence mechanisms that exist in it, which can be classified as follows:

a) Agents that act directly as antimicrobials, including oligosaccharide glycoconjugates, some prothemes such as lactoferrin, lysozyme, fibronectin, immunoglobulins, complement components and mucin.

b) Growth promoters of protective micro-organisms such as lactobacillus bifidus, created by partially digested substrates from human milk.

c) Breast milk leukocytes.

d) Anti-inflammatory agents.

e) Immunostimulatory agents.

Oligosaccharides from human milk

Oligosaccharides are complex carbohydrates, their concentration is especially high in colostrum and decreases over the course of lactation as lactose concentrations increase. Milk oligosaccharides can act as soluble homologues of cell surface receptors that are targets of specific bacterial pathogens, inhibiting bacterial adhesion to these cells. In the breastfed infant, a low level of clostridium and enterococcus and a tendency to a lower level of enterococcus are observed in the intestinal flora.

The oligosaccharides in human milk comprise a heterogeneous group of compounds of which more than 200 have been described. They are quantitatively found in greater quantities than the proteins and represent the element that marks the greatest differences currently recognised between the composition of cow's milk, human milk or adapted formula milk. The term oligosaccharides refers to carbohydrate molecules containing 3-10 sugar molecules. The general composition of human milk oligosaccharides includes the presence of terminal positions of sialic acid or L-fucose, a nuclear structure of lacto-N-biose or N-acetyl-lactosamine and a reducing end of D-lactose. Human milk oligosaccharides are grouped into two types: acidic (which include sialic acid) and neutral (which can be fucosylated and non-fucosylated). The spectrum of oligosaccharides and their content in breast milk is genetically determined and related to their secretory status and the ABO and Lewis blood group determinants. The different secretory phenotype of oligosaccharides explains a different protective effect against infection depending on the secretory phenotype of the mother; moreover, the oligosaccharides in breast milk decrease in concentration as lactation progresses and increase in preterm milk in relation to term newborn milk. Another function of breast milk oligosaccharides is to provide sialic acid, an important element of the gangliosides that form part of the membranes of neuronal cells. The sialic acid content of secretions in breast-fed infants is higher than in formula-fed infants.

98% of oligosaccharides are not absorbed, they reach the colon where they are digested by the bifidogenic flora to which they serve as a nutritional substrate, only 1-2% of the total amount ingested is absorbed and eliminated in the urine. It has been suggested that the type and quantity of oligosaccharides in breast milk determines the type and density of the intestinal bifidogenic flora, so that feeding breast milk with a higher content of 2-fucosyl-lactose determines a predominance of intestinal bifidogenic flora, while a decrease in its concentration determines a predominance of intestinal pathogens.

Breast milk microbiota

Human milk bacteria are, in the opinion of some authors, among the first to colonise the intestine of the newborn, preventing the settlement and proliferation of pathogenic bacteria and thus decreasing the risk of infectious diseases. In 2003, a spetffic microbiota of human milk was described for the first time. *Lactobacillus fermentum* CECT5716 (*L. fermentum*) is a probiotic strain isolated from breast milk in healthy women. This strain has shown anti-infective activity related to its antibacterial and immunoregulatory activity.

The composition of human breast milk is complex, containing factors that interact with the infant immune system. The microbiota plays a recognised role in human health by performing metabolic functions in the healthy individual that are lacking in humans. Dysbiosis, understood as an alteration in the function and composition of the gut microbiome, has been linked to inflammatory bowel disease, diabetes, obesity, allergy, vaginal infections, atopic dermatitis and dental caries.

Bibliograffa

1. Bauer J, Gerss J. Longitudinal analysis of macronutrients and minerals in human milk produced by mothers of preterm infants. Clin Nutr 2011 Apr;30(2):215-20.

2. Uberos J, Narbona E. Probiotics and prebiotics in very low birth weight infants. Making the difference between health and disease. 1 ed. Saarbrucken: Editorial Academica Espanola; 2017.

3. Ballabriga A. Complementary feeding of the infant: introduction to the problems it poses. Avances en nutricion de la infancia (4). 1 ed. Barcelona: UNIASA; 1991. p. 3-36.

12. Infant and pre-school nutrition

Dr. Cristina Campoy

Dr. Jose Antonio Garcia Santos Dr. Estefania Dieguez Castillo

Adequate feeding of the child during the infancy and pre-school period constitutes an initial opportunity to ensure growth and development, to establish food preferences, to progressively acquire autonomy, and to promote family interaction. During this age period, important changes occur in the child's maturational function, affecting mainly the nervous system, the digestive system and the excretory system, changes which allow us to differentiate several nutritional stages in which both the type and quantity of food are adjusted to the age and stage of maturation. The first of these stages, the **stage of the born and lactating æeaën**, covers the period from birth to two years of age, and in it we can distinguish two major pennodes: *a) Exclusive breastfeeding period,* comprising the first 6 months of life, during which the infant is fed exclusively on breast milk or, failing that, on infant formula; *b) Transition period towards adult feeding,* defined from the age of 6 months, characterised by the progressive introduction of semi-foods and solids that nutritionally complement the infant. The second major stage is established **at the pre-school age of the child (4-6 years)**, a time conceived as a key moment to establish adequate feeding habits and control their nutritional situation, thus promoting optimal health in later stages of life.

Exclusive breastfeeding period

In the first 6 months of life, the healthy infant is able to suck effectively, but its neuromuscular immaturity prevents it from making the tongue extrusion movements necessary for swallowing solid foods. In addition, the composition and quantity of the different secretions (salivary, gastric, pancreatic, biliary and intestinal), as well as the functioning of the hepatic and renal systems, favour exclusively the digestion of liquid foods, maturing in the first months towards characteristics more suited to the digestion of foods of a more solid consistency. These maturational changes mean that, during the first months of life, the healthy infant feeds exclusively on breast milk or, failing that, on infant formula, gradually beginning to introduce different types of food depending on its physiological maturity. Breast milk is considered the *"ideal food"* for the healthy infant as its nutritional composition, which varies from birth, is adapted to the nutritional and physiological needs of the infant during the first months of life (Tables 12.1 and 12.2).

The **World Health Organization (WHO)**, the American Academy of Pediatrics (AAP) as well as the Breastfeeding Committee of the Spanish Association of Pediatrics recommend **exclusive breastfeeding for the first 6 months** of a child's life, continuing this practice together with complementary feeding until the age of 2 years. These recommendations are based not only on the characteristics of breast milk, but also on the presence of **bioactive compounds** that play a key role in the development of the infant:

>   Digestive enzymes, such as amylase, trypsin and lipase, which facilitate the hydrolysis of nutrients present in breast milk.

>   Bacteriostatic compounds, mainly lysozyme, capable of breaking down certain components of the bacterial wall, or lactoferrin, with the ability to *"sequester"* the iron necessary for the growth of pathogenic bacteria.

>   Oligosaccharides with a prebiotic effect, favouring the proliferation in the intestine of a microbiota rich in *bifidobacteria* which prevent the growth of pathogenic micro-organisms, as well as favouring the synthesis of certain vitamins.

>   Prebiotics and probiotics essential for healthy intestinal colonisation (predominantly *Lactobacillus* and Bifidobacteria) and optimal immune and anti-infective function.

> Immunoglobulins from the mother, which act as antibodies against pathogens present in the infant's digestive and respiratory tract.

> Growth and development factors, as well as cytokines, with anti-inflammatory and immunomodulatory activity.

> Hormonal factors, such as calcitonin and somatostatin, essential for proper signalling between tissues and organs, regulation of the infant's appetite, as well as in the establishment of sleep patterns.

> key microRNAs for the regulation of gene expression, short-term disease prevention and immune system enhancement.

Along with these nutritional characteristics, breastfeeding is associated with numerous advantages, including: *a) psychological*, given the direct involvement of the mother in the infant's upbringing, giving her a sense of recognition and a physical-affective relationship with her child; *b) correct development of the infant's jaws*, due to the position of the mother's *jaw; c) the development of the infant's jaw*, due to the mother's direct involvement in the infant's upbringing.

c) better digestion and absorption of nutrients; *d) osmolarity* adapted to the infant's renal function; *e) optimal hygienic and thermal conditions*; and *f) protection against infections*, reduced incidence of *allergies, eczema and infant colic*, as well as prevention of *diseases* in later life (diabetes mellitus, Crohn's disease, obesity or heart disease).

Table 12.1. Nutritional characteristics and function of the main types of breastmilk.

TYPES OF BREAST MILK		
	NUTRITIONAL CHARACTERISTICS	FUNCTION
CALOSTRO (up to 4-6 days of life)	ₛHigh protein content, IgAs, lactoferrin, oligosaccharides, and intestinal growth factor ₛRich in polyunsaturated fatty acids and cholesterol, low fat content ₛHigh percentage of minerals and fat-soluble vitamins	ₛOptimal early infant growth and development ₛImmune protection ₛMaturation of the digestive tract
TRANSITIONAL MILK (6-15 days of life)	✓Lower amount of IgApproval of the intestine, ✓High levels of lactose, l^pids and vitamins digestive system and kidneys to the fat-soluble and water-solublemilk mature milk	
MATURE MILK (from the 3rd week of life)	ₛHigh energy content (700 kcal/L) ₛ80% water ₛProtein content of 0.9 - 1.2 g/dl	Nutritional support necessary for optimal growth and development during the first 6 months of life.

IgAs: Immunoglobulin A secretory; ***Ig:*** *Immunoglobulin A secretory;* ***Ig:*** *Immunoglobulin*

However, there may be special situations in both the mother and the infant that make breastfeeding difficult *(low milk production, metabolic diseases of the infant, organ alterations, maternal diseases and use of incompatible drugs,...).* In this case, the use of infant formula should be chosen, in a situation where its use is widespread, especially in developed countries. Nowadays, thanks to the knowledge about the composition of breast milk, the nutritional needs of the infant and the technological development, a great variety of infant formulas adapted to the needs of the infant can be found on the market, whose nutritional composition and effects on the growth and development of the infant try to resemble those provided by breast milk. This circumstance has led various nutrition-related committees *(AAP, European Society of Paediatric Gastroenterology, Hepatology and Nutrition (ESPGHAN) and the Scientific Committee on*

Nutrition of the European Commission) to establish a series of recommendations on the composition and quality of milk formulas, identifying two types of formulas: *i) starter formulas*, adapted to cover the nutritional requirements of infants up to 6 months of age. They are made by modifying the composition of cow's milk to bring it closer to mother's milk, reducing the amount of proteins and adjusting the profile of amino acids, fats, vitamins and minerals. Likewise, its composition is enriched with docosahexaenoic acid (DHA), lactose, oligosaccharides, maltodextrin and nitrogen compounds; *ii) continuation formulas*, used from 6 months of life, and with a more flexible composition given the progressive introduction of complementary feeding. There are also *special formulas* on the market *for* high-calorie *premature infants (*130 kcal/kg/fa), nutritionally modified to facilitate the growth of these infants and adapted to the immaturity of their digestive, metabolic and excretory functions.

Table 12.2. Nutritional composition of mature breastmilk

NUTRITIONAL COMPOSITION OF MATURE BREAST MILK			
COMPONENT	NUTRITIONAL CHARACTERISTICS	RECOMMENDATIONS	FUNCTION
Water	Total content of 88%.	150 ml/kg/day	a) Avoiding dehydration b) Facilitate the dilution of substances to be excreted.

Energy 65/70 kcal/dL 100-115 kcalkgdia , ...
(38 % fat, 48% to 54%) Optimal growth and development of the
carbohydrates, and 8%lactant
protems)

Protems	0,9 mg/100 ml *(60-65% a-lactoalbumin, 20% casei.na, dynamic amino acid profile according to infant's needs, high content of secretory IgA, lactoferrin and lysozyme)*	2,04 g/kg/day in the first 3 months 1.73 g/kg/day of 3-6 months	a) Provides the infant with the nitrogen needed to renew and synthesise the different amino acids or proteins in the body. b) Facilitate digestion (T casema) c) Benefits on the intestinal flora

Carbohydrates 7 g/dL (40-50% intake8-12 g/100 kcala) Energy intake without increase of
Carbon Caloricola Osmolarity
(90% lactose, 10%b) Absorptionof iron, calcium and
fructose-type oligosaccharides, magnesium
glusocamine, galactosamine, (c) Development of *Lactobacillusbifidus*
inositol, growth factord) Key metabolic role e
Lactobacillus bifidus) immune-boosting
e) Formation of galactocerebrosides essential for the development of the CNS.

Fats	3.5 g/dL (50% caloric intake T content in LCPUFA, essential fatty acids and LCPUFA (oleic, palmitic, linoleic, a-linolenic, arachidonic and docosahexanoic acids)	4-6 g/100 ml (40-55% of total calories) 1-3 g/100 of the caloric intake as linoleic acid *.	a) Structural function of cell membranes, involvement in oxidative phenomena and cholesterol transport. b) neurodevelopment, retinal function and eicosanoid synthesis c) regulation of inflammatory processes and allergies

Vitamins fat-soluble vitamins Recommended content in **Fat-soluble vitamins**
(ea) Vitamin A: i during lactation
water-soluble, although the concentration of water-soluble need for supplementation
certain vitamins (B1, maternal, lolochronic reaction of the
B2, B6, B12, E and A) varies in retin a, antioxidant function y
function of the maternal diet anti-infective
b) Infant vitamin D supplementation (400 IU/day)
c) Vitamin E^ cardioprotective and vision protection, anti-inflammatory, antioxidant function
d) Vitamin K

Water-soluble vitamins
a) Vitamin B6^ Neurological development and allergy prevention (atopic dermatitis)
b) Vitamin B12^ Maternal supplementation in vegan, malnourished or pernicious anaemic women^ Neurodevelopment
c) Vitamin C^ antioxidant function,

Minerals	Low content but better absorption and bioavailability of iron, zinc, calcium, magnesium and copper Low sodium, chloride and potassium content	Promote optimal kidney function of the infant

Finally, other infant formulas are specially modified and indicated for infants with certain metabolic dysfunctions, such as **lactose-free or hydrolysed formulas** (for infants with cow protein intolerance or allergy), **elemental formulas** (in cases of severe diarrhoea or intestinal malfunction) or **anti-regurgitation formulas** (with thickeners to suppress infant vomiting and regurgitation).

Transition period to adult feeding: complementary feeding

Food diversification, complementary feeding (CA) or *beikost means the* variation or introduction into the infant's diet of foods other than breastmilk or formula, whether they are liquid, semiKchid or solid. The introduction of different foods should be gradual, facilitating the transition to adult feeding. Clearly, this dietary diversification should be aimed at meeting nutritional requirements at this stage of life (Table 12.3), but also at creating healthy eating habits that will last into adulthood. It is important to note that, during the CA period, the risk of undernutrition is high, mainly due to the potential inclusion of foods of low nutritional quality and inadequate introduction, in terms of timing and quantity, of different foods. Frequent feeding or premature cessation of breastfeeding also contributes to insufficient nutrient intake and energy in infants older than 6 months. Consequently, the World Health Organisation (WHO) has established *"Guiding principles for complementary feeding of the breastfed infant"* to develop a guideline on desirable feeding behaviours, as well as recommendations on the quantity, consistency, frequency, energy density and nutrient content of foods (Table 12.4). At around 6 months of age, the infant's energy and nutrient needs begin to exceed what breastmilk can provide, so it is necessary to progressively introduce CA, while maintaining breastfeeding on demand. In the case of infants who are exclusively formula-fed, the introduction of new foods may occur between 4-6 months of age. However, the introduction of CA should be adjusted to the infant's motor development and neurological, renal, gastrointestinal and immune maturity. Therefore, it is necessary to recognise changes in the infant that indicate readiness for feeding other than breastfeeding, mainly: *i)* active interest in food; *ii)* disappearance of the extrusion reflex (expulsion of uncooked food with the tongue); *iii)* ability to pick up food with the hands and bring it to the mouth; and *iv)* maintaining a sedentary posture with support.

Respecting the recommended age of introduction of AC is key to avoid possible short and long term risks associated with early or late introduction; in this sense, **early introduction** (before 4 months of age) increases the possibility of choking as their digestive maturity is not adequate for this type of feeding.

A higher prevalence of acute gastroenteritis, upper respiratory tract infections, and problems associated with poor iron and zinc bioavailability have also been observed in the case of breastfeeding.

In the long term, this early introduction may predispose the infant to an increased risk of obesity, atopic eczema or type 1 diabetes mellitus later in life.

Table 12.3. Nutritional requirements for complementary feeding of healthy infants.

NUTRITIONAL REQUIREMENTS OF COMPLEMENTARY FEEDING IN INFANTS	
GENERAL RECOMMENDATIONS	**NUTRITIONAL JUSTIFICATION**
Energi'a ■ / Not more than 50% of the total energy intake, together with an intake of breast milk or formula of 500 ml^Ka ■ / 200 kcal/^a in children 6-8 months ■ / 300 kcal/dah children 9-11 months ■ / 550 kcal/dah children 12-23 months	Filling the gap in energy not provided by breastmilk from 6 months onwards
Protems ■/ Animal proteins should cover 40-50% of the estimated total recommended intake of essential amino acids.	1) To promote the replacement of body proteins necessary to maintain an adequate growth rate. 2) Avoid excessive protein intake: liver and kidney overload, increased risk of obesity.
Li'pidos ■ 40-60% of total ene^a needed in infants aged 4-6 months ■ / Gradually reduce their contribution to 35% of the total energy intake after 2-3 years. ■ / Saturated fatty acids: 10% of total ene^a; monounsaturated fatty acids: 10-20% total ene^a; polyunsaturated fatty acids: 610% of total ene^a ■ / Balanced supply of essential fatty acids: linoleic acid (3-4.5%), a- linoleic acid (0.5%)	1) Increasing the energy density of foodstuffs 2) Formation of organ and tissue structures 3) Improve the taste of food and therefore its acceptability in infants. 4) Enhance absorption of fat-soluble vitamins
Carbohydrates ■ / They should represent more than 50% of the total caloric intake of the diet. ■ / Monosaccharides should not exceed 10% of the intake. ■ / Limit consumption of refined sugars as much as possible.	1) Prevent infant cariogenesis 2) Prevent or reduce the risk of obesity or metabolic diseases in adulthood.
Fibre ■/ Progressive introduction of fibre up to 12 months, without exceeding 5 g AKa. ■/ Maintain a balance of soluble and insoluble fibre (25% and 75%, respectively).	1) Improved functioning of the gastrointestinal tract 2) Healthy effect on gastric emptying, satiating effect and laxative effect. 3) Regulation of glucose and cholesterol levels in the blood. 4) High fibre intake: flatulence, bloating, deficiency in mineral, vitamin and protein absorption. 5) Control the amount of water to avoid obstruction with small bowel impaction.
Water Adjusted for energy intake, water loss, urine density, dietary solutes and physical circumstances (temperature, humidity, altitude and physical exercise) 0.7 L/dah between 0-6 months s 0,8 L/dfa between 7-12 months 1.3 L/dfa between 1-3 years	1) Avoid dehydration (evaporative water loss in infants is more than 60% of the water intake needed to maintain homeostasis). 2) Maintain the necessary water supply to support the growth of the infant.
Sodium z Up to 12 months: less than 1 g of salt per day (less than 0.4 g of sodium)	1) Maintenance of extracellular fluids, regulation of osmolarity, control of the volume of body water compartments and normal blood pressure. 2) Excessive intake may increase the risk of hypertension and preference for salty foods in adulthood.

Iron	z Iron requirement of 0.78 mg/day from 4 months onwards z Iron requirement of 11 mg/day for 6-12 months	1) Preventing iron deficiency in infants 2) Supplementation in the case of vegetarian diets 3) Optimal intake of vitamin C for bioavailability and absorption
Calcium	z Calcium requirements between 6-12 months: 500-600 mg/day *(depending on the intake of other nutrients such as vitamin D, protein and phosphorus, individual rate of absorption and type of diet).*	1) Promote the consumption of milk and dairy products with an optimal calcium-phosphorus ratio. 2) Avoid consumption of plant foods high in phylates, oxalates and tannins.
Vitamins	A varied diet	1) Supplying the necessary amounts of beneficial fats 2) Consumption of foods rich in vitamins B and C

Late introduction of CA (beyond 26 weeks of age) is also discouraged as this practice may also increase the risk of nutritional problems (iron and zinc deficiency, food allergies or intolerances, poorer acceptance of new textures and tastes,...). *сДиё foods to use and in what sequence?* Guidelines or recommendations regarding the timing of introduction of CA vary widely between regions and cultures, and should never be interpreted as a "fixed schedule" (Table 12.5).

Table 12.4. Guiding principles for complementary feeding of the breastfed child.

GUIDING PRINCIPLES FOR COMPLEMENTARY FEEDING OF THE BREASTFED CHILD
1. Practice exclusive breastfeeding from birth to 6 months of age; introduce complementary foods from 6 months of age (180 days) and continue breastfeeding.
2. Continue frequent, on-demand breastfeeding until 2 years of age or beyond.
3. Practice perceptive feeding, applying the principles of psycho-social care.
4. Exercise good food hygiene and handling practices.
5. Start at six months of age with small amounts of food and increase the amount as the child grows, while maintaining breastfeeding.
6. Increase the consistency and variety of foods gradually as the child grows, adapting to the child's requirements and abilities.
7. Increase the number of times the child consumes complementary foods as he/she gets older.
8. Give a variety of nutrient-rich foods to ensure nutritional needs are met.
9. Use fortified complementary foods or vitamin and mineral supplements for infants according to their needs.
10. Increase fluid intake during illness including breast milk (more frequent breastfeeding), and encourage the child to eat soft, varied, palatable and favourite foods. After illness, feed more frequently than usual and encourage the child to eat more.

Adapted from Maternal, Newborn, Child and Adolescent Health. In: Infant and young child feeding. WHO, 2010; ISBN: 978-92-75-33094-4.

Regardless of the above factors, CA should prioritise the initial introduction of foods rich in iron and zinc, and it is important to introduce foods one at a time, at intervals of a few days, to observe tolerance and acceptance, and they should be foods to which no salt, sugar or sweeteners are added so that the infant can become accustomed to the natural flavours of the foods. These recommendations are of vital importance in the case of potentially allergenic foods and gluten, and so far there is no strong scientific evidence to promote the introduction of these foods beyond 6 months of age. *How much should be given?* Another important aspect to consider concerns the amount of food the infant should receive during CA. In this regard, it is necessary to emphasise to parents and/or caregivers that the introduction of CA is a gradual process, starting with small portions, and that feeding with breastmilk or infant formula should be maintained on demand and frequently. The food offered to the infant should be healthy, nutritious and safe, providing sufficient energy, macro- and micronutrients to meet the infant's needs at this stage, always in combination with breastfeeding or formula feeding. It is also important to recognise and respect the infant's hunger and satiety signals; this is probably the point where most emphasis should be placed, given that many parents, at the time of feeding their child, have expectations in terms of quantity of intake that are often not fulfilled. Therefore, rather than paying attention to quantity, it is important to pay attention to the variety of food provided, availability and the establishment of healthy eating habits.

How to offer food? Finally, the way foods are offered during CA will play a key role in the acceptance of new tastes and textures by the infant. It is recommended to progressively increase the consistency of foods, offering lumpy and semi-solid textures at 8-9 months, and a similar feeding to the rest of the family from 12 months onwards. Also, as mentioned above, providing a healthy nurturing environment is vital for infants to develop their nutritional skills and to be able to self-regulate hunger-satiety. Therefore, strategies aimed at pressuring, forcing or rewarding the infant at feeding time are discouraged, as they are simply a way to interfere negatively with the infant's perception of his or her own satiety, thus increasing the risk of overweight in infancy or nutritional problems. While traditionally the most commonly used method has been a progressive introduction of textures, nowadays the ***"baby-led feeding" (BLW)*** method has gained great interest, in which the infant is allowed to *"direct"* the feeding process from the beginning; in other words, parents and/or caregivers are responsible for offering a varied and healthy meal, but it is the infant who takes the food himself, deciding what to eat and how much to eat. It is possible to opt for a mixed modality, in which a combination of the infant eating by him/herself, but also offering pureed food or porridge at some of the meals. Obviously, the first foods offered to the infant in this mode of BLW are *finger foods* or foods on sticks, to encourage the infant to grasp the food with his or her finger and eat the piece that sticks out, offering foods cut into small pieces when the infant's ability improves. BLW encourages the introduction of CA at 6 months of age and the maintenance of breastfeeding, as well as promoting perceptual feeding based on the infant's hunger and satiety signals and the establishment of healthy nutritional habits. However, it is necessary to implement correct safety measures aimed at avoiding choking situations, mainly by monitoring the infant's position during feeding (always in an upright position), supervising the feeding process at all times and not offering foods that, due to their characteristics, pose a high risk of choking.

Table 12.5. Age of food introduction during the first year of life. Practical considerations

AGE OF INTRODUCTION OF FOOD IN THE FIRST YEAR OF LIFE											
		4	5	6	7	8	9	10	11	12	RECOMMENDATIONS
Cereals	Gluten-free										(a) Added to the milk in the bottle or, preferably, in the form of porridge
	With gluten										b) Use of pre-digested hydrolysed cereals because of their higher digestibility.
Fruits	Part										a) Without honey, sugar or sweeteners
	Juice										b) Strawberry and peach from 12 months

Food		Notes
		(potentially allergenic)
		c) Administer with a spoon
		d) Consumption of whole fruit is recommended rather than fruit juice to avoid inadequate weight gain or poor weight gain.
Meat	Chicken	(a) Not to exceed 25-40 g/day
	Lamb	b) Better in pureed form and with vegetables
	Veal	
Vegetables	Spinach, cabbage, beetroot	a) Start with potato and carrot, adding a spoonful of olive oil to the purée to improve its palatability.
	Other	b) Delay the introduction of green leafy vegetables until around one year of age to avoid methaemoglobinaemia.
Legumb'e'		Delay its introduction until 10 months of age due to its high fibre content, which is difficult to digest.
Fish		Delay until 12 months if there is a history of atopy or food allergy.
Egg	Yolk (cooked)	Do not eat more than 2 or 3 times a week.
	White (cooked)	
Yoghurt		
Cow's milk		From the year, introducing iron-fortified milk to avoid iron deficiency anaemia and iron deficiency without anaemia.

Information obtained from the Asociacion Espanola de Pediatria recommendations on complementary feeding (2018) and Lazaro A, Martin Lazaro JF. Alimentacion del lactante sano. Protocols of the AEP. Nutrition 2002; 2: 311

Feeding from 12 months and pre-school age onwards

The transition from a mostly liquid to a purely puree-based diet is an important change in infant feeding. The introduction of a small amount of safe, pureed foods should be started until they are fully accepted, a process in which the child's participation in family meals will play an important role. In the period from 12 to 24 months, it is advisable to maintain breastfeeding or adapted formula for continuation, and to extend the range of foods consumed by the child as much as possible, so that by the age of 2 years the child's diet is practically similar to that of an adult. It is also important to gradually replace the bottle with a cup, and to teach the child to use a spoon and fork until he/she becomes fully independent. The main handicap during this period is to face the physiological decrease in the child's appetite, as a consequence of a slower growth rate. Therefore, it is a key moment for a good nutritional education and to maintain a healthy and balanced diet not marked by the child's choice of food. Maintaining these healthy habits is of vital importance at pre-school age, a stage currently marked by a higher prevalence of overweight and obesity in children, perhaps as a result of the high nutrient requirements of this age and the misconception of consuming energy-dense foods rather than nutrient-dense foods. During this stage, it is advisable to establish an order with 4-5 meals a day, distributing the calories to be eaten between breakfast (20-25% of the total), lunch (30-35%), afternoon snack (15-20%) and dinner (25%). A diet rich in wholegrain and whole-grain cereals, vegetables, fruits, fish, eggs and dairy products should be promoted, reducing the consumption of meat and meat products, salt, fats and energy-dense foods of low nutritional value. Likewise, the idea of a balanced and nutritional breakfast should be emphasised, and mealtimes should be respected as much as possible, all of which should be associated with moderate physical activity. Only a healthy diet and an optimal nutritional situation will prevent the appearance of possible nutritional imbalances during childhood, which pose a real threat to the child's health because of their implication in the risk of insulin, metabolic syndrome, cardiovascular disease, etc., in later life. It is important to note that such actions should be established both in the family environment and in school canteens, and should always be based on correct nutritional habits and messages based on scientific evidence. Again, parents and educators have a key role to play, as they can positively influence children's nutrition through their dietary, activity and lifestyle patterns.

Conclusions and recommendations

Research in child nutrition has historically focused on the prevention of malnutrition and nutritional deficiencies. However, due to economic prosperity, the emphasis in recent years has shifted to balanced intake of protein and energy and the prevention of long-term disease risk. Most of the current thinking on complementary feeding is not evidence-based and has largely originated from cultural factors and available food. More data on specific nutrients, particularly micronutrients, are needed to clarify the effects they have on infant growth, development and metabolism. However, some data suggest that the composition of the diet during complementary feeding, as well as the type of breastfeeding during the first months of life, may have effects on the short, medium and long term. The ESPGHAN Nutrition Committee has recently issued the following recommendations on complementary feeding:

1. Exclusive breastfeeding is recommended for the first 6 months of life. CA should not be introduced before 17 weeks, and no later than 26 weeks.

2. The introduction of potentially allergenic foods does not show beneficial effects on the development of allergies.

3. During the period of CA, more than 90% of the iron requirements of a breastfed infant must be met by complementary feeding.

4. Cow's milk has a low iron content, so it should not be introduced as a main drink before 12 months of age.

5. Gluten should not be introduced before the age of 4 months and not later than 7 months. It should be introduced gradually while the child is still breastfed, thus reducing the risk of heart disease, type 2 diabetes mellitus and wheat allergy.

6. A strictly vegetarian diet is not recommended for infants and pre-school children. Otherwise, they should receive sufficient quantities (~500ml) of milk (human or formula) and milk products.

Bibliograffa

1. Delgado, J.R.; Campoy, C.; Martinez, R.G.; Mayo, E.G.; Gil-Campos, M.; et al. Advertising of unhealthy foods. Posicionamiento del Comite de Nutricion y Lactancia Materna de la Asociacion Espanola de Pediatna. In *Anales de Pediatria*, **2022**, 97(3), 206-e1

2. EFSA PANEL ON DIETETIC PRODUCTS, NUTRITION AND ALLERGIES (NDA). Scientific

Opinion on nutrient requirements and dietary intakes of infants and young children in the European Union. *EFSA Journal*, **2013**, 11(10), 3408.

3. Fewtrell, M.; Bronsky, J.; Campoy, C.; Domellof, M.; Embleton, N.; et al. Complementary feeding: a position paper by the European Society for Paediatric Gastroenterology, Hepatology, and Nutrition (ESPGHAN) Committee on Nutrition. *Journal of pediatric gastroenterology and nutrition*, **2017**, 64(1), 119-132.

4. Garwolinska, D.; Namiesnik, J.; Kot-Wasik, A.; Hewelt-Belka, W. Chemistry of human breast milk-A comprehensive review of the composition and role of milk metabolites in child development. *Journal of agricultural and food chemistry*, **2018**, 66(45), 11881-11896.

5. Gomez, M. Recommendations of the Spanish Association of Paediatrics on complementary feeding. *Comite de lactancia materna y Comite de nutrition de la Asociacion Espanola de Pediatria*, **2018**.

6. Koletzko, B.; Baker, S.; Cleghorn, G.; Neto, U.F.; Gopalan, S.; et al. Global standard for the composition of infant formula: recommendations of an ESPGHAN coordinated international expert group. *Journal of pediatric gastroenterology and nutrition*, **2005**, 41(5), 584-599.

7. Lazaro, A; Martin Lazaro, J.F. Alimentacion del lactante sano. *Protocols of the AEP. Nutrition* **2002**, 2, 311

8. World Health Organization. Infant and young child feeding. Model textbook chapter for textbooks for medical and other health sciences students, **2010**, Washington, D.C. Available online: https://www.who.int/news-room/fact- sheets/detail/infant-and-young-child-feeding

13. Malnutrition and obesity in paediatrics

Dr. Cristina Campoy Folgoso
Dr. Estefama Dieguez Castillo
Dr. Jose Antonio Gartia Santos.

Introduction

In 2020, nearly **3.1 billion** people could not afford to maintain a healthy diet, **112 million** more than in 2019, reflecting the effects of consumer food price inflation resulting from the economic impact of the EVID-19 pandemic and the measures taken to contain it. An estimated **45 million** children under five years of age suffered from wasting, the most deadly form of malnutrition, which increases the risk of child mortality up to 12 times. In addition, **149 million** children under five were stunted due to chronic lack of essential nutrients in their diets, while **39 million** were overweight. Worryingly, two out of three children lack the minimum diverse diet they need to grow and develop fully.

In addition, childhood obesity has become a global public health problem. Its incidence has been steadily increasing in recent years, manifesting itself at younger and younger ages. In fact, the prevalence of overweight and obesity has increased in children and adolescents from 4% in 1975 to 18% in 2016. The presence of this pathology early in life predisposes to the development of metabolic disorders later in life, such as type 2 diabetes mellitus. Although the development of obesity is complex and multifactorial, nutrition, metabolism and physical activity play an essential role. In fact, several risk factors have been identified during the first 1000 days of life (from conception to the age of 2 years) that may be possible determinants of obesity later in life.

The aetiology, pathophysiology, classification, diagnosis and updated treatment of these 2 nosological entities are described below.

Malnutrition

In practice, it is used to define situations in which the child does not receive, or cannot adequately use, the nutrients necessary to meet the requirements for normal growth and development.

Aetiology

1) Primary malnutrition, more typical of undeveloped countries and, therefore, closely linked to food shortages, scarce economic resources, etc. In this type of malnutrition, the essential factor is low food intake. It is still a *"silent holocaust" in which* millions of children die every year. It is currently estimated that 65% of children under 5 years of age in these countries suffer from some degree of malnutrition.

2) Secondary malnutrition, more typical of industrialised countries such as Spain, is due to the existence of a primary disorder, difficulties in absorption, poor utilisation, difficulties in ingestion, etc. It will eventually lead to a nutritional imbalance, with different manifestations depending on the fundamental disease that produced it (Table 13.1).

Table 13.1. Diseases that can most frequently lead to secondary malnutrition.

Chronic inflammatory bowel conditions (Ulcerative colitis and Crohn's disease)	The percentages range from 68 to 87%.
Chagas' fibrosis	It is one of the main causes of chronic malabsorption, due to pancreatic insufficiency leading to a variable degree of steatorrhoea and nitrogen loss through the faeces, inadequate energy intake and increased energy needs in cases with pulmonary involvement.
Celiaqrna	Malabsorption with loss of fats and proteins, as well as folic acid and iron deficiency.
Liver diseases	Anorexia, fat malabsorption, increased energy requirements and increased energy expenditure.
Neurological diseases (cerebral palsy, mental retardation, and other conditions with significant disabilities).	Inappetence, swallowing and swallowing difficulties, need for feeding through a stoma, side effects of drugs, etc.
Congenital heart disease	Anorexia, food refusal, fatigue, hypoxia and alterations in absorption with loss of intestinal proteins.
AIDS	Energy and protein malnutrition is a frequent complication, which contributes significantly to morbidity and mortality. Two different underlying mechanisms are cited: on the one hand, low energy intake (inappetence, oral pathology, etc.) and, on the

	other hand, metabolic disorders related to opportunistic infections.
Cancer	Anorexia, vomiting, opportunistic infections, pharmacological effects, toxic metabolites, etc.

Classification

In relation to its duration, malnutrition can be *acute and chronic*. In terms of intensity, it can be *mild, moderate and severe*. In turn, in the severe forms, a distinction must be made between *Marasmo* (fundamental lack of ene^a) and *Kwashiorkor* (predominant lack of protems), although intermediate forms with aspects of both types must also be admitted.

The **Gomez classification**, one of the most widely used, uses the weight-for-age index, which is very useful for children under five years of age. The severity of undernutrition is recognised clinically and is classified according to the weight deficit of children in relation to the 50th percentile weight of children of the same age. The values can be local or international, undernutrition is classified as follows: *Grade 1* (Deficit 10 to 24%), *Grade 2* (Deficit 25 to 39%) and *Grade 3* (Deficit greater than 40%). Children with oedema, regardless of their deficit, are classified as Grade 3.

For mild and moderate forms, the **Waterlow classification**, which distinguishes between weight-for-height deficiency and height-for-age deficiency, is currently preferred. Normality for this classification is set for both cases at two SD below the mean.

For severe forms, the most frequent is to find mixed forms between Marasmus and Kwashiorkor, and they are called **Kwashiorkor-Marasmatic**. In 1969 a classification was proposed for these forms based on two criteria: 1) Lack of weight (assessed in relation to weight for age) and 2) The presence of oedema. According to these criteria we distinguish between: *a) Underweight **children:** those who have between 60-80% of the expected weight for their age, without oedema. b) **Marasmus**: those who have an expected weight for their age below 60%, without oedema. c) **Kwashiorkor:** those who have an expected weight for their age between 60-80% and the presence of oedema and d) **Kwashiorkor-Marasmatic: those who** have an expected weight for their age below 60% and present oedema.

Physiopathology

In the development of malnutrition, different physiological mechanisms are set in motion to try to compensate for the lack of nutritional intake, the child reduces its physical activity (less consumption), if this is not sufficient, fat deposits are mobilised and consequently weight loss appears, if the problem persists, growth will be affected, in mild and moderate forms of malnutrition this may be the only manifestation. In cases where protein and protein deficiency is more important and prolonged, the subcutaneous fat almost disappears. Potassium depletion is parallel to protein depletion. When the lipid reserves have been consumed, a process of muscular proteolysis begins with a loss of lean mass. If the deficit persists, both brain and muscle resort to energy consumption from ketone bodies and hormonal mechanisms are set in motion to recycle amino acids and even reduce protein losses. In this way, blood glucose levels remain within normal ranges, although increased demand can occur at any time and hypoglycaemia can occur. The decrease in protein synthesis triggers adaptive mechanisms to preserve visceral proteins and their functions. In the muscle, the release of amino acids is facilitated, in the muscle the degradation of proteins is reduced and the reuse of amino acids is increased, almost eliminating the catabolic process, although a low-level metabolism persists.

Chemical forms

- **Mild or moderate forms**. Depending on the course, there are two forms: 1) Acute with preferential weight loss and 2) Chronic in which height may be affected. In the weight-for-height deficit, it occurs in a short period of time and improves after adequate nutrition. In the chronic form, on the other hand, the process can start even intrautero, and growth rate, weight and height decrease. These children end up being shorter than their genetic potential (Table 13.2).

- **Severe forms.** *Marasmus* usually occurs in children under one year of age. It usually begins with a delay in weight and later on height is affected. Physical activity, psychomotor development and affectivity are quickly affected. The skin is thin, flaccid and poorly formed due to lack of essential elements in its different layers. The limbs are very thin. Muscle is scanty and atrophic. Along with these structural changes, there are other functional manifestations: **a) Increased susceptibility to infection; b) Alteration of hydromineral metabolism; c) Endocrinological changes** (Table 13.2).

Table 13.2. Clinical manifestations of malnutrition.

Nervous system	In the acute phases, there is apathia, irritability, decay and a tendency to drowsiness. In an attempt to save energy the child seems to be easily absent and has little interest in what is happening. It is accepted that malnutrition at an early age may have repercussions on future psychomotor development.
Kidney function	Reduced glomerular filtration and renal plasma flow. Dysfunction of tubular function (in relation to Mg and K levels) occurs.
Edemas	It is a manifestation with varying degrees of evolution, usually starting in the lower limbs and extending until it becomes generalised and gives the appearance of a "cushingoid syndrome". Several factors are involved in its genesis, including hypoproteinaemia, levels of K, Na, ADH, Mg.
Dermatological lesions	Manifestations related to nutrient deficiencies (essential fatty acids, minerals and vitamins) and global malnutrition itself. We can find: a) Changes in skin colour (brownish, reddish). b) Presence of cracks in different areas (inguinal region and areas of folds). c) Dry and flaky skin. d) Hyperchromic or hypochromic. e) Bleeding lesions in certain areas.
Fan lesions	The hair is pale, devitalised, brittle and easily shed, with areas of more or less extensive alopecia in extreme cases. The nails are also brittle, dull, with irregularly coloured areas.
Visceromegaly	Hepatomegaly is described in up to 70% of cases of a certain intensity. There is a decrease in glycogen and a fatty infiltration of glycogen. Various factors have been included in its aetiology: environmental pollutants, oxidative stress, presence of toxic substances.
Digestive system	Diarrhoea is frequent, both due to intestinal infection (an important cause of dehydration and death), and secondarily due to alterations in the enterocyte and

	intestinal lactase deficiency.
Delay from growth	Growth will be affected if the nutritional deficiency is prolonged over time, if so, it is possible that future height may be affected.
Susceptibility to infection	It is common to find a depletion of the immune system with poor response to infection, secondary to; a reduction of lymphoid tissue, decreased specific cellular immunity, decreased leukocyte function, decreased serum complement. This results in an increased susceptibility to Gram-negative infections and opportunistic germs. Predominance of gangrenous rather than suppurative infections. With poor response to the inflammatory process, fever (an important defence mechanism) often does not appear.
Analytical alterations	a) *Anaemia*. More or less intense depending on the duration, degree and type of deficit. b) *Endocrinological changes*. Depending on the intensity of the symptoms and the length of time they last, various endocrinological changes can be observed. In the initial phases, there is an increase in GH and cortisol and a decrease in insulin and somatomedin C. If the situation is prolonged, an increase in thyroid function may appear. In addition, the pituitary-gonadal axis may be affected, with important influence on gonadal development. c) *Plasma hypoproteinaemia*. Decreased albumin and prealbumin, retinol-binding protein and transferrin. Decrease in amino acids. d) *Deficiency of essential fatty acids.* e) *Mineral deficiency*. Deficiencies of zinc, copper, calcium and phosphorus are common.

In ***Kwashiokor***, fortunately less and less frequent in its pure forms, at the expense of mixed forms of ***Marasmo-Kwashiorkor***, which should be interpreted as a form of improvement of socio-economic and sanitary conditions. It usually starts from the anus onwards. It is very often **affected by stature and bone maturation**, but the main clinical sign is the presence of **oedema.** It is also associated with changes in the skin (pigmentation and appearance of cracks due to lack of Kpids) and the appendages (brittle, depigmented and thinning hair). Functional alterations include hypotoma, irritability, indifference and early impairment of liver function due to steatosis. Intestinal alterations are more accentuated than in Marasmus, as well as the appearance of anaemias and micronutrient deficiencies such as copper, folic acid and vitamin B_{12} (Table 13.2).

Treatment

Initially, the patient's clinical situation, the degree of malnutrition and the possibility of the existence of risk factors must be assessed so that they can be given preferential attention (**Table 3**). Thus, in acute forms, the following should be addressed: a) hypothermia, b) restoration of blood volume, c) gastrointestinal manifestations, d) hypoglycaemia and d) correction of electrolyte imbalances and EAB. Once the normality of these aspects has been verified, the best way to provide nutrients and the rate of nutrient administration must be chosen.

In very serious cases, enteral and parenteral feeding may be indicated, but it is usual for the child to be able to ingest orally in a natural way, and for this reason, feeding guidelines have been designed; the purpose of which is to provide those quantities of nutrients that allow their metabolisation without complications appearing. It should be implemented with caution, to avoid an excess of metric, ionic and proteinic contributions. It is necessary to start by offering small amounts, in very small quantities and on a frequent basis.

Table 13.3. Assessment of nutritional status in malnutrition.

Clinical history	Perinatal history, birth weight and height and their evolution over time should be evaluated. Special attention should be paid to data suggestive of acute, chronic or recurrent organic pathology, and to the accompanying symptomatology.
Physical and somatometric examination (assessment of body composition)	This consists of measuring changes in total body mass (weight and height), or in some of its components (lean mass and fat) by anthropometry; basic measurements include: weight, height, cranial penimeter, brachial penimeter and tricipital fold; or by bioelectrical impedance (BIA). In addition, densitometry allows quantification of bone mineral content, and is of great interest in children with severe dietary deficiencies (eating disorders) or chronic diseases (cystic fibrosis, inflammatory bowel disease).
Analytical determinations	The tests to be performed must be carefully selected and adapted to the history and characteristics of each patient. Usually, haemogram and biochemistry with iron metabolism, zinc, prealbumin, albumin, immunoglobulins and liver function are determined.
Primary disease determinations	If the patient's history points to a primary disease of a gastroenterological, infectious, inflammatory, onco-haematological, metabolic, etc. type. Tests aimed at identifying and evaluating the primary disorder causing the malnutrition will be requested.

A widely accepted criterion is as follows: a) Energy intake, start with 50-55 kcal/kg^a and work up to a normal or even higher intake of 150 kcal/kg^a. b) Protein intake, start with a very low intake of 0.6 kcal/kg^a and work up to an intake of 5.7 kcal/kg^a, even higher than the required amount. In principle, the most appropriate food is milk, occasionally lactose-free in the initial stages. After the first week, if there is good tolerance and there are no complications, a diet adapted to the child's characteristics can be established, with other foods that complement the nutritional needs.

In secondary malnutrition, treatment should focus on two different aspects: 1) Treating the malnutrition, which will need individualised treatment for each patient according to the degree, characteristics and type of deficit found, and 2) Treating the underlying disease, according to the best available evidence.

Obesity

Obesity is the most common nutritional disorder in childhood and adolescence. Despite ongoing research and health policy efforts, the obesity epidemic remains a major public health problem and new strategies are urgently needed. The prevalence of obesity in children and adolescents has increased rapidly, with more than 100 million children and adolescents affected in 2015. This epidemic is a major public health problem in developed and developing countries because it increases the risk of obesity in adulthood, which has been associated with the development of chronic diseases such as type 2 diabetes, hypertension, and cardiovascular disease. Therefore, obesity in children and adolescents is associated with adult mortality and premature death.

In Spain, several studies have been conducted on the prevalence of obesity in children and adolescents, which have demonstrated the exponential progression of obesity in this age group. In 2010, in a study funded by the European Union, 24% of Spanish adolescent boys aged 13 years fear obesity and 12% of girls. More recent data from the ALADINO study (2011-2012) put the prevalence of overweight and obesity in Spanish children aged 6-9 years at 44.5% (26.2% overweight and 18.3% obese). This means that practically one out of every two children is overweight with respect to the growth patterns established by the WHO.

Classification

Excessive intake and/or reduced caloric expenditure are the cause of **exogenous or polygenic obesity** which affects the majority of obese children (95%). The remaining 5% of obese children suffer from **organic** *(intrinsic, endogenous)* **obesity** associated with dysmorphic syndrome, endocrinopathies and CNS lesions.

Obesity can also be classified according to other criteria, depending on: (a) **health risk** (normopese, overweight, obesity grade 1, 2, 3 and 4); (b) **fat distribution** (<u>android or apple type,</u> carries a higher risk of complications (*high triglyceride, cholesterol and blood glucose concentrations, as well as high blood pressure*); (c) obesity *type (android or apple* <u>*type,*</u> carries a higher risk of complications (*high triglyceride, cholesterol and blood glucose concentrations, as well as high blood pressure*); <u>*genoid or pear-type obesity*</u> with a peripheral distribution, and <u>*generalised obesity,*</u> the most prevalent in children and adolescents, characterised by no regional fat distribution); c) **the factors that trigger it** (genetics, diet, hormonal imbalance, thermogenic defect, nervous obesity, endocrine diseases, medication or chromosomal); d) the **<u>type of adipose cell referred to</u>** *(hyperplastic and hypertrophic).* The latter is worth highlighting, since the state of obesity is closely related to the growth, development and maturation periods of the human being; in this sense, **hyperplastic obesity** *is* common in childhood and adolescence, with a discouraging prognosis due to the impossibility of reducing the population of adipocytes established during precocious life; once established, this exaggerated population of adipocytes is characterised by its greed for fat and tendency not to recover its size. Hence the importance of taking into account dietary and lifestyle habits during the periods of growth known as the "*critical windows of growth, development and maturation*", such as 6 months, 18 months, 6 years and puberty, when adipose regrowth is stimulated and hyperplasia occurs, which is irreversible when treating obesity later in life. **Hypertrophic obesity** is characteristic of adults, where adipocytes are in adequate numbers, but are large in size and loaded with fat.

Another important factor related to the development of obesity is the type of colonisation of the infant's gastrointestinal tract that begins at birth. The acquisition and normal development of the neonatal microflora is vital for the healthy maturation of the immune system and has profound effects on health. Breastfeeding is also a beneficial condition related to reduced *risk of allergies, obesity, inflammatory bowel disease, cystic fibrosis, diabetes mellitus and childhood cancer.* Some studies suggest that the gastrointestinal microbiota determined by breastfeeding may be partly responsible for these benefits.

Aetiopathogenesis

In most cases the aetiology of obesity is multifactorial; the involvement and interaction of *genetic, environmental, physiological, metabolic anomata of the adipocyte itself and of the cells surrounding it, and psychosocial factors* have been identified, which condition disorders in the mechanisms that regulate the maintenance of weight and body composition.

- *Environmental factors*

The extent to which environmental factors predominate over genetic factors in the development of obesity is a matter of debate. In any case, it is clear that for the development of obesity, the interaction of both types of factors is necessary.

Nutritional imbalances during the first 1000 days of life influence the risk of developing obesity later in life. Epidemiological and experimental animal studies have shown that only early postnatal nutrition, independent of the intrauterine environment, is able to influence the risk of developing obesity, suggesting *"early nutritional programming"* effects *(*Figure 13.1 and Table 13.4). This period therefore constitutes a window of opportunity for early interventions to prevent the development of metabolic pathologies later in life. Breastfeeding is a protective factor against rapid weight gain in the newborn and infant, with an important role in preventing the development of obesity in adulthood (Figure 13.1).

It is widely described in the literature that environmental determinants are able to influence the determinism of obesity, in addition to prenatal factors, lifestyle (*sedentary lifestyle, eating habits,...*), aspects related to the socio-economic status and family environment. Sedentary lifestyle is an important component of the increasing prevalence of obesity in Western countries *(obesogenic environment)*. Family behavioural factors are also key in the development of obesity, such as time spent watching television, eating behaviour at the family table and physical activity.

Table 13.4. Risk factors during the first 1000 days of life for the development of childhood obesity.

Prenatal period (0-280 d^as)	- Higher preconception body mass index (BMI) of the mother. - Excessive weight gain during pregnancy. - Maternal diabetes (gestational; pre-gestational-type 1). - Genetic predisposition.
Breastfeeding *vs.* infant formula (280 days-6 months of age)	Formula-fed infants show: a) Accelerated growth curve. b) Increased energy intake. c) Increasing the protein content of the diet. d) Low concentration of polyunsaturated fatty acids. e) Differences in the structure and functionality of the gut microbiota.
Complementary feeding (6 months-2 years of age)	- Rapid weight gain. - Early introduction of solid foods. - High protein intake.

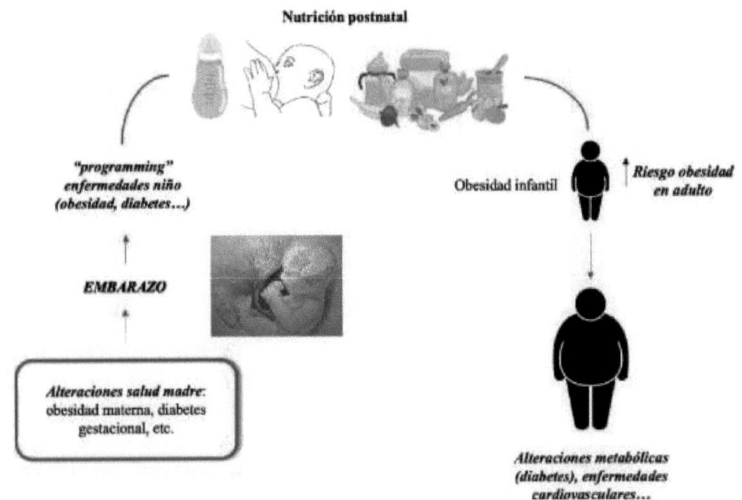

Figure 13.1. Early programming of obesity development in childhood.

Table 13.5. Complications of obesity in children and adolescents.

Psychological and cognitive development	Negative effects on cognitive development (e.g. impaired attention), low self-esteem, anxiety, depression, bullying, eating disorders, social isolation, reduced academic potential.
Endocrine	Insulin resistance, type 2 diabetes, impaired glucose tolerance, precocious puberty, polycystic ovary syndrome (girls), hypogonadism (boys).
Cardiovascular	Dyslipidaemia, hypertension, left ventricular hypertrophy, coagulopathy, chronic inflammation, endothelial dysfunction.
Pulmonary	Obstructive sleep apnoea, asthma, exercise intolerance.
Gastrointestinal	Gastro-oesophageal reflux, non-alcoholic fatty liver disease, steatohepatitis, gall bladder stones, constipation.
Musculoskeletal	Increased risk of fractures, flat feet, pain in the back, knees, ankles, etc.
Long-term risks	Metabolic syndrome, reduced occupational potential, carotid artery atherosclerosis, colorectal carcinoma, ischaemic heart disease, embolism, reduced life expectancy, premature death.

It is also important to make special mention of the consequences of other socio-cultural conditioning factors such as *television marketing, the use of smartphones, tablets and computers*, all of which are involved in the world of social networks, whose current use does not seem to be adequate, but could bring to light new potential means for obesity prevention and lifestyle modification.

- *Genetic factors*

Studies on extreme phenotypes of obesity in animals and humans have led to the identification of some mutations in genes encoding certain molecules involved in energy balance that are responsible for causing obesity of monogenic or digenic origin. In recent years, *genome-wide association study* (GWAS) techniques have made it possible to associate chromosomal regions with obesity phenotypes.

Recent research data from animal models and humans reveal that obesity can be explained by mutations linked to the mechanism of action of hormones and receptors involved in energy metabolism and defects in genes associated with the development of the hypothalamus. However, these mutations explain only a few isolated cases of human obesity, indicating that both genetic and environmental factors play a key role in the development of obesity.

Clinical exploration

Anamnesis

The anamnesis includes detailed collection of family and personal history, growth curves and dietary intake. It is of interest to know the weight, length, cranial penimeter, brachial penimeter, triceps fold and weight-height ratio, as well as whether the birth weight was adequate, low or high for the gestational age. Other aspects to remember are the type of breastfeeding and the timing of introduction of complementary feeding and dietary diversification of the infant. Some studies report the probable protective role of breastfeeding against obesity, especially if breastfeeding is prolonged for at least 4-6 months. A detailed dietary survey and physical activity surveys should not be forgotten. The weight and height of parents and siblings should also be carefully noted. A family history of diabetes, hypertension, dyslipidemia, etc. should be sought.

On clinical examination, overweight and obesity are easy to see. **Adiposity is generalised**, with a truncal predominance in one third of cases *(apple-like obesity)*; this favours the appearance of *pseudogynecomastia* (increased fat deposition in the breasts) and burial in the male suprapubic fat of the external genitalia. Frequently, pink or white skin stasis is observed on the abdomen, thorax and hips. In other cases, especially in girls, the fat deposit is located on the hips (*pear-shaped obesity*). Some obese girls often show delayed puberty, probably secondary to elevated plasma leptin levels.

Complications

Obesity is a chronic disease that causes the individual to have a poor quality of life and a high risk of severe complications, especially cardiovascular, respiratory and metabolic, among others, that compromise life expectancy (Table 13.5).

Prevention

Overweight and obese children tend to remain obese into adulthood and are more likely to develop non-communicable diseases such as diabetes and cardiovascular disease at an earlier age. Overweight, obesity and associated diseases are largely preventable, therefore the prevention of childhood obesity should be a priority.

The prevention of childhood overweight and obesity are fundamental objectives of any health programme, which includes reducing the child's energy intake in prudent and balanced terms, and establishing adequate physical activity. It is a pathology that must be treated from a multidisciplinary point of view, involving not only the child, but also parents and teachers, as well as health professionals such as doctors, nurses, psychologists, nutritionists, among others.

Treatment

There is currently no effective treatment for children and adolescents, and the multidisciplinary team programmes needed to combat obesity, including lifestyle changes, remain economically difficult to implement. The lack of effective treatments to combat obesity and intervention programmes to prevent obesity is a major public health issue. Given that eating and physical activity habits begin in the early years of life, it is very important that health care and public health experts develop early prevention programmes during childhood and adolescence.

The general outline of obesity treatment comprises several stages:

- ***Initial period***: weight loss should be achieved. Its duration will depend on the degree of obesity, the type of diet and physical exercise chosen. In the case of children, multidisciplinary treatment should also include psychological treatment, supporting the success of dietary and physical activity interventions.

- ***Maintenance period***: the impossibility of a return to the status quo must be accepted.

The duration of this stage is closely related to the understanding by the child and his parents of the importance for his future life of maintaining a healthy diet, in accordance with his tastes and nutritional needs.

- ***Adherence to treatment:*** no therapeutic strategy will be successful, in the long term, if the obese child does not comply with the recommended instructions. For this to happen, adherence to treatment is essential, as well as the full cooperation of his or her family.

Physical exercise is an important part of the treatment of the obese child as, in addition to contributing to weight loss, it increases the functional capacity of the child's body. It is recommended that this programme be maintained on a regular basis and in conjunction with dietary treatment.

Finally, if necessary, surgical treatment (bariatric surgery - exceptional in paediatrics) and pharmacological treatment will be carried out.

Assessment of nutritional status

In the **anthropometric measurement it** must not be forgotten that the child, at each moment of his life, has an adequate weight depending on his height and sex, and once the patient's measurements have been taken, it is necessary to compare them with the reference standards. In infants and small children, possible alterations occur very quickly because they are in a period of maximum growth speed.

The most useful body composition parameters are as follows:

1. **Weight/height ratio:** assesses the ratio of these measurements, regardless of age. Percentile patterns are available for this purpose. Z-scores can also be calculated.

2. **Body mass index** [weight/height^2 (kg/m^2)]: **is an** easy-to-calculate index, which has proved very useful in defining obesity and malnutrition. Its main disadvantage is that it varies with age and that it does not distinguish fat mass from lean mass. Therefore, in children it is assessed by percentile curve or by calculating Z-scores. To discriminate between excess fat (obesity) and lean mass (athletic constitution), the measurement of the brachial pentimeter and skinfolds should be carried out.

BibliograHa

1.   La desnutricion Infantil: Causas, consecuencias y estrategias para su prevencion y

tratamiento. Published by: UNICEF Spain C/ Mauricio Legendre, 36 28046 Madrid sensibilizacion@unicef.es.

2.   Carrascosa A, Fernandez JM, Fernandez C, et al. Spanish cross-sectional growth study 2008. Part II: values of height, weight and body mass index from birth to adult height. An Pediatr (Barc) 2008; 68: 552-69.

3.   Martinez Costa C, Martinez Rodnguez L. Assessment of nutritional status. In: Comite de Nutricion de la AEP, ed. Manual Practico de Nutricion en Pediatna. 1^ ed. Madrid: Ergon; 2007. p. 31-9.

4.   Malnutrition Advisory Group/BAPEN. Todorovic E, Russell C, Startton R, et al, eds. The MUST Explanatory Booklet. A Guide to the Malnutrition Universal Screening Tool (MUST) for adults. Worcester: BAPEN, 2003; 32.

5.   Han JC, Lawlor DA, Kimm SYS. Childhood obesity. Lancet. 2010;375:1737-48.

6.   Campoy C, Martin-Bautista E, Anjos T. Critical periods for the development of obesity: INTECH Open Access Publisher; 2012.

7.   Mameli C, Mazzantini S, Zuccotti GV. Nutrition in the First 1000 Days: The Origin of Childhood Obesity. Int J Environ Res Public Health. 2016 Aug 23;13(9):838. doi: 10.3390/ijerph13090838. PMID: 27563917; PMCID: PMC5036671.

8.   Lee EY, Yoon KH. Epidemic obesity in children and adolescents: risk factors and prevention. Front Med. 2018 Dec;12(6):658-666. doi: 10.1007/s11684-018-0640-1. Epub 2018 Oct 2. PMID: 30280308.

9.   Kumar S, Kelly AS. Review of Childhood Obesity: From Epidemiology, Etiology, and Comorbidities to Clinical Assessment and Treatment. Mayo Clin Proc. 2017 Feb;92(2):251-265. doi: 10.1016/j.mayocp.2016.09.017. Epub 2017 Jan 5. PMID: 28065514.

10. Mittal M, Jain V. Management of Obesity and Its Complications in Children and Adolescents. Indian J Pediatr. 2021 Dec;88(12):1222-1234. doi: 10.1007/s12098-021-03913-3. Epub 2021 Oct 5. PMID: 34609654; PMCID: PMC8491444.

14. Swallowing and digestive disorders in the infant

Dr. Cristina Campoy

Dr. Jose Antonio Garaa Santos

Dr. Estefama Dieguez Castillo

The development of feeding and swallowing involves a complex set of interactions that begin in the embryological and foetal period, continuing through infancy and early childhood. Given the immaturity of digestive function during the first months of life, the appearance of "minor" digestive disorders *(infant colic, constipation, dyschezia and regurgitation)* is common, but they are not serious and improve with the passing months. Although they do not affect the growth and development of the infant, these ailments are a cause for consultation and concern for parents due to the discomfort they generate in the infant, a situation aggravated by the lack of knowledge of some parents in infant care and the lack of clear messages to differentiate these ailments from other more serious ones. However, the feeding process is seriously affected in those cases where the paediatric patient suffers from syndromes and pathologies of anatomical or neuromuscular origin generally associated with dysfunctions in the ability to swallow food. These situations may even lead to the need for enteral nutrition in order to avoid nutritional deficiencies. Regardless of their origin, the various swallowing and/or digestion disorders should be treated under a multidisciplinary approach with special emphasis on providing evidence-based nutritional recommendations, correct postural habits during feeding and the generation of messages in the family environment on the practices to be followed in these cases.

This chapter will summarise the necessary knowledge on the pathophysiology of the main swallowing and digestive disorders affecting the paediatric population, listing the main aspects that should be included in the therapeutic approach and the most appropriate nutritional interventions.

Swallowing disorders of the infant

Swallowing is a complex neuromuscular process that requires the coordination of cranial nerves, brain stem, cerebral cortex, and 26 muscles of the mouth, pharynx and oesophagus in order to move the food from the oral cavity to the stomach, protecting the respiratory tract during this movement. Within this swallowing process, there are 4 phases: *a) Oral preparatory phase (voluntary phase),* during which the liquid and the food are manipulated to form the food bolus, the latter remaining between the tongue and the hard palate, the soft palate descending to avoid access to the pharynx; *b) Oral phase (voluntary phase),* characterised by the elevation of the soft palate and the subsequent transfer of the food, by means of peristaltic movements, towards the pharynx. The nasopharynx closes simultaneously; *c) Pharyngeal phase (voluntary and involuntary phase):* The food bolus is transported through the posterior part of the pharynx, while the larynx closes to protect the airways. The upper part of the oesophageal sphincter also opens; and *d) oesophageal phase (involuntary phase),* in which the food bolus is transported to the stomach by means of peristaltic movements. However, both during mastication and in the different phases of swallowing, disorders may occur due to anatomical and neuromuscular dysfunctions, tumours, post-surgical consequences and infections, which seriously undermine the feeding process and the health of the infant.

Dysphagia

It is defined as dysfunction in the sequence of the oral, pharyngeal and oesophageal phases of the swallowing process caused mainly by psychological, neurological, functional and/or anatomical problems at the level of the oropharynx and oesophagus, as well as by problems in the gastric retention mechanisms.

Table 14.1. Interventions or actions needed to manage nutrition in paediatric dysphagia.

Dietary assessment *(nutritional status and nutritional requirements)* by an experienced paediatric dietician.
Fluid balance *(inflows and outflows, including vomit and saliva losses)*
Recording of oral food intake and weight gain
Non-oral supplementary feeding, if necessary. *The amount of such feeding shall be recorded in the fluid balance and dietary record.*

Its physiology and aetiology make this dysfunction prevalent in individuals with upper motor impairment, cerebral palsy, traumatic brain injury, genetic disorders, stroke, Rett syndrome, Down syndrome and neuromuscular diseases *(myasthenia gravis, Duchenne muscular dystrophy)*. Also, the use of some drugs such as neuroleptics, antiepileptics or muscle relaxants can reduce the ability to swallow food. Finally, muscular alterations affecting both muscle tone and activity (dystoma, dyskinesia, hypotoma) are also associated with alterations in the child's ability to chew, manipulate the food bolus and/or swallow food.

Specific activities for the management of dysphagia

Any dysphagia care programme in the paediatric population should be tailored to the child's developmental age, the presence and degree of dysfunction in cognitive and motor skills, as well as the child's current level of functional swallowing ability. Such a programme should be developed under a multidisciplinary approach involving physicians, speech therapists, physiotherapists, dieticians and nurses, with the aim of preventing respiratory and nutritional complications in these patients. More specifically, dysphagia management should include the following activities:

1. ***Nutrition and hydration monitoring*** (Table 14.1), aimed at assessing the patient's nutritional status and implementing the necessary nutritional measures to avoid nutritional deficiencies related to oral motor dysfunction, difficulties in communicating food cravings or food preferences, inability to feed themselves, gastro-oesophageal reflux and aspiration.

2. ***Postural measures.*** It is recommended to maintain a safe body position, with the child seated, back in contact with the back of the chair, and feet flat on the floor. The head should be slightly bent and the chin down. In cases where the patient shows poor head control and/or trunk stability, appropriate and individualised positioning techniques are required. In addition, the patient should be prevented from extending the neck at all times during feeding and, once feeding is completed, the patient should be prevented from lying down immediately. Failure to comply with these recommendations significantly increases the risk of bronchial aspiration.

3. ***Dietary measures aimed*** at controlling bolus size, taste and texture. In some cases, large boluses are recommended to increase the sensitivity of the oral cavity, help bolus formation and reduce the fanngeal transit time. It is also recommended to vary the texture to facilitate swallowing, opting for semi-solid boluses or boluses with a consistent texture. However, the elasticity and viscosity of the food should always be considered when introducing texture changes. Finally, it is advisable to offer the child a *wide range of* recommended textural *flavours*, recording tolerance and texture preferences at all times.

4. ***Supportive dysphagia management devices*** adapted to the specific circumstances of each child. *Modified* feeding *utensils* are recommended for children with oral swallowing problems, the use of *spoons of different sizes and shapes* to control bolus size, and *plates with protective rims or bowls with supports* for children who are learning to feed themselves. When the need for these utensils is identified, the child should be

referred to the occupational therapist and physiotherapist.

5. ***Aspiration,*** checking before, during and after swallowing for *signs of broncho-aspiration* (coughing, choking or respiratory distress) and especially for the presence of *silent breathing* (no signs).1

Table 14.2. Therapeutic approach for parents and/or caregivers in the management of functional disorders of the infant.

Infant Colic	> Establish an adequate communication link, aimed at the spontaneous resolution of the disorder from the 3rd or 4th month of life of the infant. > Postural hygiene measures: place the infant face down on the arm, with the head resting on the crook of the elbow and the abdomen on the forearm. Perform gentle rocking movements. Abdominal massage accompanied by raising the legs.
Regurgitations	> To duly inform parents of the physiological nature of this disorder and its spontaneous resolution from the 5th month of life onwards. > Indicate the warning signs for which you should consult your paediatrician > Monitor for symptoms of nasal congestion or difficulty breathing during sleep. > Postural measures: upright or left lateral position in the immediate postprandial period. > Reduce the volume of the intake and increase the time between intakes.
Constipation and dyschezia	> To reduce family anxiety by informing about the possibility of spontaneous resolution at the age of one year. > Reinforce nutritional messages and recommendations for these disorders, mainly the intake of high fibre foods or the use of prebiotic supplements.

Functional disorders of the digestive system

During the first months of life, and given the immaturity of their digestive system, infants frequently present gastrointestinal symptoms due to functional disorders, mainly *regurgitation, constipation, and colic*. As a general rule, these usually disappear as the baby matures or when certain changes in feeding habits are made. However, despite the infant's good clinical condition, anthropometric and neuromaturative development, these complaints are the cause of frequent visits to the paediatrician, parental concern and unnecessary dietary changes and medication. It is therefore important to recognise the symptoms of these disorders and to act in a timely manner to prevent them from interfering with the infant's development and well-being. These objectives are achieved through a multidisciplinary approach in which dietary and pharmacological intervention must be accompanied by correct information to parents, who often show great concern because they do not know if they are adequately caring for their infant and because, on many occasions, they do not know how to distinguish this type of minor ailment from something more serious (Table 14.2).

Infant colic" is defined as the occurrence of paroxysmal inconsolable crying, which starts and stops without apparent cause, for 3 hours, 3 days a week, 3 weeks, or 3 hours a day for a week. It usually affects infants younger than 3 months and rarely extends beyond 6 months. During these crying episodes, infants adopt a characteristic position, flexing the thighs over the abdomen, clenching the nipples, with a flushed face and a tense abdomen. Although the symptoms are very clear, it is necessary to rule out the presence of organic causes as the origin of these cries, mainly a possible allergy to cow's milk proteins or gastro-oesophageal reflux (GOR). From a nutritional point of view, breastfeeding is recommended in the management of infants with colic, as its content in oligosaccharides and immunomodulatory factors favours the maturational development of the gastrointestinal system. If the infant receives infant formula, the transitional use of low-lactose or fermented formulas is recommended due to their content in *Streptococcus thermophilus* and *Bifidobacterium breve*, which favour lactose hydrolysis and, therefore, its fermentation in the colon. Supplementation with probiotics, mainly *Lactobacillus reuteri* 55730 *and L. reuteri* DSM 17938, is also an option. However, the use of anticholinergic drugs, muscle relaxants, H2-receptor blockers or acid production blockers is discouraged and parents are referred to appropriate dietary and postural measures (Table 14.2).

Table 14.3. Fundamental objectives of enteral nutrition.

Maintaining a positive nutritional balance
To promote the supply of nutrients necessary for normal growth rates.
Preventing malnutrition in children with long-term illnesses
To achieve sufficient calorie intake in children who tolerate only small volumes.
Avoiding the counterproductive effects of prolonged fasting
To provide substances with beneficial effects on the intestinal mucosa and its protective mechanisms.

Another frequent functional digestive disorder in the first months of infants' life is the presence of **regurgitations**, i.e. the expulsion of milk from the mouth that refluxes from the stomach with a frequency of 2 or more times a day for at least 3 weeks. Unlike vomiting, these regurgitations occur without effort and without symptoms of discomfort or difficulty in feeding, as they are due to the infant's own gastrointestinal immaturity, so they usually decrease gradually from the 5th month of life onwards. However, an optimal nutritional, anthropometric and biochemical evaluation is necessary to rule out any organic cause, mainly GOR and lesions associated with the passage of acid from the stomach through the oesophagus. Again, in this type of disorder, maintaining breastfeeding emerges as a priority nutritional measure to improve gastric emptying. Only in non-breastfed infants is it advisable to use modified formulas by adding a thickening substance, using cassema as the main source of protein or reducing the concentration of fat. Special emphasis should be placed on avoiding the use of homemade thickened formulas, as modifications in the osmolarity and concentration of the feed may worsen gastric emptying.

Finally, episodes of **constipation or dyschezia** are also frequent in infants during the first months of life, as well as a common reason for consultation in Paediatrics. In breastfed infants, it is usual to have an average of 4-6 stools per day, of soft or semi-fluid consistency, and green and/or yellow in colour. This frequency is lower in formula-fed infants, who alternate between 2-3 stools per day or every 2-3 days, depending on the period of lactation. In both cases, the frequency, consistency and colour of the stools change during the first[er] year of life, especially after the introduction of complementary feeding. With these considerations in mind, **constipation is** understood as difficulty in evacuation or the presence of hard and infrequent stools of entirely functional origin, while **dyschezia** is defined as a delay in evacuation (for 3 or more days) with pushing manoeuvres, facial flushing, no evacuation for a few minutes, and with intense crying that ceases with the expulsion of soft or semi-fluid stools. In this case, its origin is associated with gastrointestinal immaturity of the infant in terms of failure of coordination between increased intra-abdominal pressure and pelvic floor relaxation and ineffectiveness of abdominal and gluteal muscle contractions. While both cases resolve spontaneously within a few weeks without the need for therapeutic measures, a series of nutritional recommendations can be made to promote defecatory dynamics. These recommendations include the maintenance of breastfeeding, with special attention to the infant's weight gain, the offer of small amounts of water (5-10 ml/kg^a) or formulas supplemented with prebiotics (mainly oligosaccharides) in formula-fed infants under 6 months of age. From 6 months onwards, a complementary diet rich in fibre, vegetables, whole grains and legumes should be recommended, with an adjusted consumption of dairy products and derivatives, as their excess can favour these digestive disorders. In more severe cases, medical treatment with osmotic laxatives can be chosen, the dosage of which is adjusted until 1-2 soft stools per day are achieved without effort.

Table 14.4. Indications for the establishment of enteral nutrition in paediatrics.

Digestive diseases
Intractable diarrhoea and atrophyFeeding   after abdominal and oesophageal surgery vellositarianeonatal
Inflammatory diseases of the
Cystic fibrosis intestine
E, , ,   Enteropathies caused by abdominal radiation
Short bowel syndrome.   ..
and/or chemotherapy
Cardiorespiratory diseases and congenital cardiopathies
Kidney diseases
Severe neurological disorders with feeding difficulties
Hypermetabolic states
Individualised indications
"   . , ,Diseases with malnutrition disturbances
Prematurity   , .
secondary
Calorie-protein malnutrition .
.   .. Glycogenosis
severe primary
Anorexia   nervosaAminoacidopathies

Enteral nutrition in paediatrics

Enteral nutrition is understood to be the method of feeding by means of which food is totally or partially supplied to the stomach or intestine through a tube or by means of a gastrotomy or enterostomy. It is, therefore, an action aimed at contributing to the optimal growth and development of the infant, and is indicated only in those cases in which the presence of certain pathologies prevents optimal feeding (Tables 14.3 and 14.4). In this type of feeding, special formulas are used which are always adjusted to the age of the child, the degree of preservation of intraluminal digestion and absorptive surface capacity, as well as to the type of disorder involved in the use of enteral nutrition. According to their nutritional composition, these formulas are classified into: _a) complete formulas,_ consisting of whole proteins, proteins with varying degrees of hydrolysis and essential amino acids, and a general nutritional composition that covers the infant's needs; _and b) incomplete formulas,_ enriched or lacking in some specific nutrient, so that they do not cover all the nutritional requirements of the infant. Likewise, the formulas used in enteral nutrition can be classified on the basis of the complexity of the macronutrients present in them:

_1)_ _Polymeric formulations_, in which the macronutrients are in complex form; thus, proteins are present in their natural or purified form, di-, oligo- or polysaccharides are present as carbohydrates, and hydrates are present as a mixture of medium- and long-chain polyunsaturated fatty acids. Soy polysaccharides are often used as a source of fibre with a ratio of 94% insoluble fibre (increases faecal bulk and reduces transit time) and 6% soluble fibre (used for bacterial fermentation and production of short-chain fatty acids). In short, they are formulations with high molecular weight nutrients and low osmolarity.

_2)_ _Elemental formulations,_ consisting of free amino acids or proteins from casema or a-lactoalbumin, partially hydrolysed, and lactose-free. Mono- or oligosaccharides are used in their formulation as a source of carbohydrates, due to their better digestibility and lower osmolarity, and kpids in the form of a small proportion of polyunsaturated fatty acids or medium chain triglycerides, thus avoiding deficiencies in essential fatty acids.

_3)_ _Semi-elemental formulations,_ defined as those formulations with low osmolarity in which all the immediate principles have been modified to facilitate digestion and absorption and, consequently, intestinal regeneration, without affecting their nutritional quality. They are therefore formulations with highly hydrolysed proteins, carbohydrates in the form of glucose polymers or maltodextrin, and fats such as medium-chain triglycerides which are easily digested and pass directly into the hepatic portal circulation. They also contain the necessary amounts of vitamins and minerals to meet daily requirements, without the need for supplementation.

In children suffering from metabolic disorders or those receiving home enteral nutrition due to severe nutrient intolerances or deficiencies, **modular diets or nutritional modules are** often chosen. This feeding modality is based on the use of preparations usually consisting of a single nutrient, so that the combination of several modules will allow a complete enteral diet. Generally, _hydrocarbon modules_, consisting exclusively of carbohydrates, are used when there is a metabolic disorder associated with this macronutrient, or if our objective is to increase the caloric content of the diet. These preparations are based on the use of low-osmolarity carbohydrates, mainly glucose polymers from the hydrolysis of demineralised and deproteinised starches, which are easily digestible and well absorbed. In those cases of special ene^a requirements, or in situations with severe malabsorption or digestive intolerance to fats, _lipid modules_ consisting of medium or long chain triglycerides, high proportion of essential fatty acids and a low contribution of saturated fatty acids should be used. In any case, preference should be given to the use of medium chain triglycerides because of their higher solubility, energy value and easy absorption. *Protein modules* should be used both in situations of nutritional deficit in this macronutrient (whole protein modules) or in those cases in which the child shows a severe intolerance to whole protein (amino acid or peptide modules). High biological value proteins, either whole or hydrolysed either chemically or enzymatically, should always be chosen and may be supplemented with carbohydrates to improve the palatability of the product, especially in the case of amino acid and peptide modules. Finally, it is important to note the existence of *thickening modules* composed only of modified starches, which are usually in powder form and have a neutral taste. These modules are exclusively intended to increase the consistency of the liquid food received by patients with motor dysphagia, and their main objective is to avoid or delay the use of a naso-enteric tube or gastrostomy.

Conclusions

> Dysphagia or difficulty swallowing food is a common swallowing disorder in children with neurological disorders or anatomical-functional malformations in the digestive system. Its therapeutic approach has a multidisciplinary, individualised and specialised focus to avoid respiratory, nutritional and developmental problems.

> During the first months of life, functional digestive disorders are frequent due to the gastrointestinal immaturity of the infant, such as colic, regurgitation and constipation.

> The diagnosis of these digestive disorders is made by means of an adequate anamnesis and a thorough physical examination, and in exceptional cases complementary examinations are required.

> From a nutritional point of view, continued breastfeeding is recommended. However, it is necessary to stress to parents the benign and favourable evolution of these disorders as maturity and digestive function progress over the months.

> Enteral nutrition should be used as a way of feeding only in very serious cases in which the presence of pathologies prevents optimal feeding, with the growth and development of the child being seriously affected. The intervention, in any case, must be carried out in an individualised way by means of the use of special formulas adjusted in their characteristics to the age of the child, the physiological situation of the deglutition, absorption and digestion process, and the cause that provokes the use of this type of feeding.

Bibliograffa

1. Aguirre, I.N.; Bulnes, C.E.; Gomez, A.O.; Suazo, B.N.; Mercado, E.M.: et al. Functional digestive disorders in infants. *Archives of Medicine,* **2020**, 16(2), 2.

2. Constipation Guideline Committee of the North American Society for Pediatric Gastroenterology, Hepatology, and Nutrition (CGCNASPGHAN). Evaluation and treatment of constipation in infants and children: Recommendations of the North American Society for Pediatric Gastroenterology, Hepatology and Nutrition. *Journal of Pediatic Gastroenterology and Nutriton,* **2006**, 43, e1-e13.

3. Ezquerra, R.G.; Monreal, J.P.; Barriga, P.G.; Rubio, P.M.; Simao, M.D.A. Abordaje de

la disfagia pediatrico-neonatal. *Elservier Health Sciences*, **2022**, ISBN: 978-84-1382-211-2.

4. Standardisation Group of the Spanish Society of Parenteral and Enteral Nutrition (SENPE). Formulas de nutricion enteral en pediatna. Eds: Pedron-Giner, C.; Navas-Lopez, V.M. **2013**, ISBN:978-84-15351-1-92-4. Available at : https://www.aeped.es/sites/default/files/documentos/formulas denutricion enteralen pe diatria.pdf

5. Hiern, A.; Lindblom, K.; Reuter, A.; Silfverdal, S.A. A systematic review of prevention and treatment of infantile colic. *Acta Paediatrica,* **2020,** 109(9), 1733-1744.

6. Umay, E.; Evigor, S.; Giray, E.; Karadag Saygi, E.; Karadag, B.; et al. Pediatric dysphagia overview: best practice recommendation study by multidisciplinary experts. *World Journal of Pediatrics,* **2022**, 1-10.

7. Vandenplas, Y.; Rudolph, C.D., Di Lorenzo, C.; Hassall, E.; Liptal, G.; et al. Pediatric gastroesphageal reflux Clinical practice guidelines: joint recommendations of the North American Society for Pediatric Gastroenterology, Hepatology, and Nutrition (NASPGHAN) and the European Society for Pediatric Gastroenterology, Hepatology, and Nutrition (ESPGHAN). *Journal of Pediatric Gastroenterology and Nutrition,* **2009**, 49(4), 498-547.

15. abdominal pain in paediatrics. PREMIERE

Dr. Esther Ocete Hita

Pain in children is the most frequent cause of medical consultation and emergency care, constituting at least 50% of the reasons for hospital emergencies. Abdominal pain is a frequent reason for consultation, constituting 10% in the hospital setting and rising to 15% in primary care, although on many occasions it is a banal cause. Abdominal pain can be defined as an unspecific symptom of many processes, both intra- and extra-abdominal.

Pain can be:

♦   Constant: continuous over time and constant intensity (not vain).

♦   Intermittent: presents temporary intervals without pain.

♦   Colic: with variations in intensity and with a certain temporal rhythm.

It is the most common symptom in the clinic of diseases of the digestive tract, its causes are diverse, among them we will name:

♦   Mechanics

♦   Inflammatory

♦   Infectious

♦   Vascular

Causes of abdominal pain

The causes of abdominal pain can be grouped into three main groups: mechanical, inflammatory and ischaemic.

Mechanical: Traction, distension and stretching on the muscular layers of the hollow viscera, the peritoneum and the capsule of the solid viscera; it is important that this occurs abruptly as a gradual onset may not cause pain.

Inflammatory: The release of substances involved in the inflammatory process, both physical and infectious, is a powerful pain stimulus.

Ischaemic: The cessation of blood supply to a vein, whether primary due to embolism or thrombosis or secondary due to twisting of its vascular pedicle, causes pain due to irritation caused by the concentration of certain tissue metabolites.

The different sensitivity of the intra-abdominal structures must also be taken into account, e.g. the mucosa of almost the entire gastrointestinal tract does not feel pain, the hollow viscera are more sensitive to increased pressure, the visceral peritoneum is practically painless and there are so-called "silent areas" (gastric chamber and cecum) which do not cause pain until peritoneal irritation or obstruction occurs.

Depending on location:

Intra-abdominal: Pain secondary to irritation of the parietal peritoneum. Perforation of the hollow viscera. Primary bacterial peritonitis (pneumococcus, gonococcus). Non-bacterial peritonitis (ruptured ovarian cyst,...). Familial Mediterranean fever. Peptic ulcer. Appendicitis. Cholecystitis. Diverticulitis. Pancreatitis. Endometritis. Ectopic pregnancy rupture. Intestinal obstruction. Intestinal hypermotility. Acute biliary obstruction. Ureteral obstruction. Aortic aneurysm. Intestinal infarction.

Extra-abdominal: thoracic: pneumoma, pulmonary embolism, AMI, oesophageal rupture. Neurogenic: radicular pain, Tabes dorsalis, abdominal epilepsy. Metabolic: diabetes, ketoacidosis, uremia, acute intermittent porphyria, acute adrenal insufficiency. Other causes: collagenosis, Schonlein-Henoch purpura, haemophthalmic anaemia, drug intoxication (ergotamine), haematoma of the rectus sheath.)

Types of abdominal pain

Visceral pain. It originates in the abdominal organs. It is dull and poorly localised. It sometimes appears as a sensation of abdominal fullness. It may also be colicky (like a cramp), accompanied by nausea, vomiting, pallor and sweating.

Parietal pain. It originates in structures of the abdominal wall. It is aggravated by movement and increases on palpation.

Referred pain. It is perceived in anatomical regions other than the area of stimulation and is produced because this area of stimulation shares a sensory neuronal segment with the painful area. For example, one can have pain in the right shoulder and suffer from cholecystitis or biliary colic, or have pain between both scapulae and be suffering from the dissection of a thoracic aortic aneurysm, or have pain in the pit of the stomach and end up having a process of appendicitis a few hours later, locating the pain in the right iliac fossa.

Of the patients presenting with abdominal pain to the emergency department, approximately 25% will require surgery to resolve the problem. This is where the distinction between immediate, urgent and delayed surgery is made according to their speed of development:

- Sudden onset (instantaneous): Perforated ulcer. Rupture of a large vessel (trauma, assault with a knife or firearm). Rupture of abscess or haematoma. Rupture of ectopic pregnancy. Abdominal organ infarction. Spontaneous pneumothorax. Rupture of dissecting aortic aneurysm.

- Rapid onset (within minutes): Perforation of the hollow viscera. Upper intestinal occlusion. Pancreatitis. Acute cholecystitis. Renal colic. Mesenteric infarction. Diverticulitis. Ectopic pregnancy. Appendicitis (less common). Gradual development (few hours of evolution) Appendicitis (common). strangulated hernia Lower intestinal occlusion. cholecystitis Pancreatitis. Diverticulitis Perforation of gastric or colon tumour. Threatened miscarriage. Salpingitis. Urinary retention. Intestinal infarction. Gastroenteritis.

Characteristics of abdominal pain

Age: Many diseases occur in population groups of a certain age, which is in itself^ indicative. For example, we can expect an intussusception of the bowel as the cause of an occlusive condition in a young child, which is exceptional in adults.

Location and chronology of pain: The exact location and timing of the pain must be established and its radiations assessed. It is also important to consider whether displacement of pain has occurred. Many abdominal conditions have a characteristic pattern of pain such as, for example, the perforation of a duodenal ulcer, which has an abrupt onset in the epigastrium and then spreads to the rest of the abdomen.

Intensity of pain: This is a parameter that is difficult to assess, although it can be generalised that the intensity of pain is related to the importance of the disease, i.e. pain of low intensity is rarely a symptom of a serious process. Factors that modify the pain: it is necessary to analyse whether the pain varies with breathing, ingestion, vomiting, bowel movements, etc. For example, pain due to peritoneal irritation is aggravated by movement, ulcer pain is relieved by swallowing, in pancreatitis pain is relieved by leaning forward. Colicky pain that is relieved by bowel movements may be indicative of colonic pathology, vomiting relieves pain in obstructive processes of the upper gastrointestinal tract, etc.

Accompanying symptoms

Digestive: Abdominal pain is not usually presented as the only symptom in a patient but accompanied by other symptoms that help us to reduce its unspecific character.

Vomiting: Vomiting is a common symptom of abdominal diseases accompanied by nausea, depending on the cause of the vomiting. Three main mechanisms can be recognised:

a) Intense irritation of the nerves of the peritoneum or mesentery (perforation of the hollow viscera, appendicitis, etc.).

b) Obstruction of a smooth muscle conduit (intestine, choledochus, etc.).

c) Action of toxins on bulbar centres. It is also important to assess the materials vomited (alimentary, bilious, faecaloid vomit, etc.). It is also important to see the relationship between vomit and pain (it appears quickly in strangulation and later in occlusion, it relieves pain in gastric retention, etc.).

Intestinal rhythm: Changes in bowel habit help us to assess the diagnosis. A picture of diarrhoea with abdominal pain, colic, vomiting and fever leads to a diagnosis of gastroenteritis.

Anorexia

Stool characteristics (ask for data that may point to gastrointestinal bleeding).

Fever: this is related to the septic status of the patient. It is generally accepted that the presence of fever higher than 39°C in the presence of acute abdominal pain suggests an extra-abdominal origin, with urinary sepsis, pneumonia or meningitis.

Urinary symptomatology: It can appear in both urological and intestinal processes: retrocecal appendicitis, diverticulitis or perforated neoplasms. Gynaecological disorders: It is important to know the previous gynaecological history in women, theoretical date of ovulation, oral contraceptives, intrauterine devices, etc.

Nuclear Exploration

First of all, as with any other patient, it is necessary to assess the general state of the patient, determine their vital signs, state of perfusion, nutrition and hydration, their degree of consciousness, their attitude (peritoneal irritation immobilises the patient because movement causes pain, colicky pain causes restlessness and the patient cannot rest), their colouring, etc... The examination should begin with an inspection of the abdomen. The spontaneous mobility of the abdominal wall and respiratory movements should be observed (in processes involving peritoneal irritation, immobility is produced during respiration, with shallow breathing). The possible presence of scars from previous operations, the abdominal symmetry, the existence of protruding masses and whether there is abdominal distension should also be analysed. The presence of collateral circulation, vesicles (Herpes Zoster) or other cutaneous signs such as periumbilical ecchymosis (Cullen's sign) and flank ecchymosis (Grey-Turner's sign), which are characteristic of severe necrohaemorrhagic pancreatitis, should be noted. Palpation should be performed in a gentle manner to avoid provoking voluntary contraction of the abdominal muscles in the patient. It is also advisable to follow an exploratory routine by always standing on the same side of the patient and palpate the abdomen in quadrants following the same direction, leaving the painful area for last. The topography of the pain will be identified. Palpation is the most cost-effective exploratory manoeuvre, sometimes being the only thing on which we can base a surgical exploration of a patient. The following aspects will be assessed:

- Superficial palpation: the existence of areas of cutaneous hyperesthesia will be appreciated. *Deep palpation: we look for organomegaly (liver, spleen, kidney) and masses (vesicular hydrops, pancreatic pseudocysts, inflammatory plastrons, neoplasms, aneurysms, hernias).

- Abdominal contracture: reflects the existence of peritoneal irritation and appears in cases that usually require urgent surgery. It is very important to differentiate it from voluntary contracture, which is modified during the examination. It is sometimes difficult to differentiate it, especially in children, people in a state of anxiety, the insane, etc.

Acute appendicitis

Acute appendicitis is the most frequent abdominal surgical emergency in childhood. Its peak incidence is between 6 and 12 years of age, being exceptional in children under 2 years of age. The annual incidence is estimated at 4 cases per 1,000 children under 14 years of age. There is a predominance of males over females in most series. With regard to diagnosis, it is more difficult to establish the diagnosis in childhood than in adulthood, and particularly difficult in children under 4 years of age. In the 1-4 year age group, there is a higher risk of progression and perforation, the risk being as high as 75% for this age group. The clinical picture is characterised by pain initially in the periumbilical or epigastric region, with subsequent migration to the right symphysis fossa. Initially, the pain is visceral, manifesting as a dull, burning pain; the pain may also appear in other locations, such as the hypogastrium, pelvis or groin, if the appendix has a retrocecal location. On other occasions, the pain may be located in the left fossa, as occurs in patients whose appendix, due to its particular embryological development, appears in this location. The pain worsens with movement and even with coughing. Other symptoms may include nausea, vomiting, constipation, diarrhoea, fever or fever and anorexia. Also, micturition symptoms may occur. It is very important to ask if the patient is receiving or has recently received antibiotic therapy or analgesia, as the symptoms may be masked. The treatment of acute appendicitis is surgical, with increasing use of laparoscopic surgery in recent years. If perforation is present, antibiotics are also necessary.

Estrenimiento

Strenum is a delay or difficulty in passing stools for a period of at least 1 month in infants and young children, and 2 months in older children. The stools are harder and sometimes larger than normal and may cause pain during bowel movements. Strenum is very common in children. It accounts for up to 5% of children's visits to the doctor. Infants and children are particularly prone to constipation in three time periods. The first period is when cereals and solid foods are introduced into the child's diet, the second when the child is weaned, and the third when school starts.

The frequency and consistency of stools varies throughout childhood, and there is no single definition of what is normal. Newborns usually have 4 or more bowel movements per day. During the first year, infants have 2 to 4 bowel movements per day. Breastfed infants have more bowel movements than formula-fed infants, and usually have a bowel movement after each feeding. Infant stools are loose, yellow and look like they contain seeds. After 1 to 2 months, some breastfed infants defecate less frequently, but the stools are still pasty or kaqueous. After the first year of life, most infants pass 1 or 2 soft but formed stools per day. However, some infants and young children defecate only every 3 or 4 days.

Guidelines for identifying distress in infants and children include

- No bowel movements for 2 or 3 days longer than usual
- Hard or painful stools
- Large faeces that can clog the toilet
- Blood droplets on the outside of the faeces

In infants, signs of straining such as clenching and crying before passing a soft stool usually do not indicate straining. These symptoms are usually caused by lack of relaxation of the pelvic floor muscles during passage of stool and usually resolve spontaneously.

Parents often worry about their child's bowel movements, but constipation usually does not have serious consequences. Some children with constipation complain regularly of abdominal pain, especially after meals. Occasionally, the passage of large, hard stools can cause a small tear in the anus (anal fissure). Anal fissures are painful and may cause bright red strands of blood to be seen on the outside of the stool or on the toilet paper. Rarely, chronic stricture contributes to urinary problems, such as infections or bedwetting.

Causes of stress in children

Frequent causes

In 95% of the children, the strenghtening is caused by

₀ Problems related to diet ₀ Behavioural problems

Stress resulting from dietary or behavioural problems is called functional stress.

Diet-related problems that cause constipation include a diet that is low in carbohydrates and/or fibre (fibre is found in fruits, vegetables and whole grains).

Behavioural problems that may be associated with withdrawal include stress (such as that triggered by the birth of a sibling), resistance to using the toilet, and the need for control. In addition, children may intentionally delay bowel movements (called fecal impaction) because they have a painful anal fissure or because they do not want to stop playing. Sexual abuse may result in stress or injury that causes the child to withhold stool. If the child does not defecate when the physiological urge comes, the rectum eventually distends to accommodate the stool. When the rectum has distended, the urge to pass stool decreases, and more and more stool accumulates and hardens. This can lead to a vicious circle, with progressive stricture. If the accumulated faeces harden, they sometimes block the passage of faecal contents, a condition called faecal impaction. The more liquid stool above the hardened stool may leak around the impacted stool, stain the child's underwear and lead to faecal incontinence (encopresis). Parents may then think that the child has diarrhoea when the real problem is constipation.

Less frequent causes

In about 5 per cent of children, the withdrawal results from a physical disorder, drugs or toxins. These disorders may be present at birth or develop later. Strenuousness that results from disease, drugs or toxins is called organic strenuousness.

In newborns and infants, the most common disorder causing organ strenulation is Hirschsprung's disease (a disorder in the distribution of nerves in the large intestine).

Other causes of organic stress include

- Congenital malformations of the anus
- CFS
- Metabolic and electrolyte disorders, such as abnormally high calcium levels (hypercalcaemia) or low levels of potassium (hypokalaemia) in the blood (hypokalaemia).
- spinal cord problems (such as spina bifida)
- Hormonal disorders, such as hypothyroidism (poor thyroid function)
- Intestinal disorders, such as allergy to cow's milk proteins or ceKaca disease
- Pharmaceuticals, such as powerful painkillers called opioids (e.g. codema and morphine)
- Toxins, such as lead or infant botulism toxins

Children with severe abdominal diseases (such as appendicitis or a bowel obstruction) often do not pass stools. However, these children often have other, more striking symptoms, such as abdominal pain or bloating and/or vomiting. These symptoms usually prompt parents to seek medical attention before the number of bowel movements decreases.

Assessment of stress in children

It must be determined whether the stress is caused by dietary or behavioural issues (functional) or by disease, toxins or drugs (organic).

Warning signs

Some symptoms are cause for concern and should raise the suspicion of an organic cause of stress:

- Absence of bowel movements during the first 24 to 48 hours after birth
- Weight loss or stunting
- Decreased appetite
- Blood in the stool
- Fever
- Vomiting
- Abdominal distention
- Abdominal pain (in children old enough to say so)
- In infants, loss of muscle tone (the child appears flabby or weak) and
decreased ability to suck
- In older children, involuntary release of urine (urinary incontinence), back pain, weakness in the legs or walking problems

Complementary tests

If the cause of the constipation appears to be functional, no tests are needed unless the child does not respond to treatment. If the child does not respond to treatment or if another disease is suspected as the cause, an X-ray of the abdomen is obtained and tests for other disorders are performed based on the results of the scan.

Treatment of constipation in children

The treatment of constipation depends on the cause. For organic constipation, the causative disorder, drug or toxin is treated, corrected or eliminated. For functional withdrawal, measures include

- Dietary changes: Dietary changes for infants include giving them 30 to 120 mL of corn juice in the morning and afternoon. Infants and older children should increase their intake of fruits, vegetables and fibre-rich cereals, and decrease consumption of foods that cause constipation, such as milk and cheese.
- Behavioural modifications: Making some behavioural modifications may help older children: encourage children who do not use diapers to sit on the toilet for 5-10 minutes after meals and congratulate them when they make progress (e.g. by writing progress on a chart on the wall). For children who are in the process of removing the honeycomb, take a break until the constipation is resolved. Sitting on the toilet after meals can be helpful because food triggers the defecatory reflex. Often, the child ignores the signals of this reflex and postpones bowel movements. This technique uses the reflex to help retrain the digestive tract, establish a bowel routine and helps to achieve more regular

bowel movements.

- Sometimes, use of stool softeners or laxatives: If the constipation does not respond to changes in diet and habits, the physician may recommend certain drugs that help soften the stool (stool softeners) and/or increase the spontaneous movement of the digestive system (laxatives). These drugs include polyethylene glycol, lactulose, mineral oil, milk of magnesia (magnesium hydroxide), senna and bisacodyl. Many of these drugs are currently available over the counter. However, dosages should be based on the child's age and body weight, as well as the severity of the stress. Therefore, parents should consult a physician about dosage and the appropriate number of doses per day before using these treatments. The goal of treatment is one soft stool per day. If the child has a fecal impaction, options include mild enemas and oral agents (such as mineral oil or polyethylene glycol) taken with large volumes of Kquido. If these treatments are not effective, hospitalisation may be necessary to resolve the impaction. Infants do not usually require any such treatment, but a glycerine suppository is usually adequate. To maintain regular bowel movements, some children may require fibre supplements (such as ispagula), which can be obtained over the counter. For these supplements to be effective, children should drink 1 to 2 L of water per day.

Bibliograffa

1. Benito Fernandez J. Acute abdominal pain. In: Casado Flores J, Serrano Gonzalez A (eds.). Urgencias y tratamiento del nino grave. Madrid: Ergon; 2015. p. 1262-69.

2. Alonso Cadenas JA, de la Torre Esp^ M. Diagnosis and treatment of acute abdominal pain (acute abdomen) in the emergency department. Protoc diagn diagn ter pediatr. 2020;1:197-213.

3. Pena Quintana L, Beltra Pico R. Acute abdominal pain. In: Cruz. Tratado de Pediatna, 11^ ed. Madrid: Panamericana. 2014; p. 1465-8.

4. Varea Calderon V. Clinical and functional exploration of the digestive system. In: Cruz.
Tratado de Pediatna, 11^ ed. Madrid: Panamericana. 2014; p. 1381-8.

16. Early programming. Impact on adult diseases.

Dr. Enrique Blanca Jover

Introduction. Concept

Neonatal, foetal or early biological programming is defined as the process in which cells develop, function and adapt to the environment in response to an ingrained set of executable commands, usually emanating from cellular chromatin (DNA in the nucleus). Cells normally contain these programmes. Major early life events may reformulate these programmes, probably as adaptations to ensure early survival at the price of later disease.

Diseases associated with disruption in such programming include those that cost the most in terms of suffering and human resources, such as coronary heart disease, insulin resistance and obesity.

Because the perinatal period is an important window in which adult pathologies can be programmed, intervention strategies adopted before or during gestation or the early postnatal period may prevent the transmission of these traits to offspring.

Affecting early programming

An insult or stimulus to the intrauterine growth and developmental trajectory, as well as during early life, generates functional changes that lead to an increased risk of chronic non-communicable diseases in adulthood, such as diabetes mellitus, obesity, dyslipidaemia, and asthma, among others. The "developmental markers of adult disease" hypothesis, often called the "Barker hypothesis", states that adverse influences early in development, and particularly during intrauterine life, can result in permanent changes in physiology and metabolism, leading to increased risk of disease in adulthood. This process results from alterations in the natural balance of environmental factors, which, in the case of the developing foetus, come from the intrauterine environment and from the signals that the pregnant mother (from her diet, environmental exposure, pollution, drugs, etc.) passes on to her child through the placenta. This transfer will depend directly on the mother's own nutritional status, the genetic load of the foetus and the requirements of the growing foetus. At the cellular level, epigenetic mechanisms will be involved in this "programming" process during the early development of the individual. These mechanisms comprise a series of chemical modifications on DNA and DNA-interacting proteins, which shape and regulate gene expression in the short and long term, without altering the genetic code.

In tissues and their metabolism, accommodation occurs, which is a reversible modification in their composition, while *plasticity* is closely related to the phenomenon of early programming and is a permanent functional or structural adaptation, which is generated when a stimulus or aggression acts in a sensitive period of life, producing a change in the activity of expression of an organism.

It is known that growth disturbances early in life are also associated with an increased risk of cancer and other age-related diseases.

During the early stages of development, individuals show a high capacity to adapt to the environment, which is most evident in the generation, in a short period of time, of a complex multicellular organism from a single genome formed at the moment of fertilisation. This plasticity is highly sensitive to environmental factors, which in the short term define immediate development and in the medium and long term represent "predictive signals" of the biological environment in which the individual will live. As a result of this genome-environment interaction, the organism generates a repertoire of responses to "likely events" in order to present a better adjustment to the environment, while restricting initial plasticity, a process known as "foetal programming". For example, poor maternal nutrition during pregnancy generates signals that alert the foetus, suggesting a nutrient-deprived environment, to which the foetus responds with adaptations such as reduced stature and "thrifty" metabolism. In this way, plasticity allows a given species to develop short-term adaptations, in addition to the long-term genetic adaptations that occur as a consequence of natural selection. However, any event that interferes with the correct communication between the environment and the foetus can lead to the establishment of a phenotype that is not adjusted to the ecological niche, increasing the risk of generating diseases in the long term. Based on the example above, if the poor nutrition in the mother does not reflect the actual availability in the environment, the establishment of the thrifty phenotype in the offspring together with a nutrient-rich environment in postnatal life will lead to an increased risk of obesity and the multiple complications associated with this condition.

Impact on adult diseases. Significant environmental exposures.

Different noxae or causes are implicated in the genesis of adult diseases. Large epidemiological and cohort studies involving multiple generations provide the basis for understanding fetal programming. These initial studies focus on how maternal malnutrition, like fetal environmental exposures, programmes adult health and disease. These issues also become evident when looking at over-nutrition, environmental exposures, maternal stress, lifestyle, pollution, and toxic exposures.

All of the morbidities outlined in the above statement require interactions of multiple organ systems. For example, in terms of coronary artery disease, morbidity results from an interaction of the coronary arteries themselves, the immune system and the liver (through its regulation of serum fluid homeostasis).

In many cases we see common outcomes programmed by different perinatal insults. Although a variety of insults can alter the developmental trajectory and culminate in adult disease, there are a number of similarities in the outcomes resulting from the various perinatal insults. The similarity in the phenotypic outcomes programmed by different perinatal insults and the benefits gained from intervening in the noxa by a particular lifestyle to overcome the pathological outcomes of different perinatal insults suggest that common mechanisms are likely to be involved.

- **Malnutrition.**

The best known early factor in this field may be early maternal malnutrition. In pregnancy there is adaptation in foetal development, which is done by hormonal adjustments by the embryo and foetus to reset set points, so that the newborn is better prepared for an adverse environment, such as malnutrition. However, inadequate nutritional intake during the postnatal stage, which allows for accelerated growth, can lead to metabolic alterations that make the infant susceptible to disease in adulthood.

Over the past three decades epidemiological data and experimental studies have highlighted the impacts of gestational undernutrition on birth size of offspring and prevalence of metabolic disorders in adults, an issue of considerable importance in developing countries, where undernutrition is a major concern. Adverse intrauterine development, manifested by low birth weight, has been shown to be associated with an increased risk of cardiovascular disease, cerebrovascular ischaemia, pulmonary disease and polycystic ovary syndrome. Importantly, the timing of prenatal aggression plays a key role in determining adult susceptibility to disease, emphasising the importance of the critical periods of organ system differentiation. Epidemiological data from the Dutch famine showed that nutrient restriction during early gestation was associated with adult hypertension, while dietary restriction during late gestation was associated with increased adiposity, glucose intolerance and type 2 diabetes. Compensatory growth during early life is also a risk factor for the development of adult diseases in offspring. The degree of mismatch between nutrient availability before and after birth is the basis for the development of chronic diseases later in life. Experimentally in animals, the effects of maternal caloric restriction have been shown to lead to insulin resistance, reduced female fertility, hyperinsulinism, adiposity and hypertension in the adult population.

- **Overnutrition.**

At the other end of the problem, the increasing incidence of maternal obesity and associated disorders, such as gestational diabetes mellitus, has been a proven fact in recent years. This is a problem of considerable magnitude in economically developed societies.

Studies focused on the effects of maternal overnutrition and its fetal effects, resulting in large-for-gestational-age neonates. High birth weight is also associated with increased risk of obesity and metabolic disturbances during adulthood. Furthermore, epidemiological studies report a strong association between increased maternal body mass index and alterations in glucose-insulin homeostasis in their offspring. Although genetics may play a role in the transmission of these traits, the finding that maternal weight loss after bariatric surgery reduces the risk of obesity and other metabolic disorders in offspring supports the maternal environment as a contributing factor. Along these lines, the observation that weight gain between pregnancies increases the prevalence of obesity in younger children.

In the experimental setting, the induction of obesity in pregnant animals manifests an increase in general adiposity, reduced insulin sensitivity, glucose intolerance and hypertension in their offspring. On the contrary, different dietary restrictions in late pregnancy or improvement of pregestational obesity decrease the risk of obesity in the offspring.

These observations highlight the importance of dietary and lifestyle interventions in the prevention of obesity and various associated complications in the next generation.

- **Stress.**

Prenatal stress represents another insult that disrupts the intrauterine environment and the developmental trajectory of the foetus. Epidemiological studies have shown that stressors such as maternal bereavement or maternal depression during pregnancy result in offspring at increased risk of abnormal immune function, obesity and mental disorders.

The effects of stress on developmental outcomes may be due to direct changes in the hypothalamic-pituitary-adrenal (HPA) axis or indirectly through alterations in nutrient intake.

In animals, we have experimental evidence of exposure to stressful conditions during prenatal or early life leading to increased adiposity and weight gain with impaired glycaemic control in offspring. Other studies have shown that prenatal stress leads to lower birth weight and impaired feedback of HPA axis regulation, reduced glucocorticoid and mineralocorticoid receptor expression.

- **Sickness status**.

Illness is a stressor in its own right, as discussed above. But it also intervenes in the homeostasis of the maternal and foetal endocrine systems, which are important for normal development and for preventing the adverse effects of early aggressions. Disruption of this balance in disease situations leads to increased maternal insulin levels in obesity and gestational diabetes, increased maternal/fetal androgen levels in polycystic ovary syndrome, adrenal hyperplasia leading to increased fetal cortisol. Elevated androgens during gestation will lead to reproductive and metabolic disorders that emerge later in life.

The disturbed intrauterine environment, generating maternal hyperglycaemia in pathological states results in macrosom^a, glucose intolerance, development of obesity and metabolic disorders in the offspring. Pre-eclampsia complicates approximately 2% - 8% of pregnancies resulting in prematurity and intrauterine growth retardation, showing development of arterial hypertension during childhood and increased risk of stroke in old age.

Mild maternal diabetes is known to lead to the development of neonatal macrosom^a, while in severely decompensated cases it leads to microsom^a, alterations in hypothalamic development and compromised regulation of the insulin system. As adults, these patients develop diabetes when their glucose metabolism is stressed, such as during pregnancy.

These findings have been reproduced experimentally in animals.

- **Lifestyle**.

The lifestyle led by pregnant women and imposed on offspring during early life may contribute to susceptibility to disease. Lifestyle factors that influence perinatal programming include dietary choices, physical activity, substance abuse and medical interventions. With the advent of modern technology, physical inactivity is increasing at an alarming rate and is now recognised as the urgent health problem of the 20th century. Sedentary lifestyle is positively correlated with increased adiposity, fasting triglyceride levels and markers of insulin resistance. Importantly, physical inactivity during pregnancy has been shown to be associated with obesity in offspring. Physical activity during pregnancy appears to have many benefits including reduced body mass, reduced risk of impaired glucose tolerance and development of innate immunity that helps prevent adverse metabolic programming in offspring.

Substance abuse with illegal drugs, legal drugs (alcohol and nicotine), misuse of prescription drugs (hallucinogens, inhalants or psychotherapeutics) are serious prenatal assaults, which occupy a relevant percentage of pregnancies. In addition to the direct toxic effect of the effect, malnutrition and stress often accompany it.

- **Environmental exposure to endocrine disrupting chemicals (EDCs)**.

They are chemical substances that mimic hormone actions and can alter normal endocrine functions and change the maternal and fetal endocrine milieu, thereby altering the normal trajectory of development, potentially leading to the development of chronic disease. These mimics are called EDCs and are "exogenous agents that interfere with the synthesis, secretion, transport, metabolism, binding action, or elimination of natural blood-borne hormones that are present in the body and are responsible for homeostasis, reproduction and developmental processes" (US Environmental Protection Agency).

EDCs include naturally occurring compounds such as phytoestrogens, genistem and coumestrol or synthetic chemicals used as industrial solvents and lubricants (e.g. polychlorinated biphenyls, polybrominated biphenyls and dioxins), plasticisers (e.g. bisphenol A), pesticides (e.g. dichlorodiphenyltrichloroethane), fungicide (e.g. vinclozolin) and pharmaceutical agents (e.g. diethylstilbestrol). Because EDCs are present everywhere, fetal and postnatal exposure can occur during early developmental stages, through maternal-fetal transfer and lactation.

Apart from direct evidence of poisoning by such products, other disruptions associated with the increased presence of such substances in the environment have been documented, such as obesity, cardiovascular disease, type 2 diabetes, and several hormone-sensitive cancers.

Epigenetics

Epigenetics regulates the expression of genes in our cells. Conceptually, it can be defined as the set of chemical reactions and other processes that modify the expression of DNA without altering its structural sequence. They are attached to the genetic material and allow its correct activity. Epigenetic marks influence the genetic inheritance of organisms.

The epigenome is what causes a neuron to produce a neurotransmitter or a heart cell to beat. It is also responsible for repressing exogenous sequences that can damage our DNA. *This physiological epigenome, which also defines us as a species, is dynamic: it can be modulated by external factors.* Epigenetic adaptation is the capacity of organisms in their stage of organisation and immaturity to adjust the characteristics of their development to the needs imposed by the environment, generating changes that have a lasting effect and that can be manifested in later stages of life, through adjustment mechanisms based on the *plasticity of the genome.*

Epigenetics studies those phenomena that do not affect the DNA sequence of genes but do affect their expression. Epigenetic mechanisms play a fundamental role in the regulation of many biological processes. Alterations in epigenetic patterns have important physiological consequences, and are a central component in the development of many human diseases, including cancer.

The period of life during which epigenetic DNA imprinting is most active is from conception to the age of 2 years, hence it has been called "the period of the first 1000 days". Childhood and adult health risks can be programmed during these foetal-neonatal stages and this early metabolic programming can affect the later development of diseases such as obesity and other associated non-communicable diseases. Early life, because of the great plasticity that characterises it, is the ideal time to intervene and prevent the risk of these diseases (window of opportunity).

As a field we can divide it into developmental and environmental epigenetics. *Developmental* epigenetics studies the maintenance and execution of nested patterns of gene expression involved in growth, maturation, and tissue specificity. *Environmental* epigenetics studies how cells respond to the environment by changing chromatin structure or expressing small RNAs. The former can be said to "turn genes on and off" whereas the changes attributed to environmental epigenetics are due to a subtle and incremental modification of gene expression. Responses to the environment that switch off an important gene are unlikely to benefit the cell or the organism. The response is too drastic. In contrast, fine-tuning expression in response to the environment confers a survival advantage. In a broader sense, environmental epigenetics describes how the environment determines phenotype by modulating gene expression.

Epigenetic tools

DNA methylation. This is the most frequent mechanism. A methyl group (-CH3) is added to the cytosine base, which allows the closed conformation of chromatin, which is associated with gene silencing. This requires DNA methyltransferase, which is responsible for establishing and maintaining the methylation patterns, and requires the methyl-CpG-binding proteins which are involved in making the methylation marks.

DNA methylation acts by "silencing" one of the genes (maternal or paternal) by inserting a methyl group into cytosine nucleotides accompanied by guanosine (CpG), which are present in the promoter regions of a given gene. In the placenta, the expression of genes that promote foetal growth, for example, the gene coding for insulin-like growth factor type 2 (IGF2) or amino acid transporters, are of paternal origin. While those genes that restrict foetal growth, e.g. the gene coding for the soluble IGF2 receptor (IGF2R), are of maternal origin. Multiple diseases of pregnancy, in which there are alterations in foetal growth, are related to mutations in the promoter regions of these genes that change their expression pattern. The effect of nutritional and environmental factors on the epigenetic control of imprinted genes has so far not been determined. However, in experimental animals, alterations in the methylation patterns of several genes in hepatocytes and cardiomyocytes of foetuses whose mothers have been exposed to nutrient-restricted diets have been determined. These abnormal methylation patterns have been reversed by supplementing the diet with folate (a methyl group donor at the cellular level). It remains to be clarified whether similar mechanisms to those found in these cell types occur in the vascular system and placenta, whose functions are strongly influenced by epigenetic mechanisms, and whether supplementation treatments are a means of assistance in case these fail. Thus we are at the beginning of understanding how the environment, maternal nutrition, maternal stress and metabolic diseases of the father may, through epigenetic mechanisms, be defining the plasticity, the responsiveness of the foetus to particular conditions in postnatal life. Finally, we can make sense of the saying "we are what we eat", we can even say that we are what our parents and grandmother ate, given that the perinatal epigenetic effect has been described as being able to affect the third generation.

Histone modification. Each nucleosome (the structure that forms the fundamental unit of chromatin, which is the way DNA is organised in eukaryotic cells) is made up of an octamer of histone proteins and DNA coiled around them (approximately 150 base pairs).

Each histone octamer is composed of 2 histone proteases histones H2A, H2B, H3, and H4.

Histones can be modified qwmically by different enzymes at the N-terminal, C-terminal, and internal domains. These post-translational modifications are mainly acetylation, methylation, phosphorylation, although there are many others. Thus, the expression pattern of some genes can be changed by modifying the chromatin structure, activating or silencing these genes.

Non-coding RNA. RNA interference RNAs do not encode specific proteins but their sequences are complementary to DNA or coding RNA and prevent their translation; therefore, they are a form of negative regulation at the post-transcriptional level.

Use as a biomarker and target for intervention.

The concept that epigenetic characteristics can be intentionally and strategically modified is a future basis for personalised medicine. This leads to the use of epigenetics as a biomarker, whether it is a pattern through high-throughput studies or detailed characteristics of an individual gene. For example, life history variables, such as maternal intake of macronutrients and micronutrients, multiple gestations, mode of conception, mode of delivery and maternal smoking, associated with various differences in CpG DNA methylation.

Future studies will allow us to take the next steps to intervene specifically to soften the adult impact of an early life event. Because all interventions carry some aspect of risk, identifying the right intervention for the right person stands as the ultimate prize for doing real medicine in the whole population. Caution should be exercised in terms of intervention until our knowledge base increases. Interventions that aim to change the epigenetic characteristics of a specific gene or subset of genes in a specific tissue for a specific disease may have immediate or long-term unintended consequences.

Despite this contingency, environmental epigenetics represents hope for biomarkers and intervention in programme-acquired diseases. This hope lies in the primary difference between genetics and epigenetics, which has been paraphrased by several experts in the following observation, "you can't change your parents, but you can change your epigenetics".

We have different examples of fields of action. As the adult disease of early life events programme is undergoing a transition from the broad field of maternal malnutrition to the currently relevant problems of food deprivation and prematurity. Although many adult diseases and morbidities are associated with different early life events and schedules, the morbidities of insulin resistance, disease and obesity appear to be common endpoints of many early life events despite possible confounding factors. Environmental epigenetics as a mechanism becomes particularly relevant because it contains the ability to account for the complexity inherent in mammalian biology and environmental factors, while allowing for adaptation and change.

Bibliograffa

1. Avila Gamboa D, Karchmer S, Salazar Torres L. Perinatal programming and epigenetics. Rev. Latin. Perinat. 2018, 21 (3).

2. Bedregal P et al. Contributions of epigenetics to the understanding of human development. Rev Med Chile 2010; 138: 366-372.

3. Casanello P Krause BJ, Castro-Rodriguez JA, Uauy R. Fetal programming of chronic

diseases: current concepts and epigenetics. Revista Chilena de Pediatna. http://dx.doi.Org/10.1016/j.rchipe.2015.06.008.

4. Hendrina A. De Boo HA, Harding JE. The developmental origins of adult disease (Barker) hypothesis. Australian and New Zealand Journal of Obstetrics and Gynaecology 2006; 46: 4-14.

5. Lane LH. Fetal programming, epigenetics, and adult onset disease. Clin Perinatol 41 (2014) 815-831.http://dx.doi.org/10.1016/j.clp.2014.08.006.

6. Lau et al. Fetal Programming of Adult Disease. Implications for Prenatal Care.(Obstet Gynecol 2011;117:978-85).DOI: 10.1097/AOG.0b013e318212140e

7. Padmanabhan et al. Developmental Programming, a Pathway to Disease. Endocrinology, April 2016, 157(4):1328 -1340.

17. Evaluation of growth. Hypocretions

Dr. Esther Ocete Hita

Introduction

The growth and development of an individual is a continuous phenomenon that begins at conception and culminates at the end of puberty, during which time physical, psychosocial and reproductive maturity is reached. This transformation involves changes in size, spatial organisation and functional differentiation of tissues and organs. The increase in body size and mass is the result of cell multiplication and hyperplasia, a process known as growth. Changes in the organisation and functional differentiation of tissues, organs and systems are the result of the process of development or maturation.

The processes of growth and development are simultaneous and interdependent phenomena. Both processes have characteristics common to all individuals of the same species, which makes them predictable, however, they present wide differences between subjects, given by the individual character of the pattern of growth and development. This typical pattern emerges from the interaction of genetic and environmental factors, which establish, on the one hand, the growth potential and, on the other hand, the extent to which this potential is expressed. Genetic information establishes very precisely the sequence and timing in which these processes must occur, so that, if some noxa acts on these penodes, preventing an event from occurring within the established timescales, it can produce a definitive disorder of growth and/or development. These pentodes are called cytokinetic pentodes. The same noxa acting at another time in development may produce no disturbance or a reversible disturbance. Deficiency of thyroid hormones during intrauterine life and the first two years of postnatal life leaves a permanent neurological damage; on the other hand, at later ages the same deficiency can produce alterations in the nervous system which are reversible with the substitution of these hormones. This situation exemplifies on the one hand the interdependence that developmental processes can have (a thyroid disorder alters the maturation of the CNS) and, on the other hand, it is evidence of the developmental pathway of the CNS.

Hereditary heritage provides each individual with a specific pattern of growth and development, which can be modified by environmental factors. In relation to height, genetic effects are clearly exemplified by looking at the growth pattern of different ethnic groups, the most extreme example being the marked difference in height between individuals of Nordic origin and New Guinean Pygmies. The familial differences are as evident as the differences between the races. The genetic influence is clearly established by observing the similarity in height between monozygotic twins, which has a correlation of 0.94, whereas in dizygotic twins this correlation drops to 0.5. Study of correlation coefficients in families suggests that the determinants of growth come from both parents and that each parent has a theoretical influence of 50% on the height of the offspring. Clinical and experimental genetic studies show that the determination of height is polygenic, involving genes located both on the autosomes and on the sex chromosomes. Inheritance not only influences the final height and body proportions of an individual, but also various dynamic maturational processes, such as the sequence of bone and tooth maturation, the speed of growth, the age of menarche, etc.

The environmental influence is determined by various factors of the physical, psychosocial and socio-cultural environment of the individuals, particularly important being the level of education and family income, as well as the composition and stability of the family among others. The interaction of all of these creates the conditions of risk for disease. Within the environmental factors, nutrition and infectious diseases are particularly important in developing communities. This makes the assessment of growth and development a good indicator of the health conditions of the individual or population group being assessed. A good example of the influence of environmental factors on growth is represented by the shorter stature of adults from lower socio-economic levels relative to those from higher income strata within the same population.

Characteristics of postnatal growth

Prenatal growth follows an exponential curve, increasing slowly during the first 20 weeks and then increasing steadily until the end of gestation. By the end of gestation, the infant reaches approximately 5.7% of the weight, 30% of the height and 63% of the head circumference of an adult. Postnatal physical growth and development has characteristics which are common to all individuals, and which, when analysed in conjunction with the family genetic pattern, allow us to determine whether growth is normal.

In this regard, it is important to consider the normal changes in growth rate and body proportions, the concept of growth canal and genetic load.

Growth rate

Defined as the increase in height over a given period of time and has significant variations according to age, sex and season.

Depending on the age, three penodes can be distinguished:

1. A rapid growth period, comprising the first four years of life, characterised by a progressive decrease in speed from 25 cm in the first year to 12 cm in the second, 10 cm

in the third and 8 cm in the fourth year.

2. A slower and more sustained growth period, from the age of four years to the onset of puberty, with a growth rate ranging from 4.5 - 7.0 cm/year.

3. A new rapid growth spurt during pubertal development, where the maximum growth rate can reach up to 12 cm/year in males and 9 cm/year in females.

Sex-related differences are evident at birth: boys are taller and heavier than girls. However, this difference decreases progressively thereafter and is hardly noticeable at anus. The most notable sex variations are those that occur during puberty, and are related to both the timing, magnitude and duration of the increase in height.

Seasonal differences: maximum growth occurs during spring and summer, reaching speeds up to 2.5 times higher in these periods than in autumn and winter. There are children who may have imperceptible increases during some months of the year, a feature to be considered when interpreting growth velocity.

Growth channel

Birth height depends mainly on intrauterine environmental conditions such as uteroplacental function and multiple maternal and foetal factors. In contrast, hereditary factors tend to play a more dominant role in postnatal growth. This explains why height may vary from its initial percentile. Approximately 75% of children move from the percentile at birth, either accelerating or slowing growth until they reach the channel determined by their genetic load. Once this channel is reached, there is a strong tendency for the individual to remain within his or her K limits. If a noxa acts, there is a deviation of the growth channel, but once the individual recovers from the noxa, there is a compensatory increase in growth velocity that returns the individual to the original channel. If the insult is intense and prolonged, and particularly if it occurs during periods of rapid growth, this recovery may be partial or not occur at all.

Assessment of growth and development

Commonly used measures to assess physical growth and development are: weight, height and cranial circumference. These measures are easy to standardise and have sufficient sensitivity to detect alterations in the process. It is recommended, when possible, to use simultaneously other measures, such as thoracic and brachial circumference, skinfold thickness (tricipital, bicipital, subscapular, suprascapular, suprascapular) and body segments. The brachial pentimeter, together with the measurement of skinfolds, allows a more accurate assessment of nutritional status and body composition. Body segment measurement should always be performed when assessing a patient with short stature.

Low Size

Stunting is a common medical problem, accounting for about 50% of the endocrinological consultations of children and adolescents. However, only a small percentage of these children and adolescents present a disease when evaluated in the context of their family or ethnic group.

Definition

A patient is considered to have short stature when his or her height/age ratio is two standard deviations (SD) or less below the expected population average for age and sex, or below the third percentile. Eighty per cent of a population of children whose height is between -2 and -3 SD corresponds to a normal variant (familial or constitutional short stature). On the other hand, the majority of those below 3 SD have a pathological short stature. This severe stunting, with height 3 SD below the average, is called dwarfism. Stunting exists when the growth velocity, measured over a minimum period of 6 months of observation, is below the 10th percentile of the Tanner growth curves. Between the ages of 4-10 years, growth of less than 4.5 cm/year should be considered abnormal.

Postnatal onset short stature

Within the postnatal growth retardation with proportionate body segments there are normal variants, non-endocrine systemic diseases and hormonal disorders, the first two being the most frequent conditions. The following is a brief analysis of the main aetiologies of short stature.

Constitutional stunting

This term is applied to children who are small because they have a slower than normal maturation. It is preferably seen in boys with normal birth height, who slow down their growth rate after the age of 6 months, stabilising their growth curve around the age of two to three years. Subsequently they grow at normal speed, through a channel below -2 SD but parallel to the normal curve. Height and bone age are proportionally delayed by 2 to 4 years. The onset of puberty is later than that of their peers, achieving a final height in accordance with their genetic load. There may or may not be a history of delayed pubertal development in parents or other close relatives. They usually do not require treatment, as their height prognosis is normal, unless they have major emotional conflicts due to their short stature and do not respond to psychological therapy. When constitutional short stature and familial short stature coexist in a patient, the prognosis is more uncertain, and size predictions may overestimate the final height.

Family size delay

It is probably the most common cause of short stature. These children are small because their genetic load determines it. Their birth height is normal or low and then they slow down their growth in the first years of life, to continue later with low normal speed, growing in a channel between 2 SD and 3 SD below the median. Bone age is concordant with chronological age and exceeds height age. Age of height is defined as the age at which the average normal child reaches the height of the subject under study. Puberty begins at the usual age and the final height is low, but concordant with the family genetic load. All laboratory evaluation is normal. No treatment has been found to significantly modify the final height of these patients.

Psychosocial deprivation

This condition was initially described in children in institutional homes or orphanages, who presented severe growth retardation despite adequate nutritional intake and no detectable organic cause. The history of deprivation is difficult to obtain and should be sought in children in dysfunctional family environments, deprived of affection, with alcoholic or drug addicted parents or with psychiatric illnesses. Children usually present sleep disturbances (insomnia, night wandering), eating disorders such as anorexia, bulimia, pica, polydipsia. If the diagnosis is suspected, evidence of accompanying physical abuse should be sought in a targeted manner. The diagnosis is usually made by rule-out and often the favourable clinical evolution of these patients when they are hospitalised to rule out organic causes supports this aetiology. Pituitary failure is not always demonstrated.

Malnutrition

Globally, undernutrition is by far the most common cause of stunting, with two thirds of the world's population being undernourished. Nutrient deficiency can also be caused by voluntary restriction (athletes, ballerinas), psychiatric conditions (anorexia nervosa) or anorexia secondary to chronic illness. Malnutrition can also be secondary to exaggerated losses, as in malabsorption syndrome, or to a very high metabolic expenditure not sufficiently covered by a regular diet (heart disease, chronic infectious diseases).

Non-endocrine systemic diseases

Any chronic disease can interfere with growth and result in a low final height. These growth delays are proportionate, usually with subnormal growth velocity, decreased weight-for-height ratio and delayed bone age with respect to chronological age.

Gastrointestinal diseases

Malabsorption disorders and chronic inflammatory diseases cause severe growth retardation. The former through faecal leakage and the latter mainly through anorexia. There is not always a history of diarrhoea, and these diseases should be ruled out in children with short stature, especially if accompanied by significant bone age delay. Chronic liver diseases, such as cirrhosis and cholestatic jaundice, also cause growth retardation.

Heart diseases

These include cyanotic congenital heart disease and those with left-to-right shunt with pulmonary hypertension. The mechanism by which growth is affected is probably multifactorial, including tissue hypoxia, increased energy expenditure, decreased intake and frequent respiratory infections.

Respiratory diseases

Within respiratory diseases, chronic obstructive bronchial smdromes, especially when requiring corticosteroid therapy, can be an important cause of growth arrest. Another disease that should be ruled out is cystic fibrosis, which compromises pondo-sternal growth not only through bronchial involvement and bronchiectasis, but also through malabsorption secondary to pancreatic insufficiency.

Chronic kidney disease

They produce growth disturbances through various mechanisms: concentration defects (nephrogenic diabetes ins^pidus); renal tubular acidosis (there is no correlation between the degree of acidosis and the severity of retardation as mild or partially compensated acidosis can cause severe growth retardation, especially if accompanied by losses of bases, Na+ K+ and Ca^{++}); nephropathy with alterations of calcium and phosphorus metabolism (phosphatasic diabetes, Fanconi's syndrome); Bartter's syndrome; renal failure.

Chronic infections

In underdeveloped communities, chronic infections, especially tuberculosis and massive parasitosis, still cause stunting.

Anemias

Iron deficiency anaemias cause hypocrectile growths through lack of oxygen transport to the tissues.

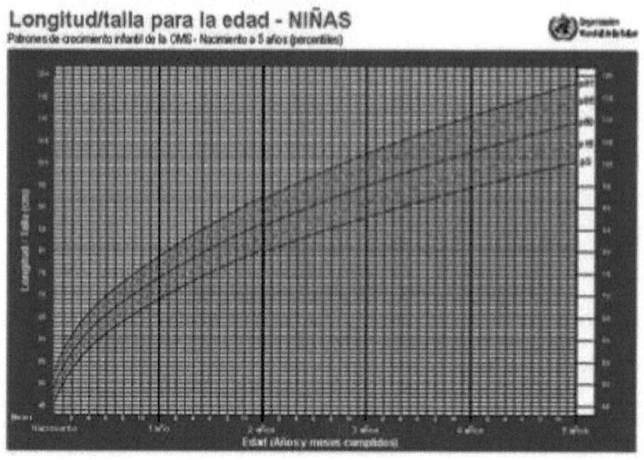

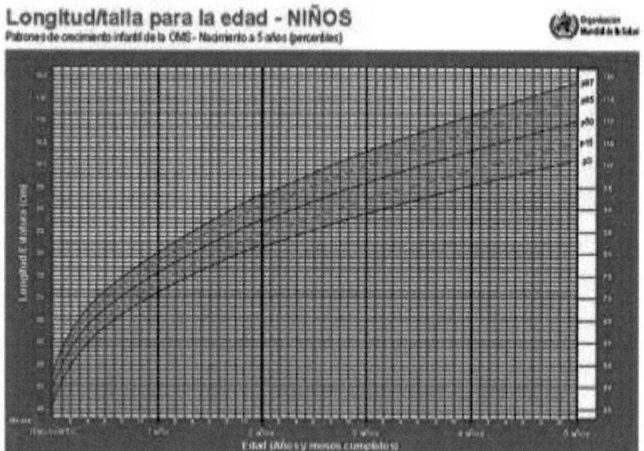

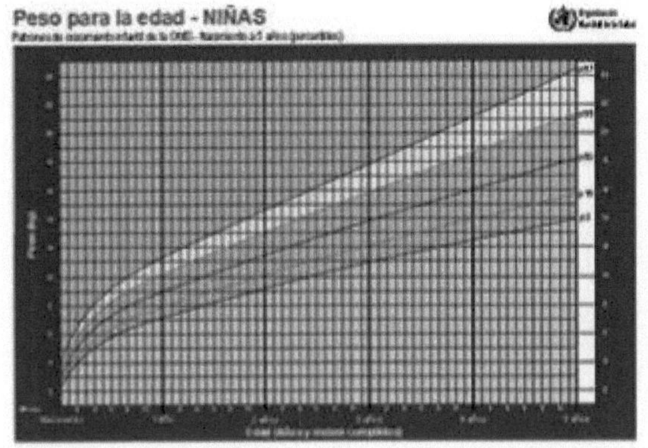

Peso para la edad - NIÑAS

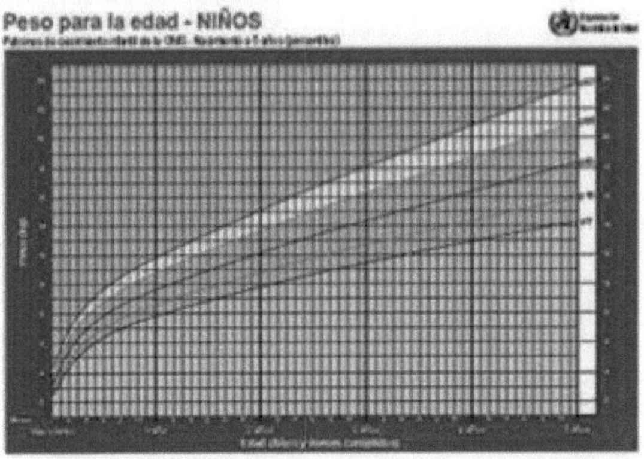

Peso para la edad - NIÑOS

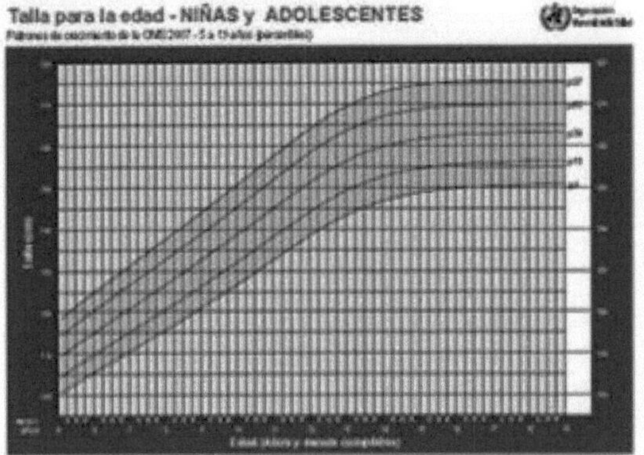

Talla para la edad - NIÑAS y ADOLESCENTES

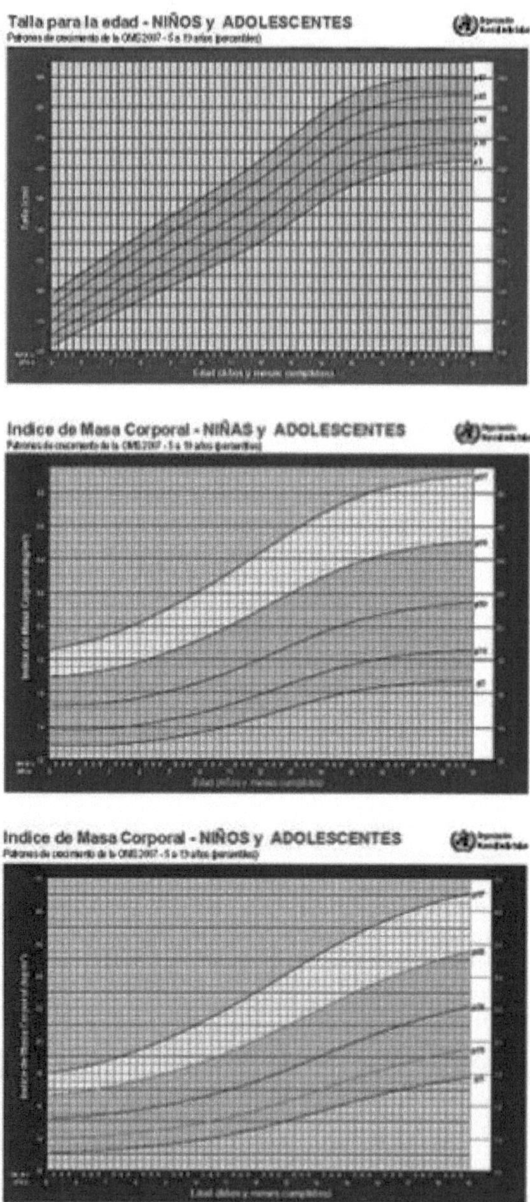

Figure 17.1. WHO charts for growth and development during infancy.

Bibliograffa

4. Karlberg J. A biologically-oriented mathematical model (ICP) for human growth. Acta Paediatr Scand. 1989; (Suppl 350): 70-94.

5. Fowden AL, Forhead AJ. Endocrine regulation of feto-placental growth. Horm Res. 2009; 72: 257-65.

6. Backeljauw PF, Dattani MT, Cohen P, Rosenfeld RG. Disorders of Growth Hormone/Insulin-Like Growth Factor Secretion and Action. In: Sperling MA, ed. Pediatric Endocrinology (fourth edition). Philadelphia: Elsevier Saunders; 2014. p. 292-404.

7. Boersma B, Wit JM. Catch up growth. Endo Rev. 1997; 18: 646-61.

8. Barker DJP. Maternal nutrition, fetal nutrition, and disease in later life. Nutrition. 1997; 13: 807-13.

9. Pozo J. Auxological assessment of growth I. Pediatr Integral. 2011; XV: 590-8.

10. Clayton PE, Cianfarani S, Czernichow P, Johannsson G, Rapaport R, Rogol A. Consensus Statement: Management of the Child Born Small for Gestational Age through to Adulthood: A Consensus Statement of the International Societies of Pediatric Endocrinology and the Growth Hormone Research Society. J Clin Endocrinol Metab. 2007; 92: 804-10.

11. Warman ML, Cormier-Daire V, Hall C, et al. Nosology and classification of genetic skeletal disorders: 2010 revision. Am J Med Genet Part A. 2011; 155: 943-68.

12. Cohen P, Rogol AD, Deal CL, et al. Consensus statement on the diagnosis and treatment of children with idiopathic short stature: a summary of the Growth Hormone Research Society, the Lawson Wilkins Pediatric Endocrine Society, and the European Society for Paediatric Endocrinology Workshop. J Clin Endocrinol Metab. 2008; 93: 4210-17.

13. Backeljauw PF, Miller BS, Dutailly P, et al. Recombinant human growth hormone plus recombinant human insulin-like growth factor-1 coadministration therapy in short children with low insulin-like growth factor-1 and growth hormone sufficiency: results from a randomized, multicenter, open-label, parallel-group, active treatment-controlled trial. Horm Res Paediatr. 2015; 83: 268-79.

18. Puberty and adolescence

Dr. Jose Uberos Fernandez

Adolescence is a transitional period in development. This stage is accompanied by intense physical, psychological, emotional and social changes. It begins with puberty and ends around the second decade of life, when physical growth and development and psychosocial maturation are complete.

Adolescence is a vague period of time, and its duration has been increasing in recent years due to the earlier onset of puberty and the lengthening of the period of school and vocational training. The WHO considers adolescence as the period between 10 and 19 years of age and youth as the period between 19 and 25 years of age. Adolescents are exposed to many risks: accidents, violence, delinquency, drug use and consumption, risky sexual behaviour, pregnancy, family problems, school problems, information technology, and mental disorders, among others. It should be noted that most of these behaviours are preventable.

Etymologically, the term puberty comes from the Latin "pubere" which means pubis with hair. It is a biological process in which the development of secondary sexual characteristics takes place, the complete maturation of the gonads and adrenal glands, as well as the acquisition of peak bone, fat and muscle mass, reaching adult height. The definition of puberty is based on statistical criteria, i.e. if the appearance of secondary sexual characteristics is within the range of +-2.5 SD (standard deviation) for the reference sex and population. The onset of normal puberty is considered to be the onset of telarche between the ages of 8-13 years in girls and the increase in testicular size between the ages of 9-14 years in boys.

Stages of adolescence

Adolescence can be schematized into three stages that overlap with each other.

- **Early adolescence.** It covers approximately 10 to 13 years of age, and is characterised mainly by pubertal changes.
- **Middle adolescence.** It is characterised, above all, by family conflicts, due to the relevance that the group acquires; it is at this time when risky behaviour is more likely to begin.
- **Late adolescence.** It covers the period from 18 to 21 years of age and is characterised by the re-acceptance of parental values and the assumption of the tasks and responsibilities of maturity.

Physiology of puberty

The onset of puberty is marked by the onset of pulsatile secretion of gonadotrophins (LH and FSH) and gonadotrophin-releasing hormone (GnRH). There are external factors that influence the timing of pubertal onset, such as nutrition, exercise, stress, social and psychological factors, circadian rhythm and daylight hours or environmental endocrine disruptors, mainly pesticides. GnRH induces, in the pituitary gonadotropic cells, the synthesis and pulsatile release of the pituitary gonadotrophins, LH (luteinising hormone) and FSH (follicle-stimulating hormone), which act in the gonad to induce the maturation of germ cells (oocytes or spermatozoa) and the production of sex steroids, as well as other gonadal peptides (inhibins, activins) and other circulating hormones (le ptin....), which exert, through feedback mechanisms, stimulatory and inhibitory actions at different levels of the hypothalamic-pituitary-gonadal axis.

Adrenarqwa or adrenal maturation (appearance of pubic and/or axillary hair) occurs between 6-8 years of bone age. It generally begins about 2 years before the increase in gonadal steroids and is independent of the hypothalamo-pituitary-gonadal axis.

There is a very close relationship between metabolism and reproduction, due to the peripheral signals that inform the brain of the nutritional status of the organism. Thus, obesity is related to pubertal advancement and malnutrition to pubertal delay. Leptin, a hormone synthesised in adipose tissue, has been shown to play a role in promoting pubertal development. The peptide ghrelin, an orex^genic factor secreted in the oxymic cells of the stomach, appears to inhibit gonadotrophin secretion. Leptin increases during puberty and ghrelin decreases.

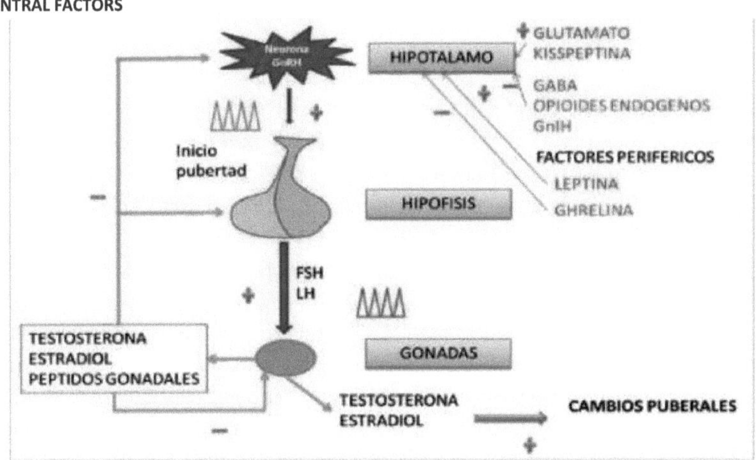

Figura 1. *1. Hypothalamic-pituitary-gonadal axis. Pulsatile GnRH secretion initiates puberty (Taken from Guemes-Hidalgo et al. 2017).*

Pubertal growth and development

There is a deceleration of growth that precedes the peak of maximum growth speed, which usually occurs between 12 and 13 years of age in girls and between 14 and 15 years of age in boys. This pubertal growth is not harmonious, it grows in "segments", with initial growth of the lower segment (lower limbs) and with an order of growth from distal to proximal, with the feet growing first. The final height is reached between 16-17 years of age in girls, and may be delayed until 21 years of age in boys. Weight gain during pubertal growth spurt is about 50% of ideal adult weight. Girls accumulate more fat than boys and, in boys, bone and muscle growth predominates. In adulthood, men have a fat percentage between 12-16%, while women have a fat percentage of 18-22%.

Brain development

In relation to brain development, we should know that the brain matures intermittently from hindbrain to forebrain and does not complete its maturation until the age of 25-30 years; it depends on three processes:

- Rapid neuronal-glial growth and the formation of new synaptic connections.
- The selective elimination or pruning of the less efficient synapses (what is not used is eliminates).
- Myelination of axons to facilitate and speed up neuronal transmission between different parts of the nervous system, which is not completed until the age of 25-30 years.

In the first 3 years of life, in order to achieve physical autonomy, the brain increases in volume by thickening its cortex at the expense of the formation of neural networks. This increases the cranial penis, which grows faster than ever before. In the later years, from 3 to 10 years of age, brain volume continues to increase, but at a slower rate, by the end of childhood the brain has almost reached its maximum size. It will still grow a little more in adolescence, but now the changes are due to other phenomena that will radically modify its structure.

The adolescent brain undergoes a reorganisation. While some areas increase in size, others decrease in size. Changes appear in the brain circuits, this happens because it is necessary for new circuits and connections to appear in order to sustain the analytical thinking that characterises the adult human being. Until now, the brain created circuits to support its most necessary functions: to give meaning to perceptions, to control posture and manipulation, to master language and communication. In adolescence, circuits must be created that allow decisions to be made based on a critical analysis of each situation. The intuition is that these circuits will be much more complex. In adolescence, the brain continues to perfect its cognitive capacities, memory, language, complex learning... those skills that it has already mastered, and continues to use, will consolidate the circuits that support them. The dendrites and axons that make them up will form faster, more mature synapses, which will be surrounded by myelin, a sheath that accelerates communication. The skills that are not practised will make less use of the circuits that support them and the synaptic junctions will be "undone" in a kind of pruning of the superfluous. **At the same time,** these new, more complex decision-making circuits appear, which require larger and sometimes more distant brain areas to be connected to each other. The main seat of these "decision-making circuits" is the prefrontal cortex, **which is in the** most anterior part of the brain and therefore the last to mature according to the established general programme.

Reward-seeking areas of the adolescent brain develop earlier than areas related to planning and emotional control (prefrontal cortex). This means that experimentation, exploration and risk-taking during adolescence are normative rather than pathological. Also, we know that the adolescent brain has a great capacity to change and adapt.

Sexual maturation

The most striking changes take place in the sexual sphere and culminate in the acquisition of fertility. The sexual maturation index, which is assessed by Tanner's stages (1962) and is based on the development of the genital organs and secondary sexual characteristics (*Figs. 18.2 and 18.3*). This allows differentiation between normal and pathological puberty.

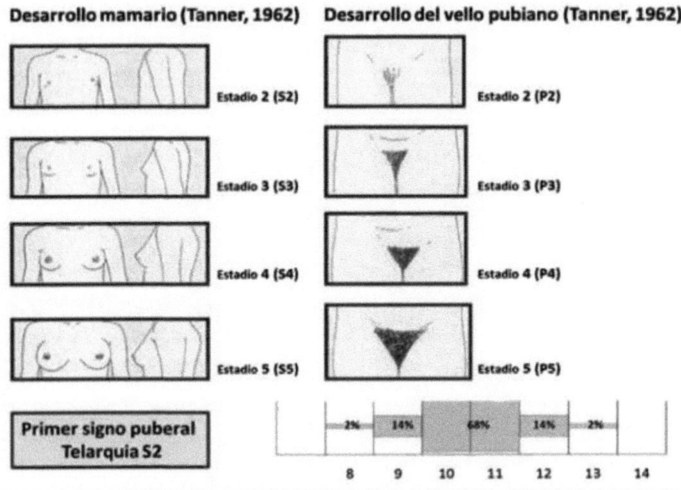

Figure 18.2. Pubertal stages in females (2).
Average duration of puberty 4 years (1.5*8 years)
Duración media de la pubertad 4 años (1,5-8 años)

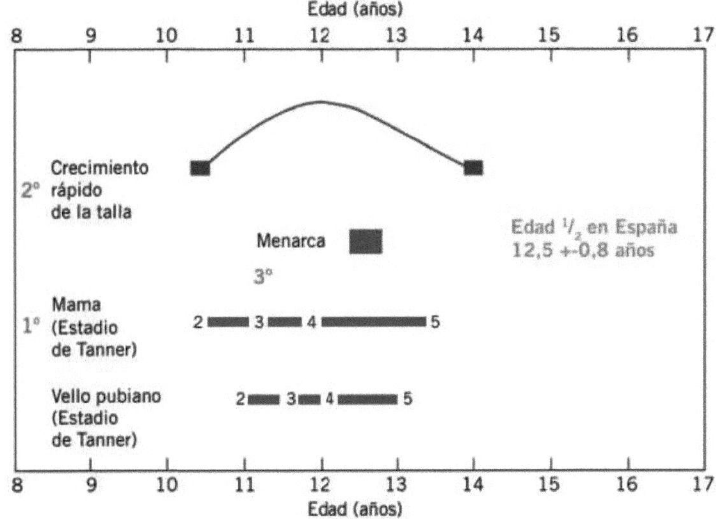

Figure 18.3. Sequence of pubertal events in girls.

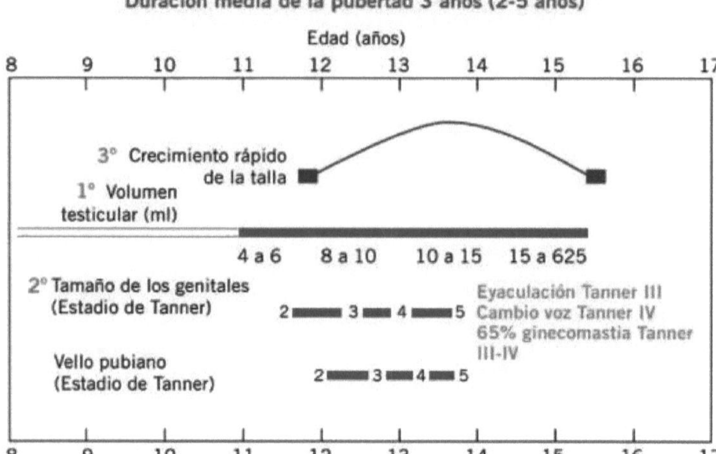

Figure 18.5. *Sequence of pubertal events in boys.*

The first sign of pubertal development in girls is the enlargement of the breast bud, which may begin between the ages of 8-13 years, together with an increase in growth rate, and occurs at the age of 11 years. Before the age of 8 years we speak of precocious puberty and after the age of 13 years of puberty ta^a.

The peak of maximum growth velocity occurs relatively early (Tanner II-III), while menarche is a late event, usually occurring about two years after telarche and generally signalling growth faltering.

The first sign of pubertal development in boys is an increase in testicular volume, as well as redness and roughness of the scrotal pouch, which may begin between the ages of 9-14 years and occurs at an osseous age of 13 years. Before the age of 9 years we speak of precocious puberty and after the age of 14 years of puberty ta^a. A volume of 4 ml (Prader's orchidometer) or a length of 2.5 cm mark the onset of puberty.

Psychosocial development

The psychosocial aspects to be achieved and which characterise the whole development of the adolescent are the following:

-    **Acquisition of independence from the family environment**. During the early phase of adolescence, there is less interest in parental activities and a greater reluctance to accept parental advice or practices. There is an emotional void that can create behavioural problems, sometimes manifested by a decline in school performance. By the end of adolescence, the young person is integrated back into the family and is better able to appreciate parental advice and values.

-    **Body image awareness and body acceptance.** During the early phase, due to pubertal physical changes, the adolescent experiences a great deal of self-doubt. During the middle phase, acceptance of his or her body is taking place, with attempts to make it more attractive. In late adolescence, pubertal growth and development is complete.

- **Relationships with friends and partners are established.** In early adolescence, there is a strong interest in friends of one's own sex, whose opinions become more important than those of parents. In middle adolescence, the role of friends is very powerful. There is an intense integration of the adolescent into the subculture of friends, in conformity with their values, rules and dress, in an attempt to further separate him/herself from the family. In the late adolescent phase, the group becomes less interested. There is less exploration and experimentation, and more time is spent in establishing intimate relationships; couples are formed.

- **Establishment of sexual, vocational, moral and self identity.** In parallel with the physical changes, the adolescent's cognitive capacity begins to improve, evolving from concrete to flexible abstract thinking. In middle adolescence, intellectual capacity and creativity increase, and they expand into the realm of feelings, with a new ability to examine the feelings of others. In late adolescence, thinking is already abstract and forward-looking, and practical and realistic vocational goals are established. Moral, religious and sexual values are delineated, and the ability to compromise and establish boundaries is established.

Socio-cultural influences. Risk and protective factors

The adolescent is a reflection of the society in which he or she is immersed and it is evident that the environment and the family have changed radically in today's welfare societies. The size and structure of households has changed: people live longer, have fewer and later children, the size of families has been reduced, mothers have started working, parents are more permissive, separations have increased and new family forms are appearing (single-parent, single-person, childless couples, homosexuals, etc.). The family, which is the main support for young people, is a social and cultural structure in crisis. All of this has important repercussions for the development and overall health of the adolescent.

Risk factors can be defined as the detectable characteristics of an individual, family, group or community that signal an increased likelihood of compromising health, quality of life and life itself, while protective factors are the opposite, as they promote successful development. In this sense the following elements can be considered protective factors during adolescence:

Of the adolescent:
- Good physical health and nutritional status
- Good body image
- Responsibility for appropriate health habits
- Adequate physical activity
- Good relationship with colleagues
- Social skills
- Experiencing hope, joy, success and love
- High self-esteem
- Managing the stress of distress
- Age-appropriate autonomy
- Development of personal identity and independence

- Responsible sexual behaviour
- Respecting the rights and needs of others
- Set educational and vocational goals
- Establishing a value system

Family members:
- Provide basic needs: food, shelter, clothing, security, etc.
- Understanding the emotional changes of adolescence
- Stimulating activities that promote the adolescent's self-image
- Spending time with the adolescent and making them feel loved
- Rewarding achievement
- Encourage the development of friendships
- Recognising the changing role of the adolescent and parents
- Providing sexuality education
- Stimulating adolescent independence and responsibility
- Develop a balance between support, tolerance and appropriate Kmites
- Supporting their educational and vocational goals
- Provide a system of values and models

Community:
- Provide quality educational and vocational opportunities.
- Provide activities for adolescents: recreational, educational, sporting and social.
- Supporting families with special needs
- Legislation to protect adolescents
- Offer comprehensive and differentiated health and education services for adolescents.
- Environment free of risks (toxics, violence, pollution, road safety, etc.).

Most pubertal problems can be followed up in primary care; as we have seen, no special tests or specific treatments are needed. Most psychosocial problems are preventable, so early detection and preventive measures on risk factors, promoting protective factors or resilience, are essential. Adolescent care must be carried out in a comprehensive manner; on many occasions, the help of other professionals will be required and the paediatrician must coordinate it with knowledge, interest and professionalism.

Bibliograffa

1. Rodnguez-Sacristan J, Masse Gartfa P. Drug use-abuse in adolescence. Pediatr Integral 1997;2(3):261-71.

2. Guemes-Hidalgo M, Cenal Gonzalez-Fierro MJ, Hidalgo-Vicario M. Development during adolescence. Physical, psychological and social aspects. Pediatr Integral 2017;21(4):233-44.

19. Malformative syndromes and genetic alterations

Dr. Jose Uberos Fernandez

Embryofetopathies refer to pathological conditions that occur or originate before birth to extrauterine life and are due to two broad categories of aetiological factors: genetic or endogenous and environmental or exogenous. The aetiology of congenital malformations can be established in about half of the cases. They occur with an average frequency of 2.6% (in a recent Spanish study). 10% are of genetic origin (chromosomal anomaKas, single mutant genes, familial cases), 23% due to multifactorial inheritance, 3.2% caused by teratogenic agents, 2.5% due to uterine factors, 0.4% associated with twinning and the remainder of unknown aetiology.

Definitions

- *Malformation.* Morphological defect of an organ or part of an organ, resulting from an inherently abnormal developmental process (e.g. cleft lip).
- *Disruption.* Morphological alteration of an organ, part of an organ and more often of a larger region as a consequence of an external failure of an originally normal developmental process. Example: amniotic flange complex.
- *Deformity.* An abnormal shape, configuration or position of a body part caused by endogenous or more often exogenous (non-disruptive) mechanical factors. For example: congenital torticollis.
- *Dysplasia.* Abnormal cellular organisation in a given tissue with consequent morphological disorders. For example, achondroplasia.
- *Defect of a developmental field.* Pattern of abnormalities resulting from disruption of a developmental field. For example, holoprosencephaly malformation complex.
- *Sequence.* A set of multiple anomaKas derived from a first known disorder. For example, fetal akinesia deformation sequence (FADS), with multiple contractures, growth retardation, facial anomaKas, pulmonary hypoplasia, short umbilical cord and redundant skin.
- *Syndrome.* Multiple anomaKas with pathogenetic relationships to each other, excluding a sequence, with idiopathic or known aetiopathogenesis. For example, Down's syndrome.
- *Association.* The occurrence, not due to chance, in two or more patients, of multiple anomaKas in a syndrome or sequence. Examples: association of Wilms' tumour, aniridia and hemihypertrophy; VATER or VATERAL association, with vertebral defects, imperforate anus, oesophageal atresia, tracheoesophageal fistula, ca^ac defects and radial and renal dysplasia; CHARGE association, with coloboma, cardiopathy, choanal atresia and growth and developmental delay.

Classification

Prenatal pathology can be systematised, according to the time of gestation at which the responsible noxa acts, into genopathies, blastopathies, embryopathies and foetopathies (Warkany). It is preferred to call the first group gametopatfas.

Gametopathies. The pathogenic noxa acts on the gametes, which is why it is generally a preconceptional pathology. This group is subdivided into: a) chromosomopathies, i.e. numerical and structural chromosomal errors; b) genopathies: hereditary diseases, resulting from mutations in genes present in the oocyte or spermatocyte, or in both at the same time, being transmitted to the offspring according to the laws of Mendelian inheritance.

Blastopathies. These include pathological conditions arising in the blastula penodo or first 18-21 days of development. From fertilisation to the early post-implantation period, the new being possesses relatively few cells and is endowed with a great capacity to replenish totipotential cells. Therefore, the effect of a toxic agent follows the "all or nothing" phenomenon, i.e. either a large number of cells are damaged (death of the product), or so few cells are affected that repair generally takes place without injury. During the third week of gestation, however, the toxic effects on the product can lead to major defects.

Embryopathies. They correspond to the pathology of the embryo and are characterised clinically by deviations in the development of the organs, giving rise to single or multiple congenital malformations. Chronologically, they are limited to the period from the 4th week of development to the 8th week of gestation.

Fetopathies. These are diseases of the foetal penis, which begin at the end of the 8th month and end at birth.

The phenotype is the result of genetic characteristics modified by various environmental agents. Gametopathies are generally endogenous in origin, although they can be influenced by environmental circumstances. Blastopathies are an aetiologically poorly understood group; in some cases (chromosomal mosaicism) they are due to endogenous factors, but most likely the causative factors will be environmental. Embryopathies and foetopathies are of exogenous or environmental origin, although in several cases these factors remain unclear. These causal factors may act in isolation, but in other cases they require predisposing genetic conditions to manifest themselves.

Chromosomopathies

The chromosome is the unit of the genome that contains numerous genes on a long double-stranded DNA chain, being visible under the microscope as a morphological unit during cell division. Its study is the focus of cytogenetics. The nucleus of all human *somatic cells* has 46 chromosomes, constituting the diploid series, represented by 2n; the *sex cells* (egg and sperm) have only 23 chromosomes: they are the haploid series and are represented by the letter n. The 46 chromosomes form 23 pairs of chromosomes. The 46 chromosomes form 23 pairs: 22 pairs of homologous autosomes and 1 pair of gonosomes or sex chromosomes, XX in females and XY in males. Each pair consists of one chromosome from the father and one from the mother. The ordered distribution of the metaphase chromosomes of a cell, according to their size and shape, constitutes the "karyotype".

Chromosomal alterations, whether numerical or structural, in single lines or in mosaics, involve a large number of genes and their consequences have a negative impact on development; their severity will depend on the type of alteration and the chromosome involved, but the clinical manifestations, considered in isolation, can rarely be considered pathognomonic for a given chromosome. When a normal cell line is present in the mosaic, the clinical repercussions are usually attenuated.

Numerical alterations. The normal number of chromosomes can be altered by excess or defect, and this alteration will affect the whole haploid series (n) or isolated chromosome pairs. If they affect the entire haploid series, they are called *euploid^as:* triploid^as (2 n + n), tetraploid^as (2n + 2n), etc. When the number is high, they are usually called polyploid^as. If they affect isolated pairs, they are called *aneuploid^as: monosoiwa* if there is a loss of one chromosome (2n - 1), *trisom^a* the increase of one chromosome (2n + 1), *tetrasom^a* if there are two chromosomes in excess (2n + 2), *hyperploid^as* the increase of several isolated chromosomes, and *hypodiploid^as* when there is a loss and increase of different chromosomes.

Structural alterations. Structural lesions of the chromosomal material mostly represent a visible alteration of the genetic material and can be detected by the morphological modification of the chromosome. *Deletion* is the loss of a chromosomal fragment by breakage; it can be terminal or interstitial. *Translocation* is the exchange of genetic material between two or more chromosomes; we speak of balanced translocation when a chromosomal region changes position in the genome, but the number of copies of this region remains the same. People with such translocations may or may not be affected. When fusion between two acrocentric chromosomes occurs, a Robertsonian translocation. The *inversion involves* the breakage of a chromosomal fragment, a 180° turn of the central fragment and its reconstruction, but altering the order of the genes. By changing the morphology of the chromosome, it is possible to detect it; if the centromere is present in the broken fragment, it is called a pericentric inversion, and if not, a paracentric inversion. *Duplication* indicates repeated genetic material on the same chromosome; it may be due to translocation of a fragment from its homologue, to an unequal *crossing over* during meiosis, or to an endoreduplication of this fragment during DNA replication. *Ring chromosome* is a chromosome that has been broken at both ends and once the fragments have been separated, they have been rejoined, forming a ring; it may also be formed by telomeric fusion, in which case there is no loss of material.

Autosomal syndromes

Autosomal disorders are consistently accompanied by growth retardation, mental deficiency, malformations of variable location and severity, and various degenerative physical features.

Trisomy 21 (Down's Syndrome)

An excess chromosome 21, which may be free (95%), translocated on another chromosome (3-4%) or form mosaics (1-2%), constitutes Down's syndrome. Its frequency in the general population is 1 in 700, but when maternal age is taken into account, the incidence ranges from 1 in 1000 before the age of 30 to 1 in 40 after the age of 45. Molecular studies show that 80% of cases of regular trisomy are due to maternal nondisjunction and the remaining 20% to paternal nondisjunction.

Clinical features. It associates psychomotor retardation and a very peculiar phenotype related to genes located in a narrow region of the long arm of chromosome 21 (critical region: 21q22.2- q22.3) which plays an important role in the facial manifestations and in the complex anatomical and functional alterations of the syndrome. At the level of the head they are brachycephalic children, with flat face and occiput, oblique eyes, with palpebral openings directed upwards and outwards, epicanthus and hypertelorism. A whitish stippling (Brushfield's spots) appears on the iris. Various ocular anomalies may be present: cataract, nystagmus, iris hypoplasia, strabismus, microphthalmia, anophthalmia, glaucoma. The nose is small, with depressed ^z. The mouth is small, with thick lips, favouring the protrusion of the tongue. The pinnae are usually dysplastic with frequent low implantation and a very narrow ear canal. In the trunk there is not infrequently a keeled or infundibuliform malformation, as well as umbilical hernia, with great hypotoma of the abdominal musculature. In the extremities, the hands are coarse, with short fingers, especially the fifth finger, which usually shows *clinodactyly,* with absence of the second flexion crease. The palmar, middle and distal flexion creases are usually fused, constituting the Knea or *four-finger crease.* In the newborn and infant, there is an intense hypotomy. In the feet there is usually a marked separation between the big toe and the second toe.

Among the malformations, the most serious and most frequent are ca^acal, followed by digestive (intestinal malrotation, Meckel's diverticulum, annular pancreas, duodenal stenosis, megacolon), renal, genital or central nervous system malformations.

Trisomy 18 (Edwards' syndrome)

The clinical picture is related to the critical 18qll band or region. The *frequency* is estimated to be about 1.3/10,000 live births, with a female predominance.

They are children with low birth weight, hypertoma and a malformation picture with microcephaly, prominent occiput, dysplastic and low-set ears, small nose, narrow palpebral fissure, frequent microphthalmia, small mouth with narrow palate, frequent lip and palatal fissures, micrognathia. In the extremities there are joint contractures, especially in the hands the flexion of the index and little fingers over the middle and ring fingers, respectively; the feet show the "rocker foot" deformity with a prominent heel and convex plantar region. The nails are hypoplastic.

Various malformations are associated: ca^acal, renal, digestive and genital malformations. Half-life is very short due to severe visceral malformations. In prolonged survival, severe psychomotor retardation and skeletal defects are evident. Mosaic cases and partial trisom^as (short arms, long arms, isochromosomes) which do not involve trisom^a for the 18q11 band, can be separated from the described picture, especially when there are remnants of other chromosomes.

Trisomy 13 (Patau's Syndrome)

The average incidence is 1 case per 5,000 foetuses or 10,000 births.

The clinical picture is dominated by malformations of the craniofacial area, with microcephaly, anomaKas of sutures at vertex level and possible defects of the scalp and even of the underlying bone, microphthalmia, anophthalmia, colobomas, cataracts, the nose may have a single orifice (cebocephaly) and when not accompanied by a cleft lip, it is large, resembling that of a boxer; Lip and palate clefts are frequent (hare's snout appearance), postaxial polydactyly, syndactylies, hand in a pinna, some narrow and convex, rocker foot. The most frequent malformations are cardiovascular and nervous system malformations with aplasia or hypoplasia of the corpus callosum and other areas.

5p- deletion (Lejeune syndrome)

Known as "cat's meow syndrome", it is caused by a deletion of the short arms of chromosome 5 (5p-), which includes the chromosome 5p14-15 coding region. Its frequency is estimated at 1/50,000 newborns. The cry in the newborn and early months resembles the meowing of a cat *(cri du chat)*.

Gonosomal syndromes

Gonosomal alterations preferentially affect the gonadal area, while the repercussions on intelligence, growth and malformations are variable.

Turner Syndrome

It is a consequence of complete (45, X) or partial (isochromosome, deletions, rings, mosaics) monosom^a of an X gonosome. Some cases may be caused by deletions of the Y gonosome with loss of testicular determinant genes.

Typical cases show female phenotype with short stature, gonadal dysgenesis (gonadal girdle) with genital infantilism, absence of puberty, hypergonadotropic hypogonadism, amenorrhoea, sterility and characteristic physical features. Coarctation of the aorta responsible for the absence of the femoral heartbeat, hearing loss, cutaneous and intestinal telangiectasias and cutaneous pigmented nevi are common. Other malformations, mild mental retardation and reactive psychic disorders, especially melancholia, may eventually occur. Treatment is aimed at compensating for growth retardation and hypogonadism (anabolic steroids, growth hormone, oestrogens), psychological measures, removal of the dysgenic gonad if there is a Knea with remnants of the Y-gonosome because of the risk of malignancy (gonadoblastoma, dysgerminoma) and correction of malformations.

associated.

Bibliograffa

1. Bueno M, Perez-Gonzalez J. Prenatal pathology. Embryofetopathies. In: Cruz M, editor. Tratado de Pediatna. 8- ed. Madrid: Ergon; 2001.

2. Ballesta F, Cruz M. Chromosomopathies. In: Cruz M, editor. Tratado de Pediatna. 8- ed. Madrid: Ergon; 2001.

PART III

20. Anomalies of sexual differentiation

Dr. Jose Uberos Fernandez

In a broad sense, the so-called "intersex conditions" consist of any discordance between the various parameters or criteria defining sex. These criteria or "sexes" are numerous. Of the various sex-defining criteria, from the clinical point of view we must consider chromosomal, gonadal, genital and somatic sex. Other aspects such as social or psychological sex are not considered in this chapter.

It is important to clarify the differences between two concepts that are often used interchangeably: intersex status, which refers to the discordance between sex-defining criteria; and genital ambiguity, which refers to the unspeakable appearance of the external genitalia.

Strictly speaking, genital ambiguity refers to a situation of the external genitalia which does not permit the unequivocal assignment of a specific sex, male or female. Intersex conditions result from the altered determination of the undifferentiated gonad into ovary or testis, and/or from the subsequent differentiation of the ducts of Wolff and Muller and the external genitalia into male or female during foetal life. Depending on the gonad, disorders of sexual differentiation fall mainly into three categories:

1. AnomaKas of gonad determination with various alterations: the fetal undifferentiated gonad is not differentiated into a normal gonad. These include true hermaphroditism, in which ovarian and testicular tissue is present; the numerous gonadal dysgenesis, in which there are histological alterations of the gonads; and agonadisms in which no gonad is found.

2. Female pseudohermaphroditism: the gonad is a normal ovary, the sex chromosome is 46,XX, but the external genitalia have been virilised to a greater or lesser degree.

3. Male pseudohermaphroditism: the gonad is a testis, normal or partially differentiated, the sex chromosome is 46,XY, or at least in one cell Knea the Y chromosome, or material from it, is present, but the external genitalia are ambiguous or totally female.

Physiological recall of sex determination and differentiation

Sexual determination

The genetic sex of an individual is determined at the moment of fertilisation of the egg, depending on the gonosomal load of the sperm (Y = male, X = female). Depending on the gonosomal endowment of the new individual, its undifferentiated gonocytes will develop male (testis) if the gonosome is Y, and therefore carries the SRY gene, or female (ovary) if it does not have a Y chromosome, and therefore lacks the SRY gene.

Sex differentiation

Once the sex has been determined and the corresponding gonad has developed, it will be in charge of carrying out the male or female differentiation (differentiation of internal and external genitalia in one direction or the other).

Until the 6th week the sexual structures are identical in both sexes. Those from which the genitalia derive are formed by two pairs of Wolff's ducts (which give rise to the ductus deferens and seminal vesicles) and Muller's ducts (which give rise to the fallopian tubes and uterus), and by the urogenital sinus, labio-scrotal and urethral folds, and genital tubercle from which the external genitalia derive.

Male or female differentiation will depend on the action of the corresponding gonad:

- **In the male**, the *Leydig cells* will release testosterone, which will stimulate the development of the Wolffian ducts (male internal genitalia), which are thought to be sensitive only to foetal testosterone or very potent androgenic stimuli. Testosterone, metabolised to dihydrotestosterone, will act on the structures from which the external genitalia originate, so that they differentiate in a male (male external genitalia) rather than female direction. On the other hand, the *Sertoli cells* will release MFI (Mullerian Inhibitory Factor), which will inhibit the development of the Mullerian ducts, preventing the formation of female internal genitalia.

- **In the female sex**, *the absence of cë/Leydig cells* conditions the absence of testosterone, so that the development of the Wolffian ducts is not stimulated (absence of male internal genitalia), and there is no dihydrotestosterone (absence of male external genitalia), and consequently the structures are differentiated in the absence of androgenic stimulus in the female sense (female external genitalia). *The absence of cë/Sertoli cells* means that there is no IFM, so Muller's ducts develop (internal female genitalia).

It could therefore be said that male genital differentiation is due to the "active" action of the testes (stimulating testosterone and inhibiting IFM), while female genital differentiation occurs "passively" when these stimuli are absent.

Classification of intersex conditions

They are divided into two main groups, depending on whether they originate from incorrect sex determination or sex differentiation:

- **Abnormalities of gonad determination:** Undifferentiated gonocytes do not differentiate normally, giving rise to what are known as *gonadal dysgenesis*, which includes dysgenesis proper, true hermaphroditism and agonadism.

Pathogenically they can be grouped into:

- Abnormal ovarian differentiation or maintenance: Turner syndrome (X0).
- Abnormal testes differentiation or maintenance: Klinefelter's syndrome (XX0).
- Presence of testicular and ovarian tissue: true hermaphroditism.

- **Anomalies of sexual differentiation:** This includes those cases in which sexual determination was normal (gonad differentiated according to the chromosomal sex), however, the genitalia are more or less tending towards the opposite sex. This classically includes *pseudohermaphroditism*.

Mixed gonadal dysgenesis

Mixed Gonadal Dysgenesis (MGD) is a disorder of sexual differentiation (DSD) characterised by the presence of immature o dysgenetic testicular tissue on one side and contralateral gonadal stenosis, often associated with a 45 X / 46XY chromosomal mosaic. It is the second cause of ambiguous genitalia in neonates after congenital adrenal hyperplasia and is characterised by short stature and Turnerian stigmata in infancy and primary amenorrhoea in adolescence. It should be diagnosed early as it is often associated with malignancy of the gonads related to the presence of a Y chromosome in one of the affected person's cell lines.

True hermaphroditism

It can be understood in a number of different spheres:

- Etymologically it means the ability to fertilise and to be fertilised.
- In certain animals: Possession of male and female genitalia (snail, oysters, etc..)
- In humans: Possession of gonadal and ovarian tissue.

It is defined by the presence of testicular and ovarian parenchyma in the same person. It is actually a form of gonadal dysgenesis, as both tissues are histologically abnormal, but hermaphroditism can be described separately, because it is an entity with its own clinical personality. Most of the cases described are sporadic, but occasionally it occurs in a familial form. The most frequent karyotype is 46,XX (70-80% of cases).

The gonads may be located in the labioscrotal formations, in the inguinal canal or intra-abdominally. According to the gonadal anatomy, hermaphroditism is classified as: 1) *alternating:* when there is ovary on one side and testis on the other; 2) *bilateral:* when there are ovotestes (ovarian and testicular tissue together) or separate testis and ovary on both sides, and 3) *unilateral:* when both tissues are on one side only. Ovotestes is the most frequently encountered gonadal structure (more than 60% of cases) and is usually bilateral; alternating hermaphroditism is the rarest form. The differentiation of the *internal genitalia* is diverse.

The reason for consultation is usually a newborn baby with genital ambiguity. At the onset of puberty, signs of virilisation may appear in a patient considered to be a girl (enlargement of the clitoris, hirsutism) or signs of feminisation in a patient considered to be a boy (gynaecomastia, urethral haemorrhage), or poor pubertal development in patients considered to be normal males or females.

Genital sex: The findings can be very variable, tending more towards female sex if there is no Y chromosome sex (which, as we have seen, is the most frequent).

Internal genitalia: Those derived from Mullerian structures are usually well developed, with tubes, uterus and vagina frequently found, while Wolffian structures are usually poorly developed (rudimentary vas deferens).

External genitalia: It is possible to find very diverse findings, sometimes very striking, being the ones that induce to study the patient, or on the contrary very little expressive, in which case the diagnosis can be difficult and late (generally due to pubertal anomaKas):

- *Penile-clitoral organ:* Structure reminiscent of a hypertrophic clitoris to a hypoplastic, hypospadic and incurved penis.
- *Labio-scrotal formations:* Simulating from a bffid scrotum without gonads inside, to labia majora containing gonads, or a labial formation on one side and scrotal on the other.
- *Common urogenital sinus:* Existence of a single cavity where urethra and vagina meet.
- *Male or female external genitalia of almost normal appearance,* in which the

warning sign leading to the study may simply be the existence of hypospadias, cryptorchidism, micropenis, other signs of virilisation or feminisation, or even haematuria at puberty (urethral haemorrhages which in fact correspond to menstruation).

Pseudohermaphroditism

Existence of ambiguous or completely normal genitalia of the opposite sex (rare) in individuals whose chromosomal and gonadal sexes are in agreement. It is therefore a disorder of sexual differentiation, which may affect both internal and external genitalia, resulting from congenital or environmental causes that interfere with the action of the (normally formed) gonads in influencing sexual differentiation.

The denomination is made according to the gonadal sex, so a pseudohermaphroditism will be male (PHM) when the gonad is a testis, and female (PHF) when it is an ovary.

Female pseudohermaphroditism

It is defined by the presence of ambiguous or all-male external genitalia in patients with female chromosomal sex (46,XX), normal ovaries and normal female internal genitalia. The usual pathogenic mechanism is virilisation of the external genitalia of a female foetus, 46XX, by the presence of androgens during gestation.

If the regression was very early, the external and internal genitalia are completely female and the picture corresponds to pure XY gonadal dysgenesis, but if testicular differentiation has begun, albeit incompletely, sexual ambiguity may result. The cause is possibly heterogeneous: vascular accident, genetic alteration or action of a teratogenic agent, etc.

The most frequent pathogenic mechanism is the abnormal presence of androgens that interfere with the normal female differentiation, which should normally take place in the absence of androgens. The origin of these androgens can be in:

- **The foetus itself**, as suffering from a form of *congenital adrenal hyperplasia* in which the androgen v^a is intact (and therefore hyperfunctioning): Deficiency of 21-hydroxylase, 11-beta-hydroxylase or 3-beta-hydroxysteroid dehydrogenase. Also due to the existence of an androgen-producing *adrenal* or *ovarian tumour* (very rare).

- **The mother**, because she suffers from *congenital adrenal hyperplasia* and sends androgens to the foetus via the diaplacental route; because she is being treated with *androgenic drugs* (androgens, smethasone progestogens, danazol, etc.); or because she suffers from *androgen-producing tumours* (arrhenoblastoma or ovarian luteoma, adrenal adenomas).

- **Unknown:** *Idiopathic* (when truly unknown), or *non-specific* (when the genital anomaKa usually presents as part of a more complex dysmorphic picture).

Prader made a classification, according to the intensity of virilisation of the external genitalia, in what is known as **Prader's Degrees of virilisation**.

Summary

- *Chromosomal sex:* 46XX
- *Gonadal sex:* Normal ovaries
- *Genital sex:* The *internal genitalia are normal female*, since the development of the Mullerian ducts is not influenced by the presence of androgens, and there is no IFM to

inhibit it (no Sertoli cells to produce it), and the development of the Wolffian ducts is only influenced by foetal testosterone, or by very potent stimuli. The external genitalia will appear virilised (ambiguous or rarely normal male).

Male pseudohermaphroditism

It is defined by the presence of ambiguous or all-female external genitalia in patients with male chromosomal sex (46,XY) and testes. The fundamental pathogenic mechanism consists of incomplete masculinisation of the external and internal genitalia of a 46,XY male foetus due to disruption of any of the steps necessary for complex male differentiation or persistence of mullerian structures: a) gonadal dysgenesis; b) pituitary disruption; c) Leydig cell agenesis or LH receptor disruption.d) inborn errors of testosterone biosynthesis; e) peripheral androgen resistance; and d) absence of Muller's duct inhibitory hormone or lack of peripheral response to this hormone. There are also cases in which the alteration of sexual differentiation is due to the action of drugs or teratogenic factors that have not been well identified.

The degree of incomplete masculinisation varies widely. Sometimes the lack of virilisation consists only of bilateral cryptorchidism and hypospadias. Other times, the lack of masculinisation is maximal and the appearance of the genitalia is totally feminine. The Wolffian structures, i.e. the epididymis, vas deferens and seminal vesicles, are often underdeveloped or absent. In cases due to gonadal dysgenesis there may be Mullerian structures, but in all other cases, except in the rare syndrome of persistence of Muller's duct, there are no Mullerian structures, i.e. no uterus and no tubes.

Summary

- **Chromosomal sex:** 46,XY or gonosomopathies with genetic material from the Y chromosome.
- **Gonadal sex:** normal or partially differentiated testes, since the maintenance of testicular trophism requires the action of the androgens produced by the testicle itself.
- **Genital sex:** The external genitalia will be shaped differently, depending on whether there is only a lack of androgens, or also a lack of IFM:

- Internal genitalia:

■ *In the absence of IFM*, female internal genitalia will be found. This occurs for example in cases of gonadal dysgenesis.

■ *Because of insufficient androgenisation*, the internal male genitalia will be insufficiently developed, or even absent, if androgen action is totally absent.

- External genitalia:

They will be ambiguous (feminised) or completely feminine in cases of total lack of androgenic action.

Some chimerical forms of male pseudohermaphroditism

Testicular feminisation or Morris syndrome (complete androgen resistance):

- **Aetiology:** X-linked recessive inheritance.
- **Frequency:** 1/20,000 - 1/60,000 live births.
- Pathogenic mechanism: Presence of normal testes that produce androgens normally, but there is a total resistance of the tissues to the action of androgens, so that the end

result is as if they are not produced in any quantity.

- **Cli'nica:**

₀ *Chromosomal Sex:* 46XY

₀ *Gonadal sex:* normal but often ectopic testes (abdomen, inguinal canal, labia majora).

₀ *Genital sex: There are no internal male or female genitalia*, as the Wolffian ducts do not develop due to the lack of the androgen stimulus, and the female genitalia do not develop because the testis has Sertoli cells which release IFM, inhibiting the development of the Mullerian ducts. *The external ones will be normal female* (there is no androgen stimulus to differentiate in the male direction), with the vagina ending in a cul-de-sac.

₀ *Somatic sex:* Normal female, even with breast development, but no hair (lack of androgenic stimulus).

₀ *Sex hormones:* Testosterone and oestradiol elevated at puberty.

Partial Androgen Resistance Syndrome (PARS)

- **Aetiology:** X-linked recessive inheritance
- **Cli'nica:**
- *Chromosomal sex:* 46,XY
- *Gonadal sex:* Normal testes, which may also be located in abdomen, inguinal canal, labia majora, or scrotum.
- *Genital sex: The internal genitalia are male with little development* (little androgenic stimulus), and there are no female genitalia (there is an IFM that prevents their development). *External genitalia are ambiguous (feminised) and highly variable*, depending on the degree of insensitivity to androgenic stimulus.
- *Somatic sex: There* may be few signs of virilisation, and even breast development at puberty, if insensitivity is very pronounced.
- *Sex hormones:* Testosterone and oestradiol may be elevated at puberty.

Persistent Mullerian duct syndrome

-**Aetiology**   : Variable, ranging from forms due to recessive inheritance linked to X, to autosomal dominant, and sporadic forms.

- **Pathogenic mechanism:** The testes do not produce IFM, not inhibiting the development of Muller's ducts.
- **Cli'nica**

₀ *Chromosomal sex:* 46XY

₀ *Gonadal sex:* normal testes

₀ *Genital sex: Normal male and female internal genitalia* (there is correct androgen stimulation, and no IFM). *Normal male external genitalia* (correct androgen stimulation). The diagnosis is most often made by the surgeon when operating on a hernia *"hernia utero-inguinalis"* as this is the most frequent location of the female genitalia (90 % of cases), in the remaining 10 % the location is intra-abdominal.

₀ *Somatic sex:* Normal male. Cryptorchidism is not uncommon in some cases.

General diagnosis of genital ambiguity

Anamnesis: Investigate consanguinity, other affected relatives (genetic aetiology).

General examination: Look for Turnerian stigmata, nephro-urological malformations which are often associated with the embryological intimacy between the genital and urinary tracts.

Examination of the external genitalia: Palpation of the gonads. When successful, it is most likely to be the testis, as it has a tendency to descend, while the ovary will remain intra-abdominal.

Examination of internal genitalia: Ultrasonography of the abdomen and genitalia will be useful, sometimes genitography with contrast or endoscopy of the common urogenital sinus. In many cases, laparotomy or laparoscopy is necessary, taking advantage of the opportunity to take a gonadal biopsy. In pseudohermaphroditism this is not necessary as the internal genitalia are known to be normal female.

Other complementary examinations: Genetic study. Hormonal study prior stimulation with chorionic gonadotrophin in those older than 5 months. Molecular biology studies and other techniques for prenatal diagnosis. Psychological report, essential to know the psychological sex, etc.

General considerations on the treatment of genital ambiguity

It is usually complex and must be personalised in each case, and is generally carried out by a multidisciplinary team (endocrinologist, surgeon, plastic surgeon, psychologist, moralist, jurist, etc.). As a general basis, the following can be considered:

- **Choice of sex:** Considering the anatomical situation of the external genitalia, and the possibility of reconstruction so that the individual can lead an active sexual life.

- **Plastic surgery:** It is advisable that at school age the genitalia are, at least apparently, appropriate to the social sex, to avoid discrimination with peers, and psychological sequelae. Clitoridoplasty is usually performed before the age of 18 months, while vaginoplasty is usually delayed until pubertal age (slower growth rate of scar tissue).

- **Gonadectomy:** Difficult decision, in which the gonad is usually assessed to be of the opposite sex to that finally assigned. The risk of gonadal malignancy is higher if the individual has a Y gonad.

- **Hormonal treatment:** Substitution treatment if there is a deficit of the hormones corresponding to the sex finally assigned.

- **Psychological treatment:** Very important, not only for the patient but also for the parents.

- **Preventive treatment:** Where possible (dexamethasone in 21-hydroxylase deficiency).

Bibliograffa

1. Audi L, Toran N, Martinez-Mora J. AnomaKas of sexual differentiation. In: Pombo M. Tratado de endocrinolog^a pediatrica. 3^ Ed. Pgs: 835-79. Interamericana:Madrid. 2002.

2. Delgado A. Ambiguous genitalia. In: Pediatna clmica: La pediatna a traves de la historia clmica. Vol 11. pp: 100-23. Boan: Bilbao. 2002.

3. Rodnguez-Hierro F, Ballesta F, Ibanez L. Smdromes of genital ambiguity. Intersexual states. In: Cruz. Tratado de Pediatna. 8- Ed. Pags: 819.37. Ergon: Madrid. 2001.

21. Neurodevelopmentally-focused care

Dr. Jose Uberos Fernandez

Developmental Centred Care (DCC) is a system of care for the premature and/or sick newborn that aims to improve the development of the child through interventions that favour the newborn and the family, understanding them both as a unit. The CCD includes interventions aimed at improving both the environment of lights, noises... and the micro-environment in which the child develops (posture, manipulations or pain). In addition, action is taken with the family to facilitate their role as the child's primary caregiver as much as possible. The correct implementation of CCD requires, therefore, the opening of doors 24 hours a day of the Neonatal Units, as recommended by the WHO.

The CCD requires the joint and close collaboration of all health personnel involved with the newborn. This task brings numerous benefits, which we will explain below. These benefits are not only reflected not only in the patient, but also in the parents and the staff of the Neonatal Unit itself, creating a pleasant and humane environment.

Influence of the environment on preterm development

The stay of the newborn in the neonatal unit has undesirable effects on both the newborn and its family. The exposure of the child to a hostile environment such as the NICU hinders the organisation of the developing brain. Behavioural, learning and emotional disturbances and social difficulties often appear in the development of children who were born prematurely. In addition, parents feel an emotional impact that changes the parenting process.

Preterm infants have to develop in an extra-uterine environment at a time when their brain is in the process of organisation and synaptogenesis, which means that it is a very active and delicate period in the developmental process. In addition to being in an extra-uterine environment, they are subjected to stress resulting from separation from the mother and the simultaneous and repeated experience of pain.

The preterm infant has a limited ability to organise his or her behaviour and adapt to the environment and is unable to reject harmful stimuli; in the NICU, the preterm infant receives an inappropriate pattern of stimulation that may alter neural development.

In the last weeks of gestation is when there is the most intense activity in the brain development of the foetus. This means that the premature newborn fulfils these stages of maximum activity and development outside its "natural habitat", i.e. in an extra-uterine environment.

Brain development in the foetus from the 25th week of gestation onwards is very rapid. At this time, astrocytes are forming and migrating into cortical layers, and the process of myelination and apoptosis begins: more than 70% of the neurons that have formed undergo apoptosis from 28 weeks to the end of gestation: 50% of the neurons created in the first 7 months die. It is important to note that the structure of the brain is as much a product of growth and proliferation as it is of cell death and rearrangement.

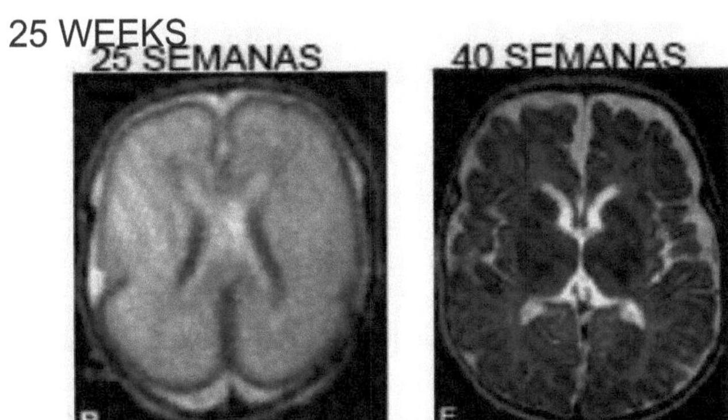

Figure 21.4. Brain imaging in a 25-week preterm infant and a term infant

Neuronal apoptosis occurs under normal conditions in an environment of "minimum stimulation": darkness, silence, with an adequate posture and in a state of foetal well-being without stressful situations. In a preterm newborn who at birth is transferred to a neonatal ward or NICU, this situation is altered, the patient not being in a physiological and adequate situation for the correct development of his central nervous system, as he is overstimulated and this alters the process of neuronal apoptosis, which can give rise to long-term neuropsychological and sensory consequences and problems.

The aim of CCDs is to enhance brain development and developmental outcome by preventing toxic sensory overload in an immature but rapidly growing nervous system.

Intrauterine environment: The ideal environment for sensory and motor development

The foetus begins its development in an environment that modulates all the stimuli that act on it during its development: the maternal uterus.

In this warm, dark and warm environment, the foetus receives the necessary stimuli for the development of the senses which appear and mature sequentially (tactile, proprioceptive/kinaesthetic, vestibular/auditory, smell/taste and vision). In addition, the uterus fulfils other basic functions such as nutrition, thermoregulation and modulation of the sleep-wake cycle.

From a postural point of view, the uterus provides flexion, which favours the middle Knea, containment and comfort of the foetus, which is in deep sleep 80% of the day.

Children who are born prematurely are dramatically deprived of this pathophysical environment and miss out on the intrauterine stimulation necessary to complete proper development.

Sensory experiences allow us to learn about and interact with the environment around us and also have a great impact on the central nervous system. The tactile, proprioceptive and vestibular systems are very vulnerable in the period of rapid brain growth and neuronal differentiation that occurs between 28-40 weeks of gestation, which is why to achieve adequate sensory integration in the preterm newborn, we must provide opportunities for the newborn to self-regulate, modulate their responses, organise themselves and produce adaptive responses to the environment.

According to the literature, many of the respiratory and cardio-circulatory problems that occur in preterm infants may be the result of the neonate's attempts to adapt to the extra-uterine environment and to the aggression of the stay in a Neonatal Unit.

Teona developmental synactive

This theona is based on the studies of Dr. Heidelise Als, included in the NIDCAP (*Neonatal Individualized Development Care and Assessment Program*), who applied to the preterm infant the methodology of observation of neonatal behaviour developed by the group of Dr. Thomas Berry Brazelton. Dr. Als' theory provides a framework for understanding preterm behaviour, according to which the infant's behaviours are interpreted according to five systems of functioning:

1. *Motor*: Assesses muscle tone, movement, activity and posture.
2. *Autonomic*: Assesses skin colour, heart rate and breathing pattern.
3. *States*: Categorises the level of the central nervous system in terms of sleep.

deep-sleep-light sleep-wakefulness-wakefulness-sleep (according to the states described by Brazelton, ampKa in practice seminar 1), demonstrating the robustness and modulation of their states and patterns of transition from one to the other.

4. *Attention-interaction*: A child's ability to interact with the environment.
5. *Self-regulation*: Values the child's efforts to achieve balance with the other subsystems.

In the healthy term newborn these subsystems are mature, integrated, synchronised and function uniformly. Preterm infants are unable to handle environmental stimuli, responding hyper-reactively and with poor tolerance to minimal stimuli. As a consequence they exhibit loss of control and stress responses.

Individualised developmental care interventions are aimed at improving physical and behavioural outcomes, reducing environmental stressors and restructuring care activities in response to the child's behavioural cues.

There are two categories of behaviour:

a) **Regulatory behaviour**

Whether the stimulus is appropriate in intensity, complexity and time.

The balance of self-regulation is demonstrated by the presence of regular breathing, rosy colour, stable visceral functions, smooth movements, modulated tone, calm gaze and gently flexed postures with periods of continuous sleep and alertness.

b) **Stress behaviour**

In response to stimuli that are too complex, intense or inappropriate in time.

We observe in the newborn: *changes in colour (pale pink), stretching of hands and feet, facial grimacing*. Unstable and stretching behaviours are considered to reflect stress while well modulated flexing behaviours may reflect self-regulation.

The preemie tries to avoid negative stimuli by turning his head, raising his hands and shielding his face with his hands.

These are signals against overloading of stimuli:

- Averting the view or turning the head away from the module
- Frowning

- Squeeze lips tightly together
- Twisting movements of the arms, legs or trunk
- Exaggerated and sustained extension of arms and/or legs
- Hyperextension or arching of the trunk
- Peripheral oxygen desaturation
- Variable respiratory rate and heart rate
- Colour changes
- Exaggerated salivation

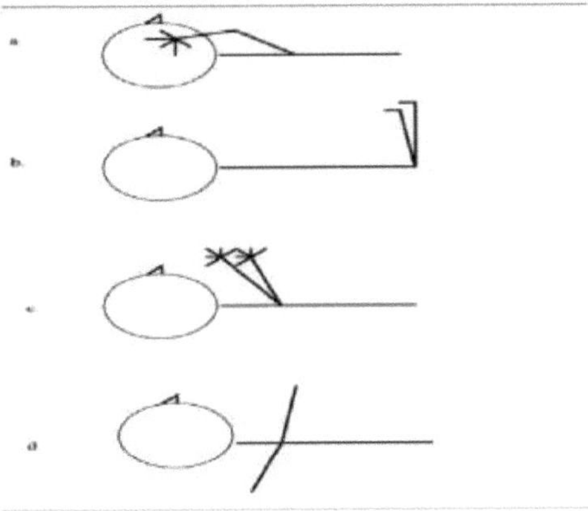

Figure 21.2. *Arm and leg movements indicative of stress.*

Brazelton Scale

The NBAS (Neonatal Behavioural Assessment Scale or Brazelton Scale) is an interactive assessment technique and is considered to be one of the best suited for both the detection of deficits and the identification of emerging abilities of the newborn, key aspects for the initiation of early intervention. This scale is considered to be the systematisation of a very detailed clinical examination of the newborn, the essential part of which is the evaluation of behaviour, but without neglecting the neurological assessment of the newborn. Until recently, the Brazelton Scale has been used primarily as a research instrument, but in recent years it has been adapted for clinical use. The aim of the clinical use of the scale is to create in the parents the ability to observe their newborn child, so that they themselves will be the ones to detect from the first days which strategies or forms of action are the most suitable at each moment of their child's development.

With its application we obtain a profile of scores that allows us to detect a possible alteration or pathology, but at the same time, within the normal parameters, to detect both the potentialities or "strong points" and the problems or "weak points" of the newborn, as well as its peculiar ways of acting and reacting to the variables of the environment. A profile of the child's behavioural characteristics is thus obtained.

The Brazelton scale assesses the newborn's behavioural repertoire in 28 behavioural items that are rated on a 9-point scale. The scale also includes an assessment of neurological status in 18 reflex items, each with a 4-point rating. The reflex items will identify gross neurological abnormalities if the scores deviate from the norm, although they are not designed for neurological diagnosis. In the second edition of the NBAS (Brazelton, 1984) a series of 7 additional items were added with the intention of better capturing the degree of frailty and the quality of behaviour of high-risk children.

The Brazelton scale can be used without any adaptation in term infants and can be applied until the end of the second month of life. With the addition of supplementary items it can also be used in apparently healthy preterm infants (less than 37 weeks gestation) and for them, depending on the degree of immaturity, application is possible up to 48 weeks post-conceptional age.

The 28 behavioural and 18 reflex ftems are administered in a particular sequence and can be grouped into "modules" that follow a set order. This grouping makes the sequence of administration easy to remember; the items have also been categorised into other groups according to their conceptual affinity; asb all the items in the habituation module are designed to assess the neonate's ability to inhibit to aversive stimuli. These items are to be administered in sequence. Those measuring visual and auditory abilities are collected in the orientation module and administered together. The other items on the scale are grouped in terms of the level of intensity of stimulation required and are administered according to the increase in intensity.

The modules are as follows:

a)   the habituation module, comprising the repeated stimulus response decrementing items. This group should be administered first and only omitted if the child is not in appropriate sleep states;

b)   the oral-motor module. This group of minimally invasive items includes the foot reflexes and the search reflex, the sucking and glabella items;

c)   the core module includes all moderately stimulating ftems: undressing and manipulation, including also tonic deviation of head and eyes;

d)   the vestibular module comprises the ftems of maximum manipulation and stimulation: defensive movements, tonic neck reflex and Moro;

e)   the social-interactive module includes all the orientation items and is linked to the state of consciousness. It can only be administered when the child is in an appropriate state of alertness and is therefore a movable group. The assessment of the ability to be comforted and the ability to be comforted can also interrupt the standard sequence if the infant becomes tearful.

As a general guideline, it is advisable to memorise the total outline of the administration. In this respect it is recommended to consult the audio-visual supplementary material on this subject (https://www.youtube.com/watch?v=F vgTelzHE.).

Before administering the scale, we must stop for 2 minutes to observe the neonate's condition:

a)   State 1: Deep sleep. Regular breathing, eyes closed, no spontaneous activity except jerking or spasmodic movements. No eye movements.

b)   State 2: Slight snoring. Irregular breathing. Eyes closed. Low level of activity. Rapid eye movements under closed eyelids.

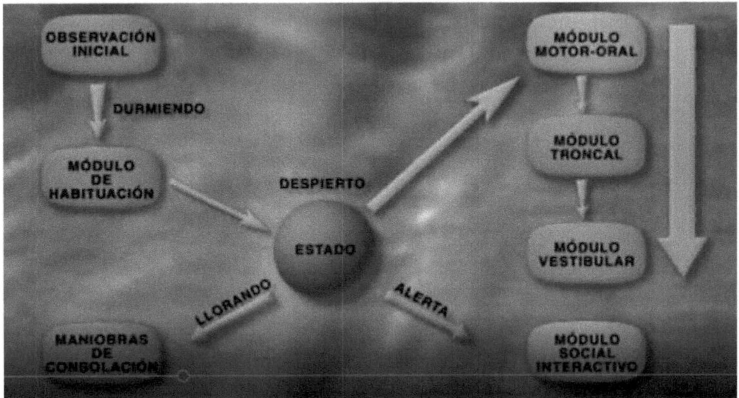

Figure 21.3. *Sequence in the realisation of the Brazelton test modules.*

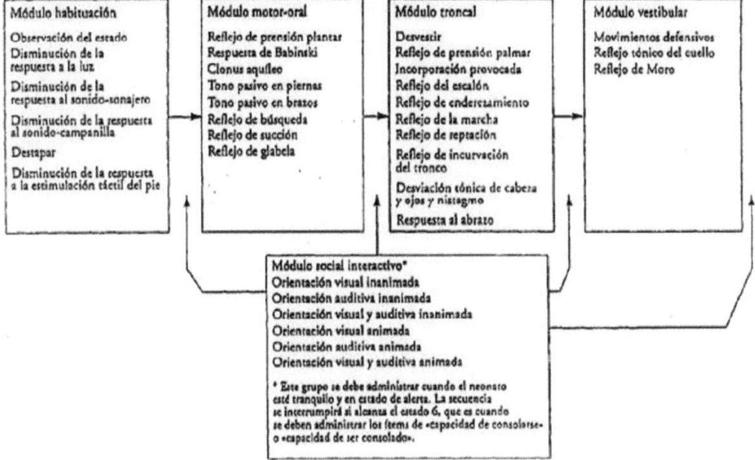

Figure 21.4. *Relation of the items included in each of the modules during the performance of the Barzelton test.*

c)   State 3: Smelly. Eyes open but fluctuating. Dull gaze. Eyelids heavy or closed. Level of activity variable.

d)   State 4: Alert. Bright eyes. Full attention to source of stimulation. Minimal motor activity.

e)   State 5: Irritability. Eyes open. Considerable motor activity. Brief vocalizations of excitement.

f)   State 6: Crying. High level of motor activity.

When the Brazelton scale is used in the clinic, it is intended to incorporate parents as active participants in the process of observing and learning more about their child's behaviour and also with the intention of developing a relationship with the family. That is, it is used to a) sensitise parents to the individuality of their child and promote a positive relationship between them; b) share parents' concerns about their child's future development; and c) promote positive collaboration between the caregiver and the clinician or health service that will continue to care for the child and the family.

Developmentally focused neonatal care

CCDs are interventions designed to reduce stress in neonatal units, reduce pain associated with diagnostic tests and invasive treatments, and facilitate parental involvement in the care of their child.

The objectives of the CCDs are:

1.   Provide appropriate medical and non-medical therapy to prevent the brain from being damaged by inappropriate and painful stimuli.

2.   Minimise and reduce energy expenditure and stress.

3.   To provide experiences that help the newborn to develop normally in the 5 areas (subsystems) that are the basis for motor, mental and social development.

4.   To provide personalised family-centred care for the child in their concept of belonging.

The consequences of CCDs are:

1.   Increased growth and weight gain in the short term.

2.   Reduction of mechanical ventilation time.

3.   Earliest suckling and feeding at the breast.

4.   Decreased incidence of intraventricular haemorrhage.

5.   They promote neuro-development.

6.   They reduce the number of days and costs of hospitalisation.

The caregiver must adapt the newborn's environment and care with the aim of reducing stressful behaviours and promoting self-regulatory behaviours. CCD interventions aim to improve the micro and macro environment of the newborn and to involve the parents in the care of the newborn. The CCD does not imply a change in the therapeutic processes, but in the attitudes of the professionals towards the newborn. The newborn becomes the centre of attention and these measures are inexpensive to implement.

Table 22.1. Some measures to be taken in CCD.

EASY TO IMPLEMENT	MEDIUM DIFFICULTY	HIGH DIFFICULTY	EXTREME DIFFICULTY
- Skin-to-skin contact - Breastfeeding Promotion - Identification and treatment of pain - Posture - Light reduction	- Limitation of Environmental Noise - Establishing "quiet hours" - Minimal manipulation - Kangaroo Method	- Free entry for parents - Entry of other family members - Spaces for parents and family members - Support groups	- NIDCAP in NICU

Interventions on the macro-environment of the neonate

This section includes interventions on:

a. Light
b. Noise
c. Activity
d. Encouraging dreaming
e. Rest

Light

Development of vision in the foetus: Vision is the last sense to develop, at around 32-33 weeks gestational age, the eyelids are closed until the 24th or 25th week, although they allow light to penetrate. The neurosensory phase of vision development coincides with synaptogenesis (late 2nd trimester) and inappropriate stimuli may interfere with its development. The relationship between light exposure and retinopathy of prematurity has not been demonstrated.

Recommendations

1. Measure the light intensity level of the unit and adjust it to the recommended levels.
2. Where possible, use natural light but regulate the entry of natural light (windows with dark curtains or blinds).
3. Use of dimmable and individualised lights. For the exploration of the infants, it is best to use the individual spotlights of the incubators, but avoid focusing on the face (protect the face from the light, e.g. by creating a shadow with the blanket). Try to ensure that the caregiver does not stand between the spotlight and the infant (so that the movement does not alter moments of light and shadow).
4. Cover the incubators with thick blankets, but leave a small strip so that the infant can be viewed and assessed periodically without having to lift the blanket.
5. Use of torches for spot observations of the child
6. Avoid direct exposure to light (cover eyes).
7. Smooth sleep-wake transition
8. If kangaroo care is used, it should be done in a darkened area or with the child protected from light.
9. Individualise light exposure according to maturity and stability.
10. Inform parents about the importance of adequate lighting so that the child can make contact with them.
11. Provide circadian rhythms for preterm infants over 32SG.
12. Use individualised lighting for the execution of therapeutic procedures.
13. Use of eye protection in premature infants undergoing phototherapy treatment

The illumination of the unit should be measured and documented, aiming for natural and gradual light, with a smooth transition in the light-dark cycles.

More mature and stable newborns are able to tolerate more visual stimulation. They may be able to visually explore toys or mobiles located within their visual field. Face-to-face interaction during breastfeeding or the newborn's alertness may be appropriate for visual stimulation.

Through a reduction of light in the neonatal units, greater respiratory stability, lower heart rate, more stable blood pressure and modulated motor activity have been achieved.

Noise

Premature infants are extremely sensitive to noise. The NICU sometimes presents an excessively noisy environment for them, with no day-night rhythm. Excessive noise or loud, high-pitched noises can damage the premature infant's delicate hearing structures, leading to some risk of sensorineural hearing loss and may affect their biorhythms.

Development of the auditory system: The human auditory system undergoes most of its development before the end of gestational age, with cochlear and auditory function beginning at 22-24 weeks with continued maturation of the auditory pathways to the central nervous system. Thus, the development and maturation of the auditory sensory system in preterm infants can occur in a neonatal unit, with airborne (as opposed to intrauterine) sounds, which can be continuous, unpredictable and loud, even by adult standards.

There is evidence of adverse effects on the child related to noise, such as interference with sleep, episodes of desaturation, and increased intracranial pressure in very unstable children.

There is a consensus that permanent exposure to a noisy environment disrupts sleep states and interferes with other physiological functions. This is particularly detrimental for neonates, because their sleep states are frequently disrupted while in the ICU. Consequently, they experience sleep deprivation as a result of spending little time in deep sleep, which causes the neonate to utilise the energy necessary for essential metabolic growth and healing procedures.

The following have been shown to be adverse effects caused by noise:

a)   Immediate adverse effects:

- Apnoea
- Bradycardia
- Heart rate fluctuations
- Dyspnoea
- Increased blood pressure
- Decrease in oxygen saturation

b)   Medium-term adverse effects

- Decrease in growth hormones
- Increased risk of hearing loss
- Increased risk of hyperactivity and attention deficit disorders

Recommendations

1.   Place ear-shaped sound level meters on room walls to raise awareness among staff and family. The AAP recommends levels < 45 dB (10-55 dB) and a maximum of 65-70 dB transiently.

2.   Posters informing about the harmful effects of noise

3.   Use of doors with silent closing mechanisms, keep them closed to avoid corridor noise.

4.   Control noise inside incubators:

i. Covered with a thick, dark blanket

ii. Do not support anything or write on the incubator

iii. Do not knock or leave objects on the incubators

iv. Careful opening and closing of the incubator doors

5. Cooperation of all professionals to reduce environmental noise:

i. Avoid crowding inside the NICU.

ii. Keep conversations away from the child and in a soft tone of voice.

iii. Keeping mobile phones in silent mode

iv. Reduce the ringing of landlines and pagers, answer them quickly v. Wherever possible, use sound and light alarms.

vi. Turn off alarms as quickly as possible, and reduce their volume.

vii. Prevent alarms from sounding prior to manipulations

6. Minimise noise generated by equipment inside the NICU (toilets, waste bins, etc.). Repair noisy equipment.

7. Move as many devices away from children as possible. Remove radios, telephones or printers from areas where incubators are located.

8. Locate the most labile patients away from high traffic areas.

9. Lowering of the light level, which helps to reduce noise.

Interventions on the neonatal microenvironment

This section includes interventions on:

a. Postural care and manipulations.

b. Minimum stimulation protocol.

c. Pain management

Table 21.2. Noise sources in the NICU.

SOURCE GENERATING NOISE	LEVEL dB
General CIN environment: voice, telephone, equipment...	45- 85
Alarms, pumps and monitors	60- 80
Close incubator door	110-120
H2O bubbling in breather circuit	62-87
Open incubator door	92
Finger drumming in the incubator	70-95

Postural care

Premature newborns admitted to a Neonatal Unit find it more difficult to maintain the flexed posture that they would have maintained in utero at the end of gestation. In addition, he/she has poor muscle tone which makes it impossible for him/her to overcome the action of gravity, forcing him/her to adopt a postural pattern in extension which moves him/her away from the midline of relaxation, favouring the retraction of the muscles of the back and hips. Poor positioning of the premature infant can cause long-term deformities such as: abduction and external rotation of the hip, eversion of the ankle, retraction and abduction of the shoulders, greater cervical hyperextension with elevation of the shoulders and progressive flattening of the head. This can affect the child's psychomotor development, the attachment relationship with parents and the child's own self-esteem as he/she matures.

The objectives of postural care of the premature infant are:

a. Stimulate active trunk and limb flexion (facilitate hand-mouth activity).

b. Achieve a more rounded skull and active rotation.

c. Achieve more symmetrical postures.

d. Facilitate anti-gravity movements.

e. Stimulate visual exploration of the environment (head in middle Knea).

f. Maintain a necessary degree of flexion, which allows for greater self-regulation and self-calming, which in turn helps in the organisation of behaviour.

The position of choice will generally be the lateral decubitus position as it keeps the limbs aligned and in the middle Knee, facilitates self-comfort movements (hand-hand, hand-mouth) and improves trunk and pelvic flexion.

As considerations we will have to try to keep arms and legs bent with hands close to the face, back bent, feet that can touch, Kmites on head and feet, as well as elements of containment around them. We will have to favour the alternation of both sides.

Table 21.3. Adverse effects of poor body positioning.

A ggf!g£.'"g	A/ftflgg/Mg
Asymmetrical head position Extensor posture y asymmetrical with tendency to neck and trunk extension y trunk extension Retract-on y shoulder rotation with scapular adduction. Abduction and external rotation of the hips. flexion of the knees torsion of the tibia e.ersion of the ankle	Cranial deformities: - Cranial anteroposterior flattening 1 Scaphocephaly). - Lococcipital flattening (Ptagiocefaiia) - Torticolrs influences ooentation y preference for visual tuning manual function y asymmetrical marking pattern has negative impact on the development of hand orientation at midline and hand-eye coordination May delay crawling and gait development

The prone posture, on the other hand, improves respiratory function. It also increases diaphragmatic movement and stabilises temperature control. It is advisable to use a ventral support and to avoid retraction of the shoulders. The arms should remain flexed and close to the mouth. The hips and knees should also be flexed with Kmites at the head and feet and restraints around them. As a disadvantage, the prone position makes alignment in the middle Knee and movement difficult. Newborns will have less visual and auditory stimulation.

The decubitus supine position is considered to be an assessment position as it facilitates procedures and observation-exploration of the infant. In addition, it seems to prevent Sudden Infant Death Syndrome. This posture contributes least to self-regulation. In order to use this posture in the infant, the head should be in midline or slightly to one side with arms flexed, knees in semi-flexion, head and foot boundaries and restraints around them. As disadvantages, this posture makes flexion more difficult, but facilitates extension. The premature infant has less respiratory capacity, with an increased incidence of apnoea, hyperextension of the neck and scapular retraction. It also favours greater temperature loss. Premature infants in the supine position are often extremely agitated, flailing limbs, tachycardic and consuming large amounts of energy and calories. All postural changes should be gentle and gradual, and should not be greater than 90°.

Restraint of the body is another measure that increases the infant's sense of security, providing stillness and self-control, and improving stress tolerance. Simple measures such as swaddling the preemie, holding hands in the midline while handling, etc. help self-regulation. The infant should be handled in a flexed position, favouring the prone or lateral position. Premature infants experience excessive handling, which is increased by the permanent procedures to which they are subjected and thus by their level of severity. As postural measures, it is important to try to change the position of the baby in the lateral cubitus position, since the supine position, raising the legs, increases the central venous pressure, which can be reflected in the intracranial pressure.

Minimal Stimulation Protocol

Research reports that the number of manipulations in newborns in intensive care exceeds 100 in 24 hours. Handling and positioning of the preterm infant should be one of the first and foremost concerns for caregivers in order to intervene in the development of the preterm infant.

When infants are in a quiet sleep, they should not be interrupted by any procedure. It is important for the infant to be allowed to continue sleeping when in a quiet sleep. Care should be taken to maintain a protocol for minimal handling of the preterm infant. These rules should be applied at least during the first week of life and thereafter should be individualised according to the condition of the infant.

This protocol consists of establishing specific times for handling the newborn, grouping non-urgent procedures and examinations within these times and coordinating the handling by the nurse, the neonatologists and the specialists. It is also important after the procedure to "accompany the premature newborn back to sleep", trying to return the newborn to the appropriate state of comfort. Constant manipulation of the newborn has been associated as a potential factor in intraventricular haemorrhage.

Pain management

We know that after 20-22 weeks the foetus is able to react to light, sound and other environmental stimuli. Preterm infants must endure many painful procedures during their stay in the NICU or in the intermediate care area. Untreated pain in the newborn contributes to morbidity and mortality, and the absence of pain is a basic right of all patients.

There are difficulties in assessing pain in newborns because of their inability to express themselves. **Pain scales** should be used to assess and record pain and to apply treatment measures. There are more than 40 scales to assess pain, none of them have demonstrated superiority over the rest (there is no gold standard), and most of them are developed for the assessment of acute and/or short-lasting pain. There is little evidence for the assessment of chronic pain.

We have a number of indicators to assess pain:

1. **Physiological indicators.** Physiological indicators of pain are heart rate, respiratory rate, oxygen saturation, vagal tone, changes in heart and respiratory rate and sweating. Some of them are useful for preterm infants, others for term infants and others for both.

2. **Behavioural indicators**. Behavioural indicators are crying, facial expression (wrinkling the forehead, squeezing the eyes, nasolabial folds and opening the mouth) and body movements (spreading fingers, squeezing fingers).

3. **Contextual indicators.** A number of factors may modify the response to pain, including: intensity of stimulation, sleep/wakefulness state (less responsive during sleep), severity of illness, state of consciousness (behavioural indicators may be absent in some infants with decreased level of consciousness or pharmacological paralysis), gestational age, postnatal age and type of pain.

When pain is prolonged, notable physiological changes and behavioural indicators occur in the infant. During episodes of prolonged pain, newborns in a state of passivity with few, if any, body movements; a facial expression; decreased heart rate and respiratory tract variability; and decreased oxygen consumption, all suggestive of a decrease in basal metabolism in order to save energy.

PIPP (Premature Infant Pain Profile, Stevens 1996)

PIPP (Premature Infant Pain Profile, Stevens 1996)

Indicador (tiempo de observación)	0	1	2	3
Gestación	≥ 36 semanas	32 a < 36	28 a < 32	≤ 28 semanas
Comportamiento *(15 seg)	Despierto y activo ojos abiertos con movimientos faciales	Despierto e inactivo ojos abiertos sin movimientos faciales	Dormido y activo ojos cerrados con movimientos faciales	Dormido e inactivo ojos cerrados sin movimientos faciales
Aumento de FC *(30 seg)	0 – 4 lpm	5 – 14 lpm	15 – 24 lpm	≥ 25 lpm
Disminución Sat O_2 *(30 seg)	0 – 2,4%	2,5 – 4,9%	5 – 7,4%	≥ 7,5%
Entrecejo fruncido *(30 seg)	0 – 3 seg	3 – 12 seg	> 12 – 21 seg	> 21 seg
Ojos apretados *(30 seg)	0 – 3 seg	3 – 12 seg	> 12 – 21 seg	> 21 seg
Surco nasolabial *(30 seg)	0 – 3 seg	3 – 12 seg	> 12 – 21 seg	> 21 seg

*Comparar comportamiento basal y 15 segundos después del procedimiento doloroso

*Comparar situación basal y 30 segundos después del procedimiento doloroso

Interpretación: dolor leve o no dolor | 6 | dolor moderado | 12 | dolor intenso

Figure 21.4. *PIPP scale.*

Pain assessment scales

One of the most widely used pain assessment scales is the PIPP scale (Premature Infant Pain Profile) developed by Stevens in 1996. The PIPP scale is one of the most widely used, as it is applicable to term and preterm infants, it is valid for procedural pain, it is valid for assessment of postoperative and/or acute condition, and it is the most complete scale for pain research. As disadvantages of this scale, its use is questionable in intubated infants and it is not useful for chronic pain.

Pain reduction mechanisms

a) **Non-pharmacological analgesia.** Non-pharmacological analgesia is a series of prophylactic and complementary measures aimed at reducing pain and which do not involve the administration of medication.

As mechanisms of action are described, but not yet well explained:

-    Release of endogenous endorphins.
-    Activation of opioid-enhancing neuropeptide systems.
-    Pain "distraction".

These measures are:

- Organisation and appropriate environment in the neonatal unit:

-    Defined analgesia protocols
-    Person in charge of analgesia for each procedure manipulation
-    Adaptation to the sleep-wake cycle
-    A suitable environment with reduced light and noise enhances the effect of pharmacological and non-pharmacological measures and modifies painful experiences.

-Administration of   24% sucrose orally, *2 min before the painful stimulus,* **0.2 cc:**

-    Safe and effective method to reduce pain (especially heel prick, venipuncture), greater effect if sucrose + suction.
-    The optimum dosage is not known, but the most widespread is 24% sucrose, ideally using pre-prepared or pharmacy-prepared single doses, or alternatively 3 sachets of ordinary sugar (8 g) in 100 ml of filtered water.
-    Store at room temperature and renew at every shift.
-    It should not be used indiscriminately to calm irritability.

More studies are needed to determine the safety of repeated dosing, especially in extremely underweight and ventilator-assisted children (Cochrane Database Syst Rev, 2010).

- Non-nutritive suction:

-    Sucking on a teat reduces pain scores.
-    The maximum effect is achieved when sucrose administration is used in conjunction with the sucking of a teat.

- Breastfeeding or administration of mother's milk:

-    It reduces pain and has a similar effect to sucrose.
-    Reduced pain and greater analgesia than with oral sucrose (not dummy) in terms after capillary punctures (breast: mean PIPP of 3; sucrose: mean PIPP 8.5).
-    There is a lack of studies in preterm infants.
-    Its use is increasingly justified by other benefits in the proper colonisation of the intestinal tract.

- Mother Kangaroo Care:

The **Mother Kangaroo Method** is a technique for the care of the newborn baby in a situation of low birth weight and/or prematurity that is based on skin-to-skin contact between the mother and the baby and the care in feeding, stimulation and protection that the mother provides to the baby. Skin-to-skin contact can also be provided by the father or another adult. This method effectively meets the newborn's needs for warmth, nourishment (breastfeeding), protection from infection, stimulation, security and love, and its effectiveness is similar to, and in some circumstances even superior to, traditional care (i.e. incubator) when compared in terms of mortality and morbidity.

This is one of the aspects that is best documented with very good evidence, therefore, the kangaroo method should be applied as an analgesic method. Whenever possible wait for the parents to come and offer them this possibility.

- **Containment measures:**

The aim is to keep the child in a flexed position with the limbs close to the trunk and towards the midline.

- **Manipulations between two people:**

Always, especially in premature infants, unless it is not possible, so that one person will be in charge of analgesia. Pharmacological pain control measures should be reserved for moderate to severe pain, or as an adjuvant in more severe cases. It requires monitoring to ensure ventilation, oxygenation and haemodynamic stability, and the dose will be defined according to the cause of the pain and the patient's response to the drug.

Pharmacological measures include:

- Opiates: Morphine, fentanyl, meperidine...
- Non-opioids: Paracetamol, NSAIDs: ibuprofen, ketorolac, indomethacin, metamizole (pharmacokinetics unknown in the newborn).
- Anaesthetics: Ketamine, topical anaesthetics (EMLA)
- Sedative-hypnotics: Phenobarbital, midazolam.

Parents as primary caregivers

The newborn baby, premature or not, is born with an urgent need to be with its mother, as she is the safest environment for it. The World Health Organisation (WHO) recommends that newborns should not be separated from their mothers, as this is detrimental to the physical, emotional and mental health of the baby and the mother. Close contact with the mother favours better psychomotor development, greater stimulation and an increased sense of security for the baby. Immediate skin-to-skin contact between newborn and mother after birth regulates the baby's heart rate, temperature, blood glucose and immune system.

The involvement of parents in the care of their children is one of the basic axes of care in neonatology. Few aspects of neonatal medicine are as important, and often as neglected, as the care of the family of a critically ill or immature infant. Parents are the mainstay of a child's development, especially during the first few years of life, and their early involvement in the care of the newborn improves the prognosis. Interactions with parents give the child confidence and security and allow the child to develop healthy emotional bonds that are important for the attachment process.

Achieving full parental involvement implies changes in the structure of the units, in timetables and, above all, in the attitudes of the caregivers, who must become aware that they are caring for families, not just the newborn. Increasing mother-child interaction helps the mother to gain greater security and self-confidence. Separation causes the newborn to feel helpless and to suffer from stress.

For parents, the birth of a premature or sick child is a traumatic situation, and they must go through a series of phases to come to terms with this situation of grief: Denial -> Anger -> Bargaining -> Depression -> Acceptance. Parents are surrounded by fears and doubts, and feel partly to blame for what has happened to their child. The birth of a premature child is an unexpected life event, for which the parents are neither physically nor psychically prepared and which provokes a crisis in the family, whose responses in each individual are determined by pre-existing personality factors, social and cultural variables. It involves a deep wound in the self-esteem of the parents, especially the mother, leading to feelings of failure, failure and guilt.

Parents should be given adequate information about what is happening to their child, conveying the truth, but with a certain attitude of "realistic optimism". We must offer them dedication, time, privacy and understanding and always give information adapted to their level of knowledge.

Adaptation to the NICU environment

The scenario of the first visit to the intensive care unit must be prepared and anticipated by the professionals. Parents find themselves in a world of which they are previously unaware. They are welcomed into an environment of lights, alarms and high technology, they meet a very young child in a very distant environment, beyond their understanding and control, and this can be overwhelming for them. The mother's anxiety increases as the child gets smaller.

Parents have to start the process of bonding with and loving their child, while preparing for the possible loss of the child, or while having doubts about their child's survival and future. We must convey the message to them that they are welcome and that their visits play a useful and important role for the child and that they should not feel excluded from the group of caregivers. Every family is different and has different needs and if we don't see them, some parents become hostile and project their frustration against the team. The process of parental involvement increases as the child improves. They move from being passive to active participants, gain confidence in their ability and stop feeling like a peripheral figure and become a central figure.

Some of the measures proposed to provide better care for families are:

- Provide prenatal care for parents of at-risk pregnancies.
- Accompaniment between pre- and post-natal care by a reference person.
- Encourage fathers to be closer to their children, integrate fathers into care. We want parents who care, not who worry.
- Teach parents to recognise the different states of their child.
- Encourage parents to interact with their child when the child's condition and the child's needs are
medical conditions permit. Teach parents to recognise signs of stress in children in order to modify stimulation and interaction.
- Teach comforting manoeuvres for the child, and positioning techniques.
- Keep parents informed about their child's condition.
- Detecting and dealing with parental stress. Ideally, parent meetings should be held to address these concerns.
- Detect and attend to socio-family situations of risk.
- Work with understanding and respect for cultural differences.
- Offer attention to the rest of the family (siblings, grandparents...).

Kangaroo care

In 1979, Dr. Rey and Dr. Martmez of the San Juan de Dios Hospital in Bogota (Colombia), concerned about the insufficient number of incubators to care for premature infants and the high rate of hospital infections, initiated a programme of care for premature infants which, in short, consisted of placing the infant in skin-to-skin contact between the mother's breasts, feeding the infant with breast milk, early discharge and continuing this type of care at home. As this method spread to other countries, studies began to appear identifying the many advantages of the kangaroo method for the child. After more than three decades, it seems clear that kangaroo care should be offered to all sick preterm or term infants as an alternative to incubator care, as it is effective for temperature control, promotes breastfeeding and allows and strengthens mother/father-child bonding.

Kangaroo care is defined as skin-to-skin contact between mother and preterm infant as early, continuously and for as long as possible with breastfeeding.

Kangaroo care must have all three components:

1. Skin-to-skin contact, placing the naked child, except for the comb, on the mother's breast, as soon and as often as possible.

2. Breastfeeding.

3. Early discharge with close follow-up.

Technique for carrying out kangaroo-type care

Once the preterm infant is considered ready for skin-to-skin contact, the parents should be properly explained the technique, reassured and informed about the advantages of this type of care. The infant is placed between her breasts so that the front wall of the infant's chest is in contact with the mother's skin. The infant's head should be turned to one side and it is advisable to keep it in a slightly extended position so that the airway is free and visual contact between mother and child is allowed. The mother's breathing will help to stimulate the infant's breathing. There is the option of securing the infant to the mother with a cloth band, so that the mother can stand up and perform all kinds of movements without the infant being at risk of falling. In many neonatal units the infant is not attached to the mother, but is simply covered with her clothes or a blanket and the mother herself holds the infant with her hands. The infant should be naked, covered with a cap and booties, and optionally with honeycomb trimmed at the front to facilitate skin-to-skin contact.

Leaving the incubator for kangaroo care involves some stress for the newborn, so it is recommended that the infant remains in kangaroo care for at least 90-120 minutes, as less time in skin-to-skin contact does not seem to offer any advantages. The practice of kangaroo care is now considered to be one of the most valuable tools available to increase the positive stimuli that the preterm infant can receive to enhance development. The newborn baby is born with the need to be with his mother, she is the safest environment for him. Skin-to-skin contact and breastfeeding represent the normal state that allows the newborn to adapt optimally to the extra-uterine environment. Skin-to-skin contact improves the newborn's heart rate, temperature, blood glucose, immune system, sleep, weight gain and brain maturation.

Benefits of the kangaroo method

a. Benefits for the premature infant.

Numerous studies, including several clinical trials, are now available that examine the benefits of kangaroo care in different aspects. Particular attention has been paid to thermoregulation, breastfeeding, apnoea pauses, pain, infections, weight gain and emotional and bonding aspects of parenting. The kangaroo position favours the reception of a series of positive stimuli: auditory through the mother's voice, olfactory through proximity to the mother's body, vestibular-kinaesthetic through the baby's position on the mother's chest, tactile through skin-to-skin contact, and visual, since placing the baby in a semi-incorporated position allows him to see his mother's face and body. All the care that favours the development of the child during admission will facilitate the adequate organisation of the brain and its subsequent evolution.

b.   Benefits for parents.

In a study on the perceptions of parents of premature infants admitted to Spanish neonatal units, the impressions of those who had used the kangaroo method were collected. First of all, parents attach great importance to the possibility of having physical contact with their child, especially close physical contact, such as that provided by the kangaroo method. Parents point to the moment when they can cuddle their child as a really important moment for them, and some say that it was in those first moments of physical contact that they recognised the child as their own. The possibility of practising the kangaroo method produces great satisfaction in the parents, makes them feel more competent in the care of their children, and in those moments they diminish the anxiety and anguish that comes with having their children admitted to the neonatal ICU. With the practice of the kangaroo method, we return the premature infant to its parents, who should be the true protagonists in the care of their children.

c.   Economic benefits.

The kangaroo method shortens the hospital stay: preterm infants experience a higher weight gain and parents feel more involved in the care of their preterm infant, thus increasing their confidence and feeling more prepared for discharge. An economic study was carried out in Tarragona on the implementation of the kangaroo method, in which an average reduction of 17 days of admission per premature infant was observed, calculating the average daily cost of a day's stay in the neonatal unit (average between the neonatal ICU and the intermediate unit) at 448 euros, the implementation of the kangaroo method resulted in an average cost reduction of 7,616 euros for each premature infant.

In a study conducted by Tessier in 2009, the positive impact of the kangaroo method was demonstrated. It was shown that both parents should be involved in the procedure and that this intervention should be targeted at those infants who are most at risk at birth. With the introduction of the kangaroo method in neonatal units, it is intended that premature infants see all their rights respected and that, together with the most appropriate and high technology they need, they can find the most humane of processes: integration into their own family nucleus, the best nourishment that the human species has prepared for them (breast milk) and early and prolonged physical contact with their parents.

Bibliograffa

1.   Vanderberg K.A. Individualized developmental care for high-risk newborns in the

NICU: Apractice guideline. Early Human Development. 2007; 83: 433-442.

2. Westrup B. Newborn Individualized Developmental Care Assessment Program (NIDCAP). Family-centred developmentally supportive care. Early human Development. 2007; 83: 443-449.

3. Als H, Duffy FH, McAnulty GB, Rivkin MJ, Vajapeyam S, Mulkern RV, Warfield SK, Huppi PS, Butler SC, Conneman N, Fischer C, Eichenwald EC. Early experience alters brain function and structure. Pediatrics 2004;113(4):846-57.

4. Perapoch Lopez J, Pallas Alonso CR, Linde Sillo MA, Moral Pumarega MT, Benito Castro F, Lopez Maestro M, Caseno Carbonero S, De la Cruz Bertolo J. Developmental Care. Situation in Spanish neonatology units. An Pediatr(Barc) 2006; 64(2): 132-9.

5. Gallegos Marfinez J, Reyes Hernandez J, Fernandez Hernandez VA, Gonzalez Gonzalez LA. Noise index in the neonatal unit. Its impact on newborns. Acta Pediatr Mex 2011;32(1):5-14.

6. Mondolfi A, Rojas I, Urbina H, Pacheco C, Bonini J, Vargas F. Pain management in intensive care and neonatology. Archivos venezolanos de puericultiura y pediatna 2002; 65(Supplement 1): S33-S43.

7. Als H, Lawhon G, Duffy FH, McAnulthy GB, Gibes-Grossman R, Blickman JG. Individualized Developmental Care Low-Birth-Weight Preterm Infant. JAMA 1994;272(11):853- 858.

8. Als Heidelise. Toward a synactive theory of development: Promise for the assessment and support of infant individuality. Infant Mental Health Journal 1982; 3(4): 229-243.

9. Als Heidelise. A synactive Model of Neonatal Behavioral Organization: Framework for de Assesment of Neurobehavioral Development in the Premature Infant and for Support of Infants and Parents in the neonatal Intensive Care Environment. 1986; 3(4):3-53.

10. Ministry of Health and Social Policy. Care from birth, evidence-based recommendations and good practice, 2010.

22. Analysis and evaluation of occupational performance in Paediatrics

Dr. Maria Luisa Fernandez Lopez

According to the Spanish Professional Association of Occupational Therapists (APETO), Occupational Therapy (OT) is a "social-healthcare profession that, by means of the assessment of the physical, psycho-sensorial and social capacities and problems of the individual, aims, with appropriate treatment, to enable them to achieve the greatest possible degree of independence in their daily life, contributing to the recovery from the illness and/or facilitating the adaptation to their disability".

The paediatric OT is currently considered an emerging field, all children who present some limitation, difficulty, problem or need some support for participation in some activity necessary for their life should benefit from occupational therapy, the diagnoses that are most frequently referred to Occupational Therapy are: cerebral palsy, psychomotor retardation, sensory processing disorders, Down syndrome, obstetric brachial palsy, muscular dystrophies, learning and attention disorders, behavioural disorders.

Based on the definition given by the APETO, the OT is the professional qualified to detect the difficulties of the individual, to improve the social participation of the minor, in accordance with the culture, society, age and level of development, aiming to promote the highest degree of inclusion and participation possible, for which he/she must have a systematic methodology of planning and intervention, thus determining the so-called Process of Intervention.

This process can be simplified into 4 blocks:

1. **Analysis and Evaluation, which includes the following sections:**

-Information gathering.

-**Examination** and complementary tests for occupational analysis and performance skills of the child.

-Occupational analysis: assessment of performance skills and child factors.

2. **Interpretation of results. Planning of objectives.**

3. **Intervention. Treatment.**

4. **Follow-up. Re-evaluation.**

Analysis and evaluation

Activity analysis is a logical reasoning process, in which the occupational therapist determines the various demands and skills in order to execute an activity. It is a technical reasoning tool through which an activity can be broken down into steps, elements, chaining sequence, materials, aptitudes and attitudes, cognitive, social and emotional skills.

In paediatrics the Occupational Therapy assessment process has to gather and interpret information from both the child's relatives and the child him/herself. The main intention is to collect information about the child's functioning, skills, abilities and possibilities.

Information gathering

The collection of information starts from the first contact with the child and the family, it is at that moment when the professional adopts an attitude of listening, observation, collection of concerns, difficulties and expectations that the parents expose. The occupational therapist takes note of the behaviour, attitude, tone of voice, attention, language used, play, reactions to an unfamiliar environment and person...

It is important to establish a relationship of trust between the OT and all the people involved in the process (the child, family, ...), in a comfortable and respectful environment. The professional will initiate an interview with appropriate questions to collect relevant information: current problem, family and personal background, weaknesses and strengths.

The most common sources to extract pre-assessment information: medical documents, school records, reports from other professionals who treat and know the child and family (paediatrician, school psychologist, educator, caregiver, social worker, physiotherapists...) and interviews with the referral source: teacher, doctor, caregiver...

Exploration and complementary tests for occupational analysis and child performance skills.

Once all the necessary data have been obtained, tools, materials and activities have to be selected to complete the assessment. The selection of tools to carry out the assessment requires a previous technical reasoning since many factors have to be taken into account: characteristics of the child and the family, skills of the child.

The most common procedure to perform the assessment:

- Observation of behaviour and skills.
- Interview with the child and carers, family, accompanying persons.
- Review of health history reports, school, specialists.
- Standardised testing, including questionnaire-type assessment.
- Activities directed at the main problem.

The application of different assessment tests provides us with information about the child's general and specific functioning (physical, mental and emotional).

Can be used:

- Standardised tools.
- Non-standardised but formal procedures, observations and interviews.
- Informal remarks.

It is important to remember that as soon as the therapist makes contact with the child and the family, the exploration begins through informal observation, taking note of each characteristic that can stimulate or inhibit the child's performance, spontaneous activity, connection with the environment, type of play, relationship and interaction with the examiner.

Occupational analysis: assessment of performance skills and child factors

In this phase we assess the skills, there is no specific sequence, but it is important to take into account the child's physical capacity and endurance, level of attention and emotional well-being.

- Motor skills   .
- Sensory skills   .
-     Communication and interpersonal skills.
- Skillsprocessing .

Assessment of motor skills, through play and various activities, fine and gross motor skills, visual-motor integration, oral motor skills, postural control and alignment, range of motion, strength, muscle tone, reflexes, endurance and coordination can be observed.

- *Gross motor skills*: the quality, form, symmetry, schemes, chaining and responses in the different movements and postural changes of the axis, lower and upper limbs are evaluated. Acquired developmental milestones: cephalic support, sitting, crawling, turning, standing, walking, going up and down stairs, jumping, running. Muscle tone, reflexes, postural control and alignment, range of motion, strength and endurance should be assessed.

- *Fine motor skills* are all those movements that require precision and coordination: grasping a small object with several fingers in opposition to the thumb (partial finger grasp) or with the thumb and forefinger (upper grip), feeding, dressing, grooming, writing, handicrafts...

- *Visuomotor integration* refers to how the eyes and hands are coordinated in order to working together.

- Oral motor skills, related to feeding, requires exploration of oral structures, swallowing skills, oral sensitivity, oral motor reflexes, oral motor skills and control including muscle forces of the face, mouth, neck, trunk and tongue.

Assessment of sensory skills. Sensory integration is responsible for organising the sensations that we receive from our body and the environment, it allows us to respond appropriately to the demands that are presented to us on a daily basis, i.e. all the information that our senses receive reaches the CNS and it is the CNS that has to process it appropriately to give an adaptive response to the environment.

The occupational therapist has to assess how information is modulated and processed from the sensory systems, and for this purpose it is sometimes necessary to carry out tests for vision and hearing as sensory problems, such as hearing loss or visual pathologies, can be identified.

- *Visual processing*: this is the dominant sense. It is necessary to ask if there is a history of visual problems. The OT can be helped by specialist reports: ophthalmologist, optometrist, and should also observe the child in play activities, functional tasks, drawing, writing.

- *Auditory processing*: the OT should assess the child's ability to respond to simple to complex verbal instructions without accompanying gestures.

- *Tactile* (somatosensory) *processing*, including:

a) Discriminatory system: perceiving and localising soft touch, deep pressure and discrimination between two points.

b) Protective system: tactile receptors are found throughout the skin and are generally stimulated and activated by touch stimuli: pain, pressure and temperature (cold and heat).

- *Vestibular processing*: The vestibular system is related to balance, movement coordination and spatial control, and is located in the inner ear. This system is activated by head movement, is influenced by gravity, and its functions are related to balance, protective reactions, muscle tone and balancing skills in order to maintain equilibrium and control posture.

- Proprioceptive processing informs about the spatial orientation of our body (position, joint movement, vibration and pressure) and has receptors in muscles, tendons and joints. This system is involved in body awareness, planning and precision of movements.

Communication and relationship skills. The area of communication can be divided into three parts:

1. Use (pragmatics) the social use of language is evaluated, i.e. the child greets when entering the consultation room, uses language to express his/her emotions, to ask for what he/she needs, respects turns, listens to others, says goodbye when leaving the consultation room...

2. Content (semantics) what words he/she uses and their meaning, vocabulary used is age-appropriate or lower, he/she understands the words he/she uses, he/she can relate words of the same family.

3. Form (morphology and phonetics) is concerned with the sentences used and understood and whether they are well structured, as well as assessing pronunciation.

Assessment of relationships with peers, familiar adults (relatives) and strangers (examiner).

Processing skills. Processing skills reflect the basic mental functions we use to plan, initiate, organise, manage, control and modify our activities of daily living. The occupational therapist should observe and analyse whether the child is able to perform activities of daily living efficiently and safely, how he/she makes decisions, whether he/she is able to solve routine problems.

Interpretation of results. Interpret, synthesise and summarise the data obtained

from both the history and the exploration carried out. Subsequently the occupational profile can be formulated, identifying the strengths and challenges occupations, performance skills and child factors that influence occupational performance and the analysed demands.

Interpretation and synthesis of the assessment data is important for intervention planning and can be done in the following steps:

- Formulation of the occupational profile: main problem of the child, characteristics of the child and his/her family, occupations, interests, school activities, extracurricular activities...

- Identification of the child's strengths and challenges.

- Identification of the performance skills of the child factors that may influence occupational performance.

Intervention. Treatment

Formulate an occupational profile to plan the activities to be carried out. Develop recommendations, determine plans and make them known to the child and family. Describe the amount of assistance required or the ranges of level of independence from being totally dependent, requiring various degrees and types of assistance, to being independent.

Follow-up. Re-evaluation

After each intervention session, it is important to make a summary of the activities carried out, evolution, challenges achieved and to give the information to the parents or carers of the child. It is also important to plan the next session.

Information gathering.

Analysis y Assessment. Exploration and complementary tests for the analysis of occupational and performance skills of the child.

Occupational analysis: performance skills assessment and

Interpretation of results. Planning of objectives.

Intervention. Treatment.

Follow-up. Re-evaluation.

Figure 23.1. *Outline of the intervention process.* **Key points**

Occupational therapy (OT) aims to promote health and well-being through occupation.

The TO tries to achieve maximum independence and improve the quality of life, adapting the child's tasks and environment such as play, relationships with peers and adults, self-care, ... as well as informing and advising the family on management guidelines and adaptations.

TO promotes the development, maintenance, recovery of abilities, aptitudes and attitudes, encourages active participation in the social environment.

The therapist addresses present and future limitations, optimising and promoting developmental maturity based on the Intervention Process.

The Intervention Process can be simplified into 4 blocks: analysis and evaluation, outcome intervention with the planning of therapy goals, intervention-treatment and follow-up-re-evaluation.

Bi bliograffa

1. Spanish Professional Association of Occupational Therapists. Definition of Occupational Therapy. Available at: https://www.apeto.com/que-es-la-to-definicion.html

2. Ayres JA. Sensory integration in children: Hidden sensory challenges. Madrid. TEA Ediciones; 2008.

3. Dommguez Jimenez I, Calvo Arenillas JI. Occupational Therapy and its role in Early Care: a systematic review. TOG (A Coruna) online journal. 2015; 12 (21): 1-22. Available at: http://www.revistatog.com/num21/pdfs/revision3.pdf.

4. Gonzalez Francisco L, Let's talk about... Occupational therapy. Anales Pediatna Continuada. 2009;7(2): 121-6.

5. Mulligan SE. Occupational therapy in paediatrics. Evaluation process. Madrid: Ed Medica Panamericana; 2006.

6. Perez Fernandez G. Pediatric Occupational Therapy. Revista Smdrome de Down. 2016; 33.

7. Polonio Lopez B, Castellanos Ortega MC, Viana Moldes I. Terapia Ocupacional en la Infancia: teona y practica. Madrid: Ed Medica Panamericana; 2008.

23. Infant cognitive and motor development

Dr. Jose Uberos Fernandez

During the embryonic and foetal period, neurogenesis takes place first, followed by cell duplication or histogenesis. The establishment of synapses between neurons that give rise to the neural network begins before birth and continues during the postnatal period, which is dominated by synaptogenesis. During this period the neural circuits that will make sensory and motor development possible are established.

Synaptogenesis is initially established in the medulla, later in the bulb and progresses upwards to the central nervous system (CNS). The maximum number of synapses is considered to be established by 8-9 months of age, and decreases with age.

In this section we will try to analyse motor skills as the code that expresses the development of the central nervous system (CNS). The body control by the CNS is realised through **global postures**. "Every movement starts from a certain posture and ends in a certain posture", that is why Vojta states that "*The posture always follows the movement like a shadow*".

The establishment of neural circuits is followed by the myelination process, which consolidates those circuits that repeatedly prove useful, thus promoting faster transmission of stimuli. The process of brain myelination begins about three months after fertilisation. Myelination follows an ascending pattern, by the third month of age myelination has reached the internal capsule, cerebellum and corpus callosum, allowing differentiation of motor and sensory responses. This process is complete by the 6th month, facilitating the development of motor automatisms.

At birth, only a few areas of the brain are fully myelinated, such as the brainstem centres that control reflexes, because survival depends on them. Once their axons are myelinated, neurons can become fully functional and can conduct rapidly and efficiently. The axons of neurons in the cerebral hemispheres are particularly myelinated, although this myelination process begins in the early postnatal period. The commissural, projection and association fibres are fibres that reach full myelination at a later time.

Newborn vision is peripheral, the development of central vision occurs after myelination of the myelinated v^as of the calcarine cortex, this aspect is important in the development of manipulation, as it allows gaze fixation, ocular convergence and tracking of moving objects. Auditory discrimination occurs when myelination of the geniculate body is complete. In the first months, postural instability predominates, with flexion of the large joints, the Moro reflex persists in the supine decubitus position and vision is still peripheral.

Different regions of the cerebral cortex myelinate at different stages. The primary sensory and motor areas begin their myelination process earlier than the frontal and parietal association areas; the latter only reach full development by the age of 15 years. It is assumed that this myelination process parallels cognitive development in the child.

The three basic components of the development of motor function are:

1. The straightening of the trunk against gravity.
2. The differentiated purposeful movement of the different body segments.
3. Balance, i.e. automatic control of the displacement of the centre of gravity within the support base.

The analysis of **postural patterns** allows us to evaluate the normality of CNS development. They allow us to evaluate "what the child does", which gives us an idea of mental age, and also "how the child does it", which gives us an idea of the degree of psychomotor development. The knowledge of the postural patterns from which the CNS expresses itself in each maturational stage, allows us to use them as a scale of normal motor development of the child.

Following Vojta (2005), we can define global postural patterns that determine each stage of psychomotor development. From the ventral decubitus, the support mechanisms of the limbs emerge for the straightening of the trunk in the face of gravity. From the dorsal decubitus, the functional differentiation of the limbs for grasping emerges (2, 3).

Tone and posture assessment

Redën newborn. The motor responses of the newborn are undifferentiated and global. Examination of the newborn should begin with an assessment of the newborn's state of consciousness. To awaken the newborn, the thorax is grasped between the thumb and forefinger of both hands and gently shaken, this manoeuvre causes the newborn to open its eyes and make facial grimaces. From 34 weeks gestation (gestational age) newborns will remain awake throughout the examination, below this age it is difficult for them to remain awake, with inability to make facial grimaces and limb movements is abnormal.

The postural function supports movement and is controlled by automatic and unconscious brain mechanisms. The performance of any movement requires prior postural adjustments that prevent the loss of balance and favour the performance of the proposed movement.

The concepts applied to describe states of consciousness in older children can also be applied to the newborn and infant:

- Lethargy awakening is easily achieved, but there is difficulty in staying awake.
- Dulling: Awakening is achieved with non-painful stimuli.
- Stupor: Awakening is only achieved with painful stimuli.
- Coma: Failure to awaken the child.

Excessive low frequency but large amplitude jerking response on awakening (shaking) is abnormal. This motor pattern can be differentiated from seizures by electroencephalogram (EEG) monitoring and because it is not associated with eye movements, changes in respiratory or cardiac pattern, and because it is triggered by stimuli. This period of hyperalertness and shivering is observed within 18 hours of perinatal asphyxia.

Cranial nerves - The perioral reflex should be complete and present at 32 weeks GA. It is characterised by a complete turning of the head on the side of the corner of the mouth stimulated. Opening of the mouth and grasping of the examiner's fingertip between the lips. At 28 weeks GA this reflex may be present but is incomplete. At 36 weeks GA a sustained force is exerted that is adequate for sucking. The perioral reflex and sucking explores the function of cranial nerves V, VII and XII. Swallowing, on the other hand, explores cranial nerves IX and X.

Most newborns open their eyelids when they begin to suckle, an opportunity to explore ocular motility. The head is gently rotated to one side causing the conjugate movement of the eyes to the contralateral side (muneye movement). The vestibular portion of the VIII pair is explored with the muneye manoeuvre and the Moro manoeuvre. The muneye reflex disappears when visual fixation is established, which coincides with the development of central vision with myelination of the calcarine cortex. The Moro reflex disappears by the third or fourth month.

Exploration of tone and arcuate reflexes. Tone is the resistance of the muscle to stretch. The nervous system distinguishes between two types of stretch: phasic and postural. Phasic tone is the response to short-term, high-amplitude stretching, which consists of an equally brief but energetic muscle contraction. If the postural stretch is a sustained, low-amplitude stretch, such as that imposed by gravity, it triggers a long-lasting, low-amplitude postural response. The distinction is important because both types of tone must be explored separately in the newborn.

Spasticity is an abnormal sensitivity of phasic tone, where the pull of gravity is sufficient to activate phasic tone, triggering in infants cross-crossed legs when performing ventral suspension. In newborns the signs of spasticity are more subtle and are expressed as fisting and sustained clonus.

Phasic tone - This is explored by the resistance of the limbs to stretching and by the activity of tendon reflexes. From the 32nd week of GA a flexed position of the lower limbs is observed, which in the upper limbs is observed from the 36th week of GA.

Of the reflexes present in the adult, the patellar reflex is the only tendon reflex constantly present at birth. To explore the patellar reflex, the child's head should be positioned with the face in the midline or interference with the cephalic neck reflex will occur, exalting the patellar reflex on the side towards which the head is turned.

A few jerks of malleolar clonus may occur in normal newborns; however, sustained clonus is abnormal. Activation of the clonus requires a state of constant stretching of the muscle which can be achieved by abrupt dorsiflexion of the foot with the hip and knee in flexion.

All newborns from 32 to 40 weeks GA lie with some degree of abduction of the thighs and flexion at the elbows, hips and knees. Full extension of the limbs at any gestational age should be considered abnormal, as should full abduction of the thighs and arms.

Two arm positions are equivalent to batrachian legs, indicators of severe hypotoma:

a) Elbow flexion with the backs of the hands resting on the support surface b) The flexion of the elbow with the backs of the hands resting on the support surface.

Under normal conditions the hand is kept loosely closed with the thumb outside the other fingers. A tightly closed hand where the thumb is enclosed by the other fingers is abnormal (fisting).

Straightening of the head: With the child in the decubitus position, the child is held by the wrists and slowly raised to a sitting position. If the tone is normal, the arms remain flexed and the head upright for a few seconds.

Straightening of the lower limbs and trunk: The infant is held by the armpits while the feet are placed on the plane of the table. After flexing, the child extends the lower limbs and straightens the trunk.

Floating attitude: In prone position, the neonate is held by the thorax and lifted into the air. Normally the head is held for some time and the lower limbs remain in flexion.

Galant reflex: With the newborn suspended in prone position, the skin is stimulated parallel to the spine. The stimulated muscles contract.

Palmar grasp reflex: also called *Darwinian reflex*, it is observed that, when a newborn baby touches the palm of the hand, he/she closes his/her hand and grasps it tightly when he/she notices something. This reflex is present from birth and lasts until the infant is four or five months old.

Peeper reflex: when the cheek of a newborn baby is stroked, it turns its head to look for food and starts sucking (sucking reflex). The peeper reflex lasts about four months and the sucking reflex two months.

Moro reflex: also called startle response or hug reflex. It is named after the paediatrician who discovered and popularised it, Ernst Moro. The infant is placed on a cushioned surface, its head is picked up and dropped, holding it before the end of its fall. The child reacts by opening its eyes and arms due to the startle. This reflex begins to weaken after the infant is three months old.

Plantar pressure reflex: if we press on the sole of the foot, the baby reacts by closing it, as in an attempt to grasp it.

Babinski reflex: If we stimulate the external margin of the sole of the foot in the direction from the heel to the toes, flexion of the first toe is produced and extension of the rest of the toes in a fan shape. It is the most long-lasting reflex, lasting up to **nine** to twelve months.

Postural patterns

First trimester

Global pattern of the newborn in prone decubitus. The newborn is very unstable in this posture, with global mass movements. The contact surface is: the cheek on the nuchal side, nuchal sternoclavicular joint, distal third of the forearm.

Global pattern of the newborn in decubitus supine position. The head is rotated, reclined to the nuchal side. Greater weight bearing on the facial side. The limbs are flexed as in prone position.

Global pattern of support on the middle third of the forearms. The support surface is shifted to the upper abdomen and middle third of the forearms. The centre of gravity falls on the navel. The spine is more extended in the axial axis.

Global pattern of the fencer. Postural pattern at the service of optical orientation. The fixation of the gaze is accompanied by rotation of the head, constituting a facial side and a nuchal side. On the facial side, elbow extended, shoulder in external rotation and hand closed. On the nuchal side the elbow is flexed and the hand is closed.

Global pattern of symmetrical elbow support. This is the postural pattern that defines the 3-month-old infant in ventral decubitus. At three months in ventral decubitus the infant's arms have advanced further upwards and find the support of the elbows as a stable posture. In this position he can keep head and shoulders straight against gravity. This support of the elbows is the condition for the whole spine to be aligned in the axial axis of the body and the head can be held straight out of the base of support and rotated through 180° (cephalic control).

Global hand-hand coordination pattern. The dorsal decubitus position also becomes a stable posture at 3 months, the child can play with his hands in the centre of the visual field, keeping the lower limbs elevated at 90° (hand-hand coordination pattern). The spine is completely aligned on the axis, the shoulder and hip joints completely centred. Only after this posture has been established can the differentiation of the limbs for grasping begin.

The newborn in dorsal decubitus shows an asymmetrical and very unstable posture. From the age of 2 months in ventral decubitus, the infant begins to extend the hips, hitherto flexed, and the arms begin to come closer to the head. Transitory support of the forearms to raise the head and direct the gaze begins to appear. This means that at this age the child is better able to fixate the gaze. This is the beginning of the support function of the arms in the service of orienting the head towards the visual or auditory stimulus that attracts the child's attention.

Second quarter

Global pattern of lateral prostration. In dorsal decubitus the support surface continues to be the trunk and the nape of the neck. The prone position is associated with a global response of the body with opening of the mouth, flexion of the legs.

Global pattern of asymmetrical one-elbow support. From the age of 4.5 months the child is able to shift the weight of his body on one arm to extend the other arm in search of an object placed further away (***asymmetrical support on one elbow***). This gaze-guided motor action means a further step in postural control, it means control over the lateral displacement of the weight towards one of the elbows without losing balance. This results in a differentiation in the muscular functions of one side of the body and the other. One arm performs a tonic function of support and the other a phasic function of transporting one arm towards the object.

Global swimming pattern. This pattern is momentary, arising from the frustration of not being able to reach objects placed in front of him. It is a simultaneous movement of all limbs with trunk extension.

Global pattern of grasping in medial tinea. An object is grasped in the middle knea of the visual field with both hands. At this time the grasping of an object in each hemibody was only performed with the hand corresponding to that side.

Global support pattern on palms of hands with elbows outstretched. The support surface consists of both hands and proximal thighs. The centre of gravity is shifted towards the legs. The hands are supported open, with dorsal and radial flexion of the wrist. For this, the hand-pressing reflex has had to disappear completely. The dorsal and lumbar spine are completely aligned on the axis. The lower limbs are held with the knees bent and 90° apart. This position allows the child to look into the distance, but the hands are trapped in the support function. If he wants to manipulate an object, he must lower the support to the elbows.

At the end of this trimester, complete opening of the hand with dorsal and radial flexion of the wrist appears. ***Hand unfolding is*** understood as maintained, isometric abduction of the metacarpals with extension of the fingers.

Global pattern of coordinated dorsal to ventral rolling. Flipping appears because the CNS is already able to control weight shifting laterally.

Third trimester

Global pattern of oblique sedimentation. During the third trimester verticalisation will begin. The infant straightens up by leaning first on the elbow, then on the hand, thus straightening to ***lateral sedation***. The entire spine, including the lumbar spine, is now out of the support base.

At the age of 7-8 months, he is able to move from the lateral sitting posture to the ***four-legged posture***, which allows him to stabilise the straightening of the pelvis on the knees. From the oblique (lateral) sitting position, the hand is fully extended, allowing the opposition of the thumb to the other fingers. Also at the age of 9 months he is able to manipulate objects with his hands while sitting with his legs half extended (*biisquiatic sedation*).

Global crawling pattern. At 9 months from the four-legged position, *crawling* appears. Normal crawling includes the following features:

- The limbs are loaded alternately and equally.
- The hands rest on the palm of the hand, with the fingers relaxed and understood.
- The shoulders are kept in external rotation and centred.
- The trunk does not lean to either side and the spine remains aligned, without lordosis or kyphosis.
- The pelvis remains horizontal, without deviating towards the striding leg.
- The feet are kept in the axis of the leg.

Fourth quarter

Global pattern of standing, side walking and free walking. After a few weeks, the child will use the same crawling mechanisms to achieve standing and lateral walking with hand support.

From the point of view of neurological maturation, locomotion involves the ability of the CNS to coordinate and control three motor functions:

1. Balanced displacement of the centre of gravity around the body axis.
2. Straightening of the trunk on points of support on the limbs, which change tfclically with walking.
3. Stepping movements (support and swing) of the limbs, maintaining defined trajectories.

Detection of motor pathology

The whole development of posture up to the acquisition of the ttpeda gait has been built on basic motor acquisitions:

- Extension and maintenance of the spine in the axial axis of the body. In motor pathology there is always a deficit in the axial extension of the spine, especially at the level of the cervico-dorsal hinge (reclination of the head) and in the dorsolumbar area (round back in sedation).
- Geometric centring of all joints. Especially hips and shoulders.
- Pattern of resting on the points instead of the hand remaining open, implying that the palmar grasp reflex has not yet been abolished. Hemiparesis, where the axial rectification of the spine is disturbed.

Knowledge of these patterns helps to detect anomaKas in their onset and to plan early action plans.

Development of the press function

To initiate propositional grasping, the newborn at 6 weeks must have begun to fixate the gaze on near objects. At 8 weeks the hands meet each other at the midline. At this time (6-8 weeks) hand-mouth coordination is established for the oral recognition of objects. The development of propositional grasping takes place during the second trimester.

Directed grasping with one hand can only appear if postural stability in the dorsal decubitus position and axial extension of the spine have been achieved by the end of the first trimester. The child can direct the hand towards an object placed in the visual field of that hand. If the object moves into the other visual field, the child ceases activity with that hand and engages the other hand to reach for it. By the middle of the second trimester, the child will be able to pursue the object with one hand beyond the middle Knea.

The development of the grasping function presupposes the development of the visual function, as it must spatially orientate the object, recognise the size and orientation before directing the hand towards the object. The ability to direct the arm towards an object assumes that capacities have been previously achieved, which can be summarised as follows:

- Stabilisation of the cervico-dorsal spine.
- Coordination of finger movements.

The precise motor couplings are:

- Coordination of eye, head and arm movements.
- Coordination of proximal and distal movements of the upper limb.
- Coupling of eye-head-hand movements

The fine functional differentiation of the hand appears within the framework of the global postural pattern of lateral sedation, when the shoulder has reached full freedom of joint movement, the shoulder is straightened and held vertically and the child is interested in the upper space.

Assessment of children's mental development

Psychological development is the result of interactions between different areas that interact with each other. The family, social and cultural environment will influence the affective and emotional development of the child and in the first years of life the psychomotor development. The term *psychomotor development* designates the acquisition of skills that is observed in the child continuously throughout childhood, it is due to the maturation of the nervous structures as well as to learning, as a result of which the child develops a behaviour, a system of relating and interacting with his environment. Nowadays most psychologists accept the definition created by Passer and Smith: "Intelligence is the ability to acquire knowledge, to think and reason effectively and to manage in the environment in an adaptive way".

The initial psychological interview is the first contact of the family with the professional, during this first contact the demand that the parents have towards the hospital and towards the services that take care of their child is determined and also the degree of knowledge that they have, the latter will be appreciated through their questions and concerns. The interrelationship between them and the child is evaluated, then the psychometric evaluation is carried out by means of the Brunet and Lezine test or the Bayley test.

The assessment of psycho-affective development is carried out through different stages. The notion of stage is not limited to a specific age, but to a series of moments, characterised by a series of traits, more or less common, as long as that stage, with its characteristics, has not been overcome, the child is not ready to move on to the next one.

- **Up to 6 months:** Undifferentiated or pure impulsive stage. Defenselessness, dependence. Satisfaction or frustration of demand shapes the infant psyche.

- **6-12 months:** Identification stage. Beginning of the first relations with objects and the first emotional reactions. Establishment of stable emotional ties.

- **3-18 months (approximate):** Beginning of the organisation: timetables, repetitions of situations. The child learns what to follow and becomes distressingly disoriented when the normal sequence does not occur or is interrupted. The existence of several caregivers can lead to inconsistent responses. In this period, sociability begins, the first negative emotional reactions (grief, sadness, fear or anxiety and anger or aggression) and positive ones (feelings of pleasure, smiles, laughter; pride and affection) begin.

- **Between 1 and 3 years:** the child undergoes a vertiginous transformation. In addition to his growing motor skills, which enable him to expand his research, he is increasingly able to represent the world to himself, the cause-effect relationships and the possibility of representing an action and anticipating its results. These words are less precise than in adults, but in a certain sense richer. Stern calls them "word-phrases", which express, more than our concepts, an affective state, they can be used in many different situations and their value can vary from one situation to another. The use of the object often replaces its name (water=drinking, glass=I am thirsty, etc.).

- **From 3-6 years:** Discovery of external reality takes place. Sexual investigation and the perception of differences begin. In this period, according to psychoanalytical conceptualisation, the problem related to the Oedipus complex develops: sharing his mother is equivalent to losing her. The child perceives that there is an external reality, independent of him, which he must take into account if he wants to achieve his goals. Affective emotions develop: envy, feelings of hostility, guilt. Primitive moral conscience appears.

- **From 6-10 years: The** overcoming of subjectivity takes place. At this stage, from the age of 6 years, the child acquires the experience of an affectively neutral environment, where he will have to build his own place under the sun, without benefiting from the favourable prejudice of parental love. In these pre-adolescent stages, the social, affective and cognitive complexities are of great magnitude, but they are necessary in development, on the way to becoming integrated adults, enduring life's setbacks and learning to be magnanimous, to win or lose with sportsmanship, to play fair.

Schooling means the insertion of the child in a social life different from the family life, it means his insertion in a group similar in physical and mental possibilities, among whom he will be measured as an equal. In this period the child begins to understand that there are other points of view different from his own.

Between 6 and 7 years, the teacher, heir to paternal omnipotence, is the axis of the social group.

Between the ages of 7 and 8 years, group loyalty increases. The child becomes very sensitive to the opinions of peers.

Assessment of cognitive development

The assessment of child psychological development began to gain importance at the beginning of the 20th century with the work of Alfred Binet (1911) and Arnold Gesell (1945). The latter author conducted studies on the normal course of behavioural development of infants and pre-school children. As a method of observation, the design of the cabinet with the camera that would bear his name (Gesell Camera) stands out, in order to make observations without the presence of the examiner in the same environment as the examined child. Gesell's work prompted other authors to develop assessment methods, among which Brunet and Lezine (1951) for the assessment of the age of mental development from birth to 30 months and the Bayley child development scale (Bayley-III) for the assessment of child development (1969) from 1 to 42 months of age.

Brunet and Lezine scale. The Brunet and Lezine scale is the result of a comparative study of other baby-test scales such as the Bulher-Hetzer and A. Gesell scales. It is intended to evaluate the child in his spontaneity, within his family environment to which he remains attached. This scale was revised in 1994 by Denise Josse, who made modifications in the evaluation of language development and maintained an important part of the original content based on the following areas: postural development, oculo-manual co-ordination, study of comprehension-expressive language, social relations and adaptation.

Bayley-III Scale. With excellent psychometric properties, its quantitative scoring system is ideal for monitoring performance throughout the assessment. It globally assesses the most important developmental areas, allowing to determine in a simple and precise way the level of child development and to identify developmental delays and obtain valid information for treatment planning.

It identifies the child's competencies and strengths, as well as areas for improvement, making it an ideal tool for evaluation in interdisciplinary teams. Reference for assessing the functional development of the child between 1 and 42 months.

Bibliograffa

1.   Gomez-Andres D, Pulido-Valdeolivas I, Fiz-Perez L. Normal neurological development of the child. Pediatria integral. 2015;19(9):640-7.

2.   Vojta V. [Early diagnosis and therapy of cerebral movement disorders in childhood. B. The developmental diagnosis]. Z Orthop Ihre Grenzgeb. 1973;111(3):257-68.

3.   Vojta V. [Early diagnosis and therapy of cerebral motor disorders in childhood. A. Postural reflexes in developmental kinesiology. I. Normal developmental stages]. Z Orthop Ihre Grenzgeb. 1972;110(4):450-7.

Developmental language disorders.

Dr. Enrique Blanca Jover

Language is a capacity that allows us to communicate between two or more interlocutors by means of a conventional code of articulated sound signals. It comprises three dimensions, each with its own process of comprehension and expression: *form*, which refers both to phonology (proper processing of sounds) and syntax (ordering and combination of words in sentences); *content*, directly related to the lexicon whose meaning of words refers to semantics; and *communicative functions*, related to conversational competence, the ability to adapt language to context and non-verbal language, among others. The process of language acquisition is universal and involves perception, attention, memory and thinking. Children acquire it implicitly as they are endowed with an "innate capacity" that allows them to discover and incorporate the registers of spoken language in their immediate environment in a natural and almost effortless way.

For oral language to appear and develop, neurological brain structures, cognitive capacities for symbolisation, affective and social stimulation, competence to interact and the ability to receive and reproduce sounds are necessary.

Neuroanatomical basis of language control

The cognitive regions in the control of language functions are concentrated in two main cortical areas. A posterior, primarily receptive and integrative, and an anterior area devoted primarily to expressive language; occupying the posterior superior temporal gyrus and extending to the end of the Sylvian fissure, this is Wernicke's area and represents the area in which auditory perceptions are integrated with thought and memory to generate the fundamental abstractions of language. In the inferior and lateral part of the frontal lobe, in front of the primary motor cortex, is Broca's area; this area is critical for expressing both spoken and written language (figure 24.1).

Language-related functions are strongly lateralised in the human brain from the foetal period, with greater development in the *left* hemisphere. Brain lesions in children that affect language centres, while producing aphasia, can recover function more frequently than in adults. Aphasia or dysphasia is described as the loss or impairment of language as a result of the involvement of areas of the brain intended for that function. This disorder must be distinguished from dysarthria which is due to a disorder in the articulation of language and/or to sensory disorders that prevent perceptual stimuli from reaching the language areas. Motor, cerebellar or phonatory disorders disrupt the flow of words, but do not produce aphasia. Gnosia refers to the brain's ability to recognise previously learned information.

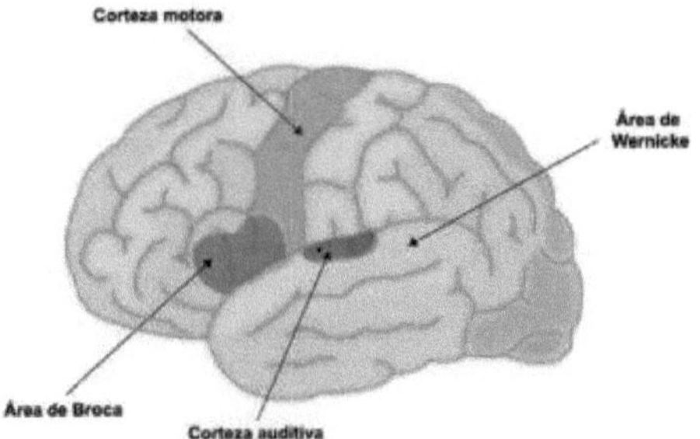

Figure 24.1. Brain areas involved in language.

Language has three basic properties; firstly, the understanding of symbols. Secondly, the ability to transform thoughts into words. Finally, we must have the ability to express these symbols.

In Wernicke's aphasia there is a severe impairment in the understanding of spoken or written language, the patient can speak with normal fluency and rhythm, although his language lacks meaning. In Broca's aphasia, spontaneous and commanded spoken and written language is impaired. Language comprehension is preserved, although as a rule, what is heard is better understood than what is read.

Mutatism describes the inability to speak; it is observed in lesions of the left frontal lobe, which includes part of Broca's area, and is often associated with right hemiplegia. It must be differentiated from anarthria, or inability to articulate words, due to alterations in the innervation or mechanics of the phonatory apparatus, and differs from mutism because the patient is able to emit sounds with difficulty.

Language development requirements

For oral language to appear and develop normally, the following are required:

- Normal neurological structures (left hemisphere)
- Cognitive abilities: object permanence.
- Social stimulation: Interlocutors.
- Ability to receive and reproduce sounds.
- Ability to interact: Communicative intent.

Language development

In order to understand language pathology, it is essential to understand normal language development, the different ling^stic dimensions and the clinical expressivity of language impairment. Table 24.1 shows the most common pattern of language development, taking into account that there are variations between individuals and deviations influenced by the socio-cultural environment. Two main stages can be distinguished: a *prelinguistic* stage, from birth to about 12 months, in which children begin to have fun with the emission of sounds and to discover their possibilities, and then a *linguistic* stage, from the age of one year to six years, with the development of the different components of language.

Table 24.1. Chronological development of normal language.

PRE-LINGUISTIC STAGE	LINGUISTIC STAGE
0-2 months. Production of vocalisations: reflex and vegetative sounds (cooing, yawning, sighing).	**12-24 months.** Expansion of the lexicon, one word at a time. nouns, global sense with overgeneralisation (holophrases).
1-4 months. Production of archaic syllables: imitation of melodies and adult sounds, increased vocalisation due to social reinforcement.	**24-36 months.** Two-word association, intonation, noun-verb-adjective order.
3-8 months. Rudimentary babbling: higher voice frequencies, low-pitched sounds (grunts), very high-pitched sounds (squeaks).	**3-4 years.** Mastery of the basic structure of the mother tongue, sentences with "than", vocabulary up to 600-1000 terms.
5-10 months. Canonical babbling: identical consonant-vowel syllables (mamama, papapa) y successive (patata).	**4-6 years.** Development of pragmatic and metalinguistic functions, expanding vocabulary, complete grammar, mature expressive form.
9-18 months. Mixed babbling: syllables y words. acquire meaning from 12-15 months onwards.	

As a guideline, from the age of one year children begin to pronounce their first words, holophrases and combinatory language (telegraphic speech) will emerge and gradually gain the characteristics of adult speech.

Receptive language development

At 26 weeks of pregnancy the foetus is able to perceive sounds. The term newborn recognises its mother's voice and at 9 months of age it is possible to understand some words, in particular the meaning of the refusal "No". At the age of 2 years the child obeys commands of 2 consecutive steps "take off your shoes and stay seated".

Expressive language development

At 4 months the infant can modulate sounds to express emotions such as pain or pleasure. At 5 months he can distinguish monosHabos and laughter and at 6-8 months he emits polysyllabic babbling sounds. At 12 months one new word per week can be acquired, so that by 18-20 months a minimum of 20 words can be used. Combined sentences of 2 words do not appear until a minimum of 50-100 words are mastered.

There are two patterns of language development, one *analytic, where there* is the evolution from simple to more complex forms of language; the other *hotistic*, where there is large use of words in familiar contexts with stereotyped phrases. Both are accurate for normal language development.

Formal aspects of language

Phonology: phonological discrimination and phonological programming

The phonological level is the first level of language organisation. The child acquires the phonological system between the ages of two and four years. Difficulties with complex syllables (pla, ter, fri, gru) are normal until the age of five and the pronunciation of /r/ may be physiologically delayed until the age of six.

The speech decoding process takes place in Wernicke's area (in 86% of the population). Phonological analysis takes place in both cerebral hemispheres (left for phonemes and words; right for intonation and accent) and the left hemisphere (right-handed), the basal ganglia and the cerebellum are involved in expression. The impairment of this area manifests itself in heterogeneous clinical forms. For example, a child with simple language delay shows phonological reduction and simplification. They make omissions ("api" for pencil), substitutions ("tote" for car) and assimilations ("nane" for big). In contrast to these, children with developmental language disorders or dysphasia show phonological disorganisation and distortion.

Lexicon and vocabulary

Lexicon involves understanding language (identification) and selecting vocabulary to convey what you want to say. Children increase their vocabulary from 10-13 months, and learn words that have familiar phonemes better than words that have different phonemes. This is due to phonological awareness, which is the ability to be aware of speech units. The left prefrontal, temporal and parietal cortical areas (in right-handers) are responsible for lexical recognition and syntactic relations. Children with lexical processing impairment have difficulties in understanding and expressing concepts of space and time, remembering the name of an object or relating it to its category. This lack of vocabulary leads to comprehension problems and influences the fluency of their speech, which becomes hesitant and full of repetitions.

Syntactic understanding and programming

The programming of morphosyntax takes place in the anterior part of Broca's area and includes word classes (noun, verb, etc.), relations between words (conjunctions, prepositions), prosody (rhythm and intonation), sentence structure and its compositions. Between the ages of 2-3 years, the child begins to associate two or more words. He produces new words, deduces the rules of language and learns them by applying them to new situations, as well as imitating and repeating. From the age of three and a half, the healthy child masters the basic structure of the mother tongue and can reproduce it intelligibly. This chronological fact is basic to understand that any child with language delay should be assessed before this key age.

Functional aspects of language

Cognitive or semantic use

The meaning or representation of the messages produced is semantics. Receptively, it is the extraction of meaning through the linguistic code, and expressively, it is the selection of the most appropriate vocabulary depending on what is to be communicated.

This function relies on the two temporo-parietal regions. Children with difficulties in this area have problems with verbal perseveration because they are unable to perceive or express an idea, and so information seems redundant and unnecessary. Their speech contains pauses, little coherence because they use few adjectives, adverbs, conjunctions and prepositions. This can be seen when asked to formulate a demand or deliver a complex message.

Pragmatic use

Pragmatics is concerned with the organisation of discourse in a conversation. It also has to do with the ability to identify the context of a conversation and make sense of it; and with the intention to communicate and adapt to the interlocutor. This language function is located in the perisylvian region of the right temporal lobe. The child with impairment in this dimension does not present relevant phonological or lexical problems, but has difficulties in constructing sentences, which are poorly elaborated, stereotyped, with little coherence and inappropriate to the context.

Language disorders

Language disorders affect 20% of children up to the age of 2 years; by the age of 5 years this percentage drops to 5%. This is because language development may be delayed in 10-14% of these children. In other words, the latter percentage corresponds to articulatory delay and simple language delay, which will show a spontaneous remission or after minimal speech therapy during the pre-school stage. From the school stage onwards, 0.3% have an instrumental hearing or phonoarticulatory organ deficit, 2.2% have mental retardation and/or autistic spectrum disorder, and 1.5% of this school population has dysphasia.

Table 24.2. Clinical classification of speech and language disorders in children, (based on Chevrie-Muller and Narbona 2001).

Disorders secondary to structural defects.
- Hearing deficit.
- Mechanical and articulatory deficits:

198

- ■ Dysglossia (anatomical): velopalatine, labial, lingual, laryngeal, maxillodental malformation.
- ■ Dysarthrias (motor): isolated pseudobulbar syndrome, cerebral palsy, muscular dystrophies, congenital paralysis, progressive **diseases.**

Speech and language disorders.
- Pronunciation **disorder:** dyslalia.
- Rhythm and fluency disorders: stuttering, mumbling.
- Specific developmental language disorders (dysphasia): **expressive or mixed.**
- Developmentally acquired aphasias:
- Aphasia-epilepsy **syndrome** (Landau-Kleffher).
- Infantile aphasia **due** to unilateral hem ispheric lesion.

Psycholinguistic disorders.
- Specific pragmatic y semantic-pragmatic disorder.
- Autistic **spectrum** disorders: childhood autism, **Asperger's,** autistic disorders not otherwise specified, childhood disintegrative disorder.
- Socio-affective deficiencies.
- Mutism o selective.
- Mental impairment: homogeneous o disharmonic (verbal ability more affected than non-verbal).

Genetic factors play a prominent role, with 30% of first-degree relatives reported to be affected. Other factors such as nutrition, hormonal and environmental disturbances may act as epigenetic factors and contribute to its occurrence.

There are different ways of classifying language disorders, but the most complete way is the one proposed by Chevrie-Muller and Narbona in 2001 (Table 2). This classification is practical because it is based on linguistic criteria and takes etiology into account. The most relevant speech-language pathologies in the child according to this classification scheme will be developed below.

They constitute early warning elements for the exploration of a language disorder:

- At 10 months: lack of or poor babbling
- At 15 months does not   use 3 words
- At 18 months: utterance of less than 10 words
- At 24 months: absence of two-word utterances
- At 30 months: absence of two-word utterances, one of which is a verb.

The failure to pronounce intelligible words at the age of 2 years and, above all, to have a vocabulary limited to a few words at the age of 3 years constitute criteria for urgent psycholinguistic action.

Disorders secondary to instrumental deficits

Hearing deficit

Hearing loss is the main organic cause of language impairment and it is imperative to ensure auditory integrity in this context. Hearing damage can originate prenatally, perinatally or postnatally. Prenatal causes include: cytomegalovirus infection, congenital rubella, toxoplasmosis and teratogenic substances. The most frequent perinatal causes are foetal distress, prematurity, anoxia and obstetric trauma. The most relevant postnatal causes are: labyrinthitis and meningitis, acoustic trauma and ototoxic substances (aminoglycosides), but repeated ototubaritis and serous otitis media are the most frequent causes of hearing loss in general.

Among the risk indicators associated with hypoacusis, the following should be explored:

family history, maternal infection during gestation, craniofacial malformations, birth weight less than 1.500 g, severe hyperbilirubinaemia, ototoxic drugs, alcoholism in the pregnant woman, bacterial meningitis, hypoxic-ischemic accident, use of prolonged mechanical ventilation for more than 5 days, genetic syndromes or diseases associated with hypoacusis (Waardenburg, Goldenhar, CHARGE, retinitis pigmentosa, mucopolysaccharidosis), severe cranioencephalic trauma and neurodegenerative disorders.

It should be borne in mind that a hearing impairment may initially manifest itself as a behavioural problem. Ëeste sera de dos vertientes: con agitacion, desobediencia, oposicionismo y agresividad; o con una conducta excesivamente tranquila, con aislamiento y defectos en la socializacion.

Otoacoustic emission screening has been crucial for early detection, but some retrocochlear sensorineural hearing loss may escape universal screening for deafness.

Treatment of hearing loss depends on the cause. In chronic or recurrent otitis, antibiotics, mucolftics and/or antihistammics will be administered depending on the patient. They may often require a surgical approach or the fitting of hearing aids depending on the type of conductive hearing loss. In sensorineural hearing loss, the time of onset of hearing loss (prelocution or postlocution stage) and whether it is cochlear or retrocochlear is key for management and prognosis. The use of cochlear implants is becoming increasingly widespread in patients with severe or profound sensorineural hearing loss who do not benefit from conventional hearing aids. After cochlear implantation, it is essential to continue a psycho-linguistic re-education programme in a specialised centre.

Mechanical articulation deficit

Dysglossia

These are articulatory alterations due to anatomical anomaKas of the articulatory organs: cleft lip, cleft palate, dental malposition, macroglossia, prognathism, retrognathia, etc. They can affect very mildly, such as a submucous fissure that produces rhinolalia (nasal voice). The treatment involves orthodontics, maxillofacial surgery and speech therapy, which is adapted to the surgical and developmental calendar of the child.

Dysarthrias

These are anomata of pronunciation due to involvement of the central motor veins, the cranial nerves or the muscle groups of the oropharyngolaryngeal region. There are muscular diseases which produce, for example, rhinolalia with an amJmic facies which should lead us to suspect Steinert's disease; or, if the amJmic facies is associated with oculomotor paralysis, we could be dealing with a Moebius syndrome.

Salivary incontinence or drooling is a frequent problem with great physical and social repercussions. It can lead to dehydration in hot weather, oesophagitis due to lack of clearance and chin dermatitis due to humidity. Social effects are evident, especially in patients with normal learning and communication skills. Drooling may be associated with spastic cerebral palsy, pseudobulbar syndrome due to congenital or acquired damage to both temporal lobes (cortical malformations or after herpetic encephalitis) and verbal dyspraxia. In its management, speech therapy training with motor practice is essential.

The application of botulinum toxin in salivary glands is very effective, but requires specialist management and administration by ultrasound, and repeat doses every 4-6 months.

Speech and language disorders

Dyslalia

These are alterations in the voicing of phonemes, a developmental disorder of pronunciation without underlying anatomical, motor or neurolingual defects.

The persistent immature emission of certain phonemes beyond the age of four years requires a specific approach and study. The most frequently affected phonemes are /s/, /r/, /l/ and /d/. The disorder may consist of an omission to simplify a consonant combination such as "gobo" for "balloon". Sometimes the dyslalia is multiple and impoverishes speech, making differential diagnosis with developmental dysphasia difficult. In cases of multiple dyslalia, verbal fluency is normal or clearly superior to that of a dysphasic child, and the phonemic error is maintained in different words and repetitions (this changes in the child with dysphasia). The response to speech therapy is favourable.

Rhythm and fluency disorders.

Tachypalatelic mumbling is rapid, rapid, rapid speech that is difficult to understand. It is important to explore the behaviour, which may be impulsive; if it is associated with multiple dyslalia, non-verbal intellectual capacity should be measured, as it may be associated with mental retardation and fragile X syndrome.

Stuttering or spasmophemia is a speech fluency disorder of unclear origin. It causes blocking and repetition of one or more syllables and may be accompanied by movements of the face, neck and limbs, and a hoarse voice or changes in timbre or pitch. Its nature is, in most cases, benign and with spontaneous remission, especially in cases of disfluencies in the third and fourth year of life. Stuttering that persists at school age should be evaluated and followed up, and exposure to stressful and insecure situations should be improved. The usual age of onset is around 3.5 years, only 5% after the age of 7 years, and it is more frequent in boys than in girls. Criteria for deciding to initiate therapy include the presence of prolongations of sounds (audible or blocked) constituting more than 25% of the disfluencies produced by the child on a sample of 100 words; and repeated occurrences of sounds or slurs, or prolongation of a sound in the first slur, irrespective of the length of the word. The severe form of persistent stuttering will generate a social problem and will require a special and prolonged speech-medical and psychological approach.

Practical advice to parents of children with stammering includes:

- Be more attentive to what the child says than to the way he/she says it and help him/her to make himself/herself understood rather than waiting for him/her to say it well.
- Talk to the child about his or her difficulties and help him or her to identify the circumstances in which he or she has the most difficulty.
- Reinforce their self-esteem at times when they speak fluently.
- Speak more slowly and with longer pauses, in a melodious and gentle tone.

- Train "rag doll" type relaxation.
- Encourage a sense of security through play and reading time at home with the family.
- Talk about new things before they happen, encourage turn-taking and waiting during a conversation.

Specific language development disorders.

Specific language development disorder (SLD), or dysphasia, is a difficulty in the acquisition and management of the decoding (comprehension) and coding (expression) skills of the language system. It is specific, because it is not dependent on a sensory, neuromotor, cognitive or socio-emotional deficit, but is an inherent language processing problem. The prevalence of SLI, whether or not associated with mental retardation, is 2% at 3 years of age. It is more frequent in males (2.4:1). The origin is genetic. MRI imaging studies identify white matter volume loss and ventricular enlargement with focal heterotopia of the parietotemporal grey matter.

It manifests itself from the very beginning of the child's language development, which is delayed and distorted. It is persistent and can last a lifetime in some severe cases or undergo transformations during its evolution. During the school years, it can interfere with learning to read and write and with the construction of more complex verbal discourse, such as telling a story or carrying on a conversation. The developmental characteristics of SLI allow it to be differentiated from simple language delay; although, in younger children, it can be a difficult differential diagnosis because it may coexist with intellectual disability or autistic spectrum disorders. There is a discrepancy between unaffected general cognitive level and functional language development. Often, there is a predominance of high language development with little analytical development. Language impairment is a source of difficulties in social interactions, making this disorder initially difficult to differentiate from autistic spectrum disorders (ASD).

There are useful linguistic markers that can differentiate SLI from normal development, such as average utterance length and pseudoword repetition lists - meaningless words such as "trophagama", "antomena", "lifanosa". Failure in this task of repeating pseudowords highlights difficulties in ling^stic processing. Measurement of non-verbal IQ, and exploration of sociability, play and empathy, are important to rule out mental retardation or associated autism. There are no medical tests that allow diagnosis, which is based on psycholinguistic examination, non-verbal IQ and exclusion of other causes.

Developmentally acquired aphasias

Unlike dysphasia, *aphasia acquired in childhood* occurs after normal initial language development in the first two years, and there is a loss or delay in its progression. This may be secondary to various causes of brain damage: infections (bacterial, herpetic encephalitis), vascular damage, traumatic brain injury, epilepsy, brain tumours, metabolic diseases, etc.

Landau-Kleffner syndrome is an age-related epileptic encephalopathy in which there is a developmental regression (3-7 years), especially in the language domain, and where the EEG abnormalities are mainly located in the temporo-parietal regions.

Psycholinguistic disorders

Autism Spectrum Disorders (ASD)

Communication impairment is one of the most important features of autistic disorder. Language difficulties are the most striking symptom and the most common reason for initial consultation.

According to the DSM-IV-TR classification, there must be a qualitative impairment in communication manifested by at least one of the following features:

- Delay or complete absence of oral language development (not accompanied by attempts to compensate through alternative modes of communication, such as gestures or mimicry).
- In subjects with adequate speech, significant impairment in the ability to initiate or maintain a conversation with others.
- Stereotyped and repetitive use of language or idiosyncratic language; or absence of spontaneous, varied, realistic or social imitative play appropriate to developmental level.
- There is a deficient use of the signalling and contact gesture.
- There is poor co-ordination of eye contact with gestures and actions.

In some children, verbal language development may be quantitatively rich, but with qualitative deficits in semantic and pragmatic aspects. Where there are quantitative deficits, there may be echolalia (repetition of sounds or words without communicative function), single words and, in the most severe cases, absence of expressive language. Most have significant deficits in the understanding of language, symbolic forms and social situations.

Asperger's disorder

These are children (more frequent in boys) with early and complete formal language development, normal or high intellectual capacity, but with motor clumsiness, difficulties in social interaction and behavioural patterns. Tone of voice is monotone, robotic, speech is pedantic and not accompanied by gesticulation or eye contact. They have difficulty understanding and processing jokes and colloquial language jokes, and are obsessive about topics of restricted and extravagant interest, such as planets, castles, maps, cars... and accumulate a large amount of information on that particular topic.

Bibliograffa

1. Aguilera Albesa S, Orellana Ayala CE. Language disorders. Pediatr Integral. 2017; XXI: 15-22.

2. Artigas-Pallares J, Paula Perez I, Ventura Mallofre E. Language disorders. Pediatr Integral 2022; XXVI (1): 12-20.

3. Crowe K, Cuervo S, Guiberson M, Washington KN. A Systematic Review of Interventions for Multilingual Preschoolers With Speech and Language Difficulties. J Speech Lang Hear Res. 2021 Nov 8; 64(11):4413-4438. doi: 10.1044/2021_JSLHR-21-00073. Epub 2021 Sep 23.

4. Crowe K, Guiberson M. Evidence-Based Interventions for Learners Who Are Deaf and/or Multilingual: A Systematic Quality Review. Am J Speech Lang Pathol. 2019 Aug 9; 28(3):964-983. doi: 10.1044/2019_AJSLP-IDLL-19-0003. Epub 2019 Aug 9.

5.   Feldman HM. How Young Children Learn Language and Speech. Pediatr Rev. 2019 Aug; 40(8):398-411.

6.   Plug MB, van Wijngaarden V, de Wilde H, van Binsbergen E, Stegeman I, van den Boogaard MH, Smit AL. Clinical Characteristics and Genetic Etiology of Children With Developmental Language Disorder. Front Pediatr. 2021 Jul 1; 9:651995. doi: 10.3389/fped.2021.651995.

25. Infantile Cerebral Palsy

Dr. Antonio Molina-Carballo

Introduction

Infantile cerebral palsy (CP) is the most frequent, most severe and most costly socio-economic motor disability in the paediatric age group. Consequently, its prevention is a public health priority, although its aetiology is very complex.

CPI is a syndrome of motor impairment due to a lesion in the developing brain, occurring before the age of 2 years. In mild forms of ICI, the patient presents with mild spasticity and contracture of the arm and leg on the same side, which interferes with fluidity of movement and fine manual dexterity. There may be associated decreased sensation and visual field disturbance on the same side, together with focal epilepsy. In severe forms, all four limbs are affected, with a mixed picture of spasticity and dyskinesia; with significant scoliosis and contractures, requiring a wheelchair to move around. They can be associated with significant learning difficulties, cortical visual blindness and propensity to pneumomas; with clinical severity depending on the time of occurrence of the lesion, clinical presentation and location. The first description of ICH is attributed to orthopaedic surgeon William Little in 1862.

Definition

According to the initial definition, ICH is a *persistent, non-progressive, motor manifestation*. It is not a disease in the traditional sense of the term, but a term describing the clinical condition suffered by children and adults who share a history of pre-, peri- or postnatal acquired brain damage.

In the current definition "Cerebral palsy encompasses a group of permanent developmental disorders of movement and posture, resulting in limited mobility, which are attributed to <u>non-progressive </u>disorders occurring during foetal or infant brain development. Motor disorders are often accompanied by sensory, perceptual, cognitive, communication, behavioural, seizure disorder and secondary musculoskeletal disorders" (Rosenbaum et al., 2007).

The proposed new definition and classification of ICH, which replaces the paragraph "non-progressive disorders occurring in the developing brain of the foetus or infant" by "<u>defect or lesion of the immature brain</u>", leading to a broader pathological spectrum, including e.g. "Developmental Coordination Disorder" or "Motor Dyspraxia". With this modification, it will be possible to diagnose ICH in 5-9% of live births, instead of 2 per thousand with the current classification, and it will also mean a change in the prevalence of the different aetiologies, and in the allocation of resources for treatment. Although the lesion is not progressive, the symptomatology of ICH changes over time, reflecting the maturational process of the CNS.

Epidemiolog^a

ICH is the most common physical disability in childhood. With a reported prevalence of 1 per 500 newborns, it accounts for an estimated 17 million people affected worldwide. Although the prevalence of ICH initially declined due to advances in obstetric and neonatal care, it increased again from the 1960s onwards due to increased survival of very low birth weight preterm infants. The birth prevalence of pre/perinatal cerebral palsy in high-income countries is decreasing and currently stands at 1.6 per 1000 live births. It is much higher in low- and middle-income countries, even with imprecise data, higher and with more intense physical disability, due to higher incidence of infectious diseases and differences in prenatal and perinatal care.

The set of aetiologies leading to ICH is not well defined in 80% of cases, but there are known risk factors identifiable from conception to the postnatal period. The key indicator of effective prevention of ICH is a decrease in its prevalence. Fetal monitoring during labour to detect the presence of acute fetal distress (loss of fetal well-being, as it is now called) has increased the number of caesarean sections by up to 40%, but has not reduced the incidence of ICH. In addition, % of ICH patients had no anomaKas on cardiotocographic recording, although the frequency of detected anomaKas is higher among ICH patients.

The aetiological cascade results from the complex interaction between risk factors at different stages, including at least 14% of cases with a genetic component. Preterm delivery and prolonged and/or dystocic labour resulting in neonatal asphyxia are the most important risk factors for ICH. Thus, the risk of ICH is 50 times higher in neonates <28 weeks gestation than in term infants.

Aetiology

The popular belief [and still held by many professionals today] that the main cause of ICH is acute intrapartum foetal anoxia dates back to the biblical scriptures in which ICH is referred to as "crippled from the mother's womb". However, we must not forget that up to 80% of the pathology diagnosed at the time of delivery has its origin in the pre- and perinatal period. The Apgar test score at one minute of life correlates with the quality of resuscitation, while the scores at 5 and 10 minutes have prognostic value, in relation to both perinatal causes and prenatal factors that are exacerbated during delivery, as the foetus is not able to withstand the added stress that all childbirth entails. On the other hand, there are a large number of aetiologies that can injure the brain postnatally (before the age of 2 years) and lead to ICH. Although unknown in most cases, it appears to be of prenatal aetiology (e.g. malformations and genetic causes).

Although the risk of ICH is relatively low in term neonates, in absolute values it accounts for up to 50% of cases. Cerebral infarction occurs in the first month of life in 1 in 4000 full term infants, and although it does not always cause cerebral infarction, it is estimated to be the most frequent cause of hemiparetic cerebral infarction (13-37% of all cases) and also of some cases of quadriplegia. Other causes are some factors of vulnerability to cerebral infarction such as genetic or acquired thrombophilia in the mother or her child, placental thrombosis, infectious conditions, surgery (caesarean section quadruples the risk of infarction in the mother); because the majority of those affected by ICH are born by caesarean section (indicated by fumculo-placental problems) and by the use of intravascular catheters. Choriamnionitis increases the risk of ICH in infants weighing more than 2500 g, with less evidence in preterm infants. Non-TORCH infectious processes [toxoplasmosis, rubella cytomegalovirus, herpes simplex and HIV] together account for up to 12% of the causes of ICH. On the other hand, there is an increased risk of ICH in relation to extreme neonatal weights, both overweight and underweight, across the entire gestational age range.

Predictors and related factors

Half of all children with ICH have high-risk indicators of identifiable disorders in the neonatal period, allowing early detection with pathogenic mechanisms developing before 5 months of corrected age (CE). In the other half, pregnancy and delivery may have been uneventful, and parents, caregivers or health professionals find a delay in developmental motor milestones (e.g., asymmetry in the use of hands or absence of standing at 9 months). This form of detection tends to occur especially in unilateral ICH, in infants who acquire early rudimentary motor skills (social smiling, swallowing and head control), and in whom asymmetry is not detected until they must acquire more complex motor skills (e.g. manual grasping).

PCI at or near term

In infants with ICH born near term or at term (> 35 weeks), four main risk factors are identified: 1) an intrapartum event potentially causing asphyxia (10%), 2) evidence of inflammation (5%), 3) fetal growth restriction (neonatal weight less than minus 2 SD (standard deviations) of mean weight for GA, sex, maternal height and parity), (8%); and 4) major congenital malformation (25-30%), with almost 10% additional if associated with fetal growth restriction.

Genetic causes

Various mutations in the ApoE gene, genes responsible for thrombophilias and the Osteopontin gene (involved in axonal regeneration and synaptogenesis after injury) have been described as susceptibility genes for ICH. In addition, there are monogenic causes of ICH (ataxic ICH genes, and others), as well as copy number variations (10-20% of cases), and other candidate genes (to be defined). Differential diagnosis with hereditary spastic paraplegia (HSPP) is sometimes quite difficult, since there are also HSPP genes involved in hereditary forms of ICH.

Physiopathology

ICH has a great etiological and pathophysiological heterogeneity. In most cases, ICH is the consequence of processes that damage healthy brain tissue, but it can also be due to congenital brain malformations. The type of lesions, their location and the response to injury all depend on the stage of development at which the lesion occurs. Although the primary lesion occurs in the motor neuron, symptoms are seen more in the peripheral neuromuscular system, especially in the skeletal muscles. The muscles are shorter and have smaller fibre diameters.

Upper motor neuron syndrome.

In ICH, upper motor neuron lesions (MNSs) located in the cerebral motor cortex give rise to two types of symptoms. The predominant and most important involves the loss of connections of the cortico-spinal tract that starts in the MNSs (cortex) and ends in the motor neurons of the anterior spinal cord (MNIs). The loss of connections causes paresis (partial paralysis), which is usually more pronounced in distal than in proximal muscles. In contrast, hyperthymia is due to the loss of the central inhibitory impulse descending to the MNIs, which causes hyperactivity of the muscle stretch reflexes (formerly known as osteo-tendon reflexes); resulting in hyperreflexia and hyperreflexia. The consequences of brain injury can extend to the entire locomotor system, especially in children with greater motor deficits, causing typical abnormal postures and deformities in the upper limbs, spine and hips, and in the lower limbs (contractures and twisting of the long bones). Signs of MNS syndrome are often classified as 'positive' (excess function, e.g. increased tone) and 'negative' for functional deficit (including poor strength and poor selective motor control).

Classification

Four components have been defined on which the classification of ICH is based:

1.   Motor Abnormalities

A.   *Nature and typology of the motor disorder:* these are the abnormalities in tone observed during examination (e.g. hypertome or hypotome) as well as the presence of movement disorders, such as spasticity, ataxia, dystome, or athetosis.

B.   *Functional motor skills:* degree of limitation of the individual's motor function in each of the body areas, including oromotor function, both chewing/swallowing and speech.

2.   Associated disorders

Non-motor neurodevelopmental or sensory problems; such as seizures, hearing or visual impairments, or attentional, behavioural, communication, and/or cognitive deficits, and the degree to which such disorders interact in individuals with ICH.

3.   Anatomical and radiological findings.

A.   *Anatomical distribution:* parts of the body affected by the motor disorder or its limitation.

B.   *Radiological findings:* neuro-anatomical lesions found on imaging tests.

4.   Cause and time of occurrence.

Whether there is a clearly identified cause, as is often the case with postnatal ICH (e.g. meningitis or head injury) or brain malformations, and the time interval in which the injury is presumed to have occurred.

When classifying ICH there are four sections to be assessed: Type, Topography, Tone and Degree:

Typology - Incidence

There are four distinct types of motor impairment <u>that can appear and change</u> during the first 2 years of life; they are: Spasticity (85-91%), Dyskinesia (4-7%; with Dystoma and/or

Athetosis; Ataxia (4-6%); or Hypotoma (2%).

Typology. Tone: Isotonic, Hypertonic, Hypotonic or Variable.

Topography. Dyskinesia, Ataxia and Hypotoma usually affect all 4 limbs, while spasticity is classified topographically as (1) unilateral (hemiplegia) (38%) or (2) bilateral, including Diplegia (with greater involvement of the lower limbs than the upper limbs - which are also affected, usually for fine motor skills), (37%), and Tetraplegia (involvement of the trunk and all 4 limbs), (24%).

Severity. Grades (Perlstein): Mild, Moderate, Severe; using the Gross Motor Function Classification System expanded and revised for children with cerebral palsy [GMFCS, grades I to V], which is the gold standard for the classification of motor function in children with cerebral palsy. The ordinal descriptors (I to V) are used according to the age of the child.

GMFCS: 6-12 years: Type I: ambulant in all contexts (no clinical gross motor limitation). II: walks unaided but has limitations in community functioning. III: walks with aids. IV: Requires wheelchairs or adult assistance to get around. V: complete dependence to move around. Approximately 2/3 of cases maintain walking, with significant motor limitations in the remaining third (grades IV or V).

Chemical manifestations

1. *Spastic ICH* (with pyramidal signs): in the form of Little's spastic diplegia, congenital hemiplegia, pure paraplegia, monoplegia or triplegia.

2. *Dyskinetic ICH* (with extrapyramidal symptomatology): atonic athetosis, athetosis, chorea, choreoathetosis, ballismus, torsional spasms, cerebellar ataxia, tremor.

3. *Atonic-asthenic syndrome* (lesion of the nuclei of the base): Initial lasting and generalised hypotoma, with flexion of the hips when the child is suspended by the arms (Foester) and mild intellectual disability, with evolution to a hypertonic picture at 3-4 years of age.

4. *Choreoatheto-athetosis syndrome*; with proximal choreic movement and unilateral or bilateral, distal, creeping type athetosis.

5. *PCI ataxic.* With static ataxia (does not keep head and trunk in an upright position), dysarthria, dysmetria of the upper limbs, with little cognitive capacity affected.

6. Mixed forms

Diagnosis

Cerebral palsy is a <u>clinical diagnosis</u> based on a combination of clinical and neurological signs, usually established in the second year of life. The type of movement disorder, the limitations and degree of impairment of functional abilities and the parts of the body affected vary widely among different patients. The type of motor dysfunction depends largely on the location and severity of the brain injury. Structural imaging (brain MRI) is recommended to confirm the clinical diagnosis. Movement impairment is characterised by spasticity (excessive contraction of muscles to rapid movement) and dystoma (sustained or intermittent muscle contractions or twitches causing abnormal, repetitive movements or postures).

Adequate motor development requires a progressive decrease in hyperflexion of the limbs, together with a simultaneous increase in trunk (body axis) tone. At birth, the term neonate presents a flexed posture of the four limbs, with very little tone of the trunk. In the first weeks, the flexed posture of the upper limbs (together with the progressive opening of the hands) will disappear, and later the hyperflexion of the lower limbs will disappear.

In the 1990s, Prechtl observed an alteration in the quality of general movements (GMs) during the neonatal period and in the first months of life in infants who subsequently develop ICH. He designed his method of qualitative assessment of general movements as a tool for assessing brain function and neurological integrity in neonates and young infants; a method that has been incorporated into structured neurological assessment schemes of the neonate, as it achieves a sensitivity of 98%. Even higher with sequential observation. The diagnostic sensitivity of encephalic MRI does not reach 90%.

The GMs assessment consists of observing the child for a period of 5-20 minutes and assigning a numerical value to the quality of the spontaneous movements. Three types of spontaneous movements are assessed:

1. Voluntary and anti-gravitational.
2. Harmonic, tangled, dancer-like (Fidgety movements).
3. Writhing movements.

GMs in preterm infants appear from ±28 weeks and persist until 36-38 weeks. They are extremely variable, including frequent pelvic rocking and trunk movements.

GM *writhing* appears between 36-38 weeks and disappears between 46-52 weeks.

Between 6-9 weeks later, both the form and characteristics of the MGs of the normal infant change from a pattern of meandering movements to a 'harmonic, entangled' pattern of small amplitude and moderate speed circular movements of the neck, trunk and limbs in all directions. In wakefulness they are present continuously, except when he focuses his attention. FM can be seen as early as six weeks later, but usually appears by 9 weeks and remains until 15 or, at most, 20 weeks. This age range remains constant for both term and preterm infants after age correction.

At any age, the basic characteristics of normal GMs are the involvement of all parts of the body, and the complexity and variation of movement with fluidity and fluency.

There are three patterns of pathological MG during the preterm, term and postterm stages (the first 2 months of age):

-   *MG of poor repertoire*. The sequences of movements are monotonous and the movements of the different parts of the body do not have the normal complex morphology.

-   *Spasmodic-synchronized* (CS, from *cramped-synchronized*) MG. They appear abruptly or spasmodically, without their normal smooth and fluid typology; in addition, the limbs and trunk contract and relax en bloc, almost simultaneously.

-   *Chaotic MG*. They are of large amplitude and in chaotic order on all limbs, with no hint of flow and fluidity; of continuous abrupt appearance.

It is abnormal if FM is absent or if the amplitude, velocity and abruptness appear moderately or severely exaggerated. There are two spastic markers for the later development of spastic CP:

1.   Presence of persistent spasmodic-synchronous type MG; over several weeks during preterm or term labour.

2.   Absence of entanglement-type MG at the usual age (9-20 weeks postnatal).

Therefore, the diagnosis of ICH can be made before 6 months of corrected age (CE) by Hammersmith Infant Neurological Assessment of General Movements (GMA) or by Hammersmith Infant Neurological Examination; together with encephalic MRI. After 5-6 months of CD, diagnosis requires Hammersmith Infant Neurological Examination, or Developmental Assessment in Young Children; in conjunction with MRI encephalic imaging. Repeat encephalic MRI at 2 years is recommended for patients with normal MRI at 12-18 months, combined with standardised motor assessment.

Evolution

The degree of motor impairment is difficult to predict in children under the age of 2 years because of the following reasons:

1.   Almost half of children over 2 years of age are subsequently reclassified according to the GMFCS,

2.   The natural history of ICP (e.g. later onset of dyskinesia, spasticity and contractures) is not well understood. Spasticity may appear after 12 months of age, and spasticity and dystoma may coexist.

3.   Motor skills are developing,

4.   Hypertoma may be present, initiate or evolve, and

5.   There is rapid brain growth with <u>use-dependent neuronal reorganisation </u>in response to therapy and care. With increased voluntary movement some symptoms may disappear (e.g. non-use of a limb), while others may worsen (e.g. increased dystonic postures simultaneous with voluntary movement). It is important to distinguish early on between unilateral vs. bilateral involvement because the treatment is different.

Comorbidities and functional limitations are common and disabling, including chronic pain (75%); intellectual disability (49%); epilepsy (35%); bone and muscle problems (e.g. hip dislocation) (28%); behavioural disorders (26%), sleep disorders (23%); cortical blindness (11%) and hearing impairment (4%). Digestive complications are very frequent, due to motor problems in sucking, chewing and swallowing; as well as respiratory complications, due to hyperextension of the neck, and derived from aspiration of food content. Approximately 10% of patients require a gastrostomy. Severe intellectual disability should be considered as the main diagnosis in children with spastic tetraplegia.

Prevention

Understood as the "set of measures that prevent the progression of a disease", it starts with primary prevention with elimination of known risk factors, such as Rh isoimmunisation, hyperbilirubinaemia, maternal iodine intake or thyroid hormone deficiency. Secondary prevention requires strategies to reduce preterm births and the development of drugs to delay labour. Administration of magnesium sulphate and antenatal corticosteroids reduce the incidence and severity of ICH in preterm infants, as therapeutic hypothermia does in high-risk term infants.

The Newborn Individualised Developmental Care and Assessment Programme (NIDCAP) aims to prevent the iatrogenic sequelae induced by intensive care and to maintain the intimate connection between parent and infant. One expression of this is kangaroo care. NIDCAP incorporates the infant into the parent's natural niche, avoids overstimulation, stress, pain and isolation, while supporting self-regulation, competence and goal orientation. NIDCAP improves brain development, functional competence, health and quality of life.

In infants with risk factors for ICH, follow-up should be close and specialised. The combined use of general movement assessment together with serial cranial ultrasonography and encephalic magnetic resonance imaging allows early diagnosis. Although 11-17% of children with a clinical diagnosis of ICH have a normal MRI. In this group of children, genetic and metabolic studies should be performed; and the scheduled follow-up of all infants ("Control del Lactante Sano" in Primary Health Care) includes the early detection of alarm symptoms in motor development such as delayed head control and balance, persistence of innate reflexes (3-4 months), lack of correlation between the different areas of development, as well as signs of neuromotor impoverishment. Other symptoms are delayed unassisted sitting up at 9 months, standing (12 m) or walking (18 m), early use of only one hand, asymmetry in crawling or walking, absence of full plantar support (persistent tiptoeing), or altered muscle tone.

Activity-dependent neuronal plasticity.

Effective tertiary prevention requires early diagnosis in order to initiate measures that take advantage of the plasticity of the maturing brain to avoid the establishment of abnormal movement patterns by means of an individualised protocol of action. Consequently, early intervention (prevention 3^) improves: 1) motor skills, 2) cognitive ability and 3) communication skills.

Treatment

There is no specific treatment for cerebral palsy. Clinical interventions are aimed at improving function and minimising factors that may worsen symptoms, such as epilepsy, feeding, scoliosis and hip pathology. These strategies include improving neurological function during the early stages of development; treatment of medical comorbidities, weakness and hypertension; use of rehabilitation technologies to improve motor function; and prevention of secondary musculoskeletal problems.

Therefore, treatment depends on the characteristics of the patients. All treatment protocols, within a multidisciplinary treatment team, aim to support innate adaptive motor development, but the anatomy and physiology of the muscles in cerebral palsy tends inexorably towards the development of muscle contractures with fixed and irreversible deformity.

By early stimulation of active and passive movements, rehabilitation treatment with physiotherapy and occupational therapy aims to inhibit abnormal reactions and enhance normal ones, thus preventing the development of deformities. The analysis of the clinical gait by means of camera and computer technology makes it possible to adapt the appropriate prosthetic aids and orthoses to the patient.

Evidence from neuroscience indicates that brain development and refinement of the motor system continues into postnatal life, driven by the activity of the motor cortex. Early intervention by introducing active movement is essential in order not to lose cortical connections and the specific function assigned to them. In addition, motor behaviour induced by the discovery of and interaction with the environment controls and generates the growth and development of muscle, ligament and bone, as well as regulating the ongoing development of the neuromotor system.

Occupational therapy

It is one of the disciplines of rehabilitation for children with ICH. Different approaches are used, including neurodevelopmental, and sensory integration. The aim is to improve the skills necessary for activities of daily living. OT focuses on several areas of intervention: play, self-care (feeding, dressing and grooming), fine motor skills such as writing, cognitive and visual-spatial problems.

Early cognitive development includes attention (and shared attention), memory, object relations, causality, imitation, problem solving and object classification. Children at risk of cognitive delay need intervention especially on early cognitive skills, such as shared attention, eye gaze and imitation.

During preschool, children are trained in language, spatial reasoning, problem solving, categorisation, physical causality, human interactions and numbers. There is a strong association between children's cognitive skills before they enter kindergarten and later achievement in primary and secondary school. Executive functioning (including self-regulation, behavioural sequencing, flexibility, response inhibition and planning) emerges during early childhood. Children with physical pathology and cognitive delays struggle with additional barriers (e.g., difficulty finding a toy or giving a parent a hug). Delayed cognitive skills confer significant risk for children's learning, behaviour and social interactions.

The provision of physiotherapy and occupational therapy should always include the participation of family and caregivers. Cognitive development and executive functioning should be addressed within the daily living skills of preschoolers and their families. Therapy leads to improved quality of life and social participation.

Parents play an important role in the rehabilitation process and are an important factor in facilitating the therapy process. Parent-centred care is important in the care of children with ICH, and adherence significantly affects the ability to achieve a good outcome. Adherence is defined as the extent to which a person's behaviour corresponds to the recommendations agreed with their health care provider. It is measured by the number of appointments and attendance, adherence to treatment recommendations, completion of prescribed programmes at home, and the level of parental or caregiver involvement in treatment. Adherence of parents with children with ICH is the main determinant of treatment efficacy.

Behavioural problems, common in children with ICH, may decrease parental cooperation in repeating therapeutic exercises at home. Predictive factors for behavioural problems among children with ICH include pain intensity, anxiety, stress and parental support, level of executive function, better gross motor function, lower intellectual ability, living in the city, and having a disabled or ill sibling. Family socio-economic status, environment and emotional environment also influence adherence to treatment. Along with the central role of the competence of health professionals such as physiotherapists, occupational therapists and physicians. Providing the community with information and the treatment it receives through the media can help reduce the cultural stigma of disability and increase positive attitudes towards treatment.

In summary, early and targeted intervention maximises neuroplasticity and minimises deleterious changes in bone and muscle growth and development. By providing a stimulating family environment, the ultimate goal is the patient's Functionality, Independence and Social Integration.

Forecast

Parents and caregivers may mistakenly assume that a diagnosis of ICH means that their child will require a wheelchair and have an intellectual disability. However, in developed countries, data indicate that 2 out of 3 children with ICH will walk, speak 3 out of 4, and 50% will have normal intelligence.

Summary

Although the frequency of cerebral palsy has hardly decreased and there are relatively few modifiable risk factors, assessment and attention to some of them may help to prevent its development. With current means, infantile cerebral palsy, especially those cases related to intrapartum asphyxia, is not preventable.

Bibliograffa

1. Als H, McAnulty GB. The Newborn Individualized Developmental Care and Assessment Program (NIDCAP) with Kangaroo Mother Care (KMC): Comprehensive care for preterm infants. Curr Womens Health Rev 2011;   7:   288-301. doi: 10.2174/157340411796355216

2. Ashwal, S. et al. Practice parameter: diagnostic assessment of the child with cerebral palsy: report of the Quality Standards Subcommittee of the American Academy of Neurology and the Practice Committee of the Child Neurology Society. Neurology 2004; 62: 851-863.

3. Cioni G. Observation of general movements in newborns and infants: prognostic and diagnostic value. Rev Neurol 2003; 37: 30-5.

4. Frolek CGJ, Schlabach TL. Systematic review of occupational therapy interventions to improve cognitive development in children ages birth-5 years. Am J Occup Ther 2013; 67: 425430. Doi: 10.5014/ajot.2013.006163

5. Graham HK et al. Cerebral palsy. Nature Rev Dis Primer 2016;2: 1-25.doi 10.1038/nrdp.2015.82

6. Novak I et al. Early. Accurate diagnosis and early intervention in cerebral palsy advances in diagnosis and treatment. JAMA Pediatr 2017; 171:   897-907. doi:10.1001/jamapediatrics.2017.1689

7. Prechtl, H. F. et al. An early marker for neurological deficits after perinatal brain lesions. Lancet 1997; 349: 1361-1363.

8. Rezaie L, Kendi S. Exploration of the influential factors on adherence to occupational therapy in parents of children with cerebral palsy: A qualitative study. Patient Preference

and Adherence 2020:14 63-72. Doi: 10.2147/PPA.S229535

9.   Rosenbaum et al. A report: the definition and classification of cerebral palsy. DMCN 2007; 49 (Suppl. 109): 8-14.

26. Intellectual Disability

Dr. Antonio Molina-Carballo

Introduction

The TIQ [Total Intelligence Quotient] is a score derived from different tests. There are many different types of intelligence tests to measure general or specific abilities: vocabulary, reading, arithmetic, memory, general knowledge, visual, verbal, abstract reasoning, etc. Traditionally, IQ is obtained by dividing the mental age of the test-taker (the age group that on average obtained this result in a random population sample) by the chronological age multiplied by 100. Currently the tests are standardised for a representative sample of the population: IQ scores for children are compared with those of children of the same age. The median is defined as 100 and one standard deviation (SD) is 15 points, so 95% of the population falls within two SDs of the mean (i.e. within an IQ range of 70 to 130). For an IQ to be reliable, it must be normalised against a population culturally similar to that of the person being assessed.

Although IQ can change with increasing age, it is a surprisingly robust concept because it predicts achievement with great strength (correlation). It has a large heritable component, but environmental factors are also involved. Heritability increases with age: it can be as low as 0.2 in childhood, 0.4 in school and up to 0.8 in adulthood. Although IQ is an apparently simple concept, it is subject to controversy. For some, for example, intelligence is a learned combination of many different skills and abilities, while for others intelligence is a single trait strongly determined by genetics, and still others believe that there are large ethnic or racial differences.

IQ tests should not be confused with knowledge tests, which attempt to measure skills and knowledge typically learned through schooling (e.g., language, arithmetic). IQ tests measure aptitude (potential ability) rather than actual achievement. Beyond the previously called "general intelligence", current theories see intelligence as a complex set of skills in a variety of areas (musical, mechanical, physical, social) that may differ substantially from each other in a given individual.

Intellectual Disability

The WHO defines Intellectual Disability (ID) as "a state of arrested or incomplete development of the mind, characterised especially by the impairment of skills that are manifested during the developmental period, and that contribute to the overall level of intelligence, i.e. cognitive, language, motor, and social skills".

The ICD-11 defines *Disorders of intellectual development'* as a group of pathologies of various aetiologies originating during the developmental period, characterised by intellectual functioning and adaptive behaviour significantly below average, approximately two or more standard deviations below the mean (below average), or at least two or more standard deviations below the mean (below average), or at least two or more standard deviations below the mean (below average).

2.3 percentile), based on appropriately normed and individually administered standardised tests.

The current, practical definition of ID includes the key symptoms of low intellectual functioning, IQ< 70 (i.e. 2 SD below average) together with adaptive behavioural disturbance. It is classified as mild (IQ 50-69), moderate (IQ 35-49), severe (IQ 20-34), and profound (IQ 0-20). Even so, there is consensus that the current model of defining intelligence, based on IQ, is of limited utility for intellectual disability, given the variety and variability of both cognitive functions and adaptive capacities. Assessing individualised levels of impairment in specific cognitive functions may be a more useful alternative.

Categories of Intellectual Disability (ID)

Kmite Intellectual Functioning (FIL) was a subcategory (or Disorder) of ID, referred to in DSM-III and DSM-IV, as "Borderline Mental Retardation". The 1961 classification manual of the *American Association of Intellectual and Developmental Disabilities (AAIDD)* proposed five levels of severity of ID: Borderline, Mild, Moderate, Severe and Profound, all defined by their own CIT range: Borderline (70-84), Mild (55-69), Moderate (40-54), Severe (25-39) and Profound (< 25). This classification scheme was adopted in 1952 by the *American Psychiatric Association* and subsequent editions of the DSM have largely followed the AAIDD grading, with the partial exception of the DSM-5. ID can occur in isolation or in combination with congenital malformations or other neurological features such as epilepsy, sensory disturbance and Autism Spectrum Disorders (ASD).

Borderline Intellectual Disability (LID) / Borderline Intellectual Functioning (LFI)

As for other psychiatric categories (e.g. Borderline *Personality Disorder)*, the prefix *'Borderline'* or the term FIL indicates the likelihood of having problems in daily functioning, but not so severe as to be unable to perform age-appropriate social functioning (work and independent living). Since 1973, DIL is not considered a disorder, and is defined only as a risk factor (which may be of current relevance or require future care) that adds nuances to the characteristics of people with Kmite intelligence and their functioning problems, as Intelligence remains an important concept in understanding human capacity.

Therefore, IDF is included within the average. A CIT of 70 is the ceiling for a diagnosis of mild ID; although "Mild" is a misnomer since the Disability can be substantial. Since IDF is not a primary diagnosis in DSM-5, its definition as a descriptive code does not require the presence of deficits in adaptive functioning. The elimination of this range implies, for example, that some individuals with FIL, such as those diagnosed with Fetal Alcohol Spectrum Disorder, who meet DSM-5 criteria for deficits in adaptive functioning, should be able to be diagnosed as ID despite achieving TIQ scores >75. In order to eliminate these mismatches, it has been proposed to remove the category of FIL and to increase (again) the range (up to 84) for diagnosing these patients as ID.

Epidemiolog^a

ID is the most common developmental disorder and affects 1-2% of the population in industrialised nations. A meta-analysis of published studies puts its prevalence at 1% of the population, which is higher in males. In adults, the female/male ratio ranges from 0.7/1 to 0.9/1, while in children and adolescents it ranges from 0.4/1 to 1:1. Given the heterogeneity of the causes of ID, estimates of its frequency worldwide are highly variable. The prevalence also varies depending on the age of the patients, e.g. 3.3/1000 between 20-50 years and 14.3/1000 in the age range 6-15 years. Prevalence is higher in low- and middle-income countries (almost twice as high as in rich countries), due to the important role of nutritional factors. In urban areas the prevalence is about half as high as in rural areas. In addition, ID is often part of a malformation syndrome affecting other organs and their functions (syndromic ID).

Aetiology

Factors influencing brain development and function can act prenatally, perinatally or postnatally, and can be divided into three groups: genetic, organic and socio-cultural, with a relevant overlap between the three groups. In up to 2/3 of mild cases (IQ 50-69) and 1/3 of severe cases (IQ < 50), the causes are not found.

The aetiology of ID is heterogeneous. Trauma, infections and toxins have decreased in incidence due to improved prenatal care, with genetic factors gaining prominence. As of today (2022), no definite cause is found in up to 40% of cases, particularly in mild ID. Environmental influences (e.g. malnutrition, emotional and social deprivation) can also cause or aggravate ID. In children in residential care, in addition to the cognitive impairment itself, Affective Deficiency Syndrome, in its most severe expression, can lead to Non-Organic (i.e. endocrine-metabolically normal) Failure to Thrive. Aetiological diagnosis opens up the possibility of specific treatment (very rare), or prevention in some severe cases, as well as allowing prediction of future occurrence of specific difficulties. Predisposing factors for genetic causes are advanced age of the parents, consanguinity and the presence of compensated chromosomal anomas in the parents.

Genetically aetiologic ID is subdivided into syndromic and non-syndromic (or unspecified) forms, depending on the presence or absence of additional distinctive clinical features. The genetic basis of the syndromic forms has been well studied, with the characterisation of the role of several genes involved, such as FMR1 (Fragile X syndrome) and MECP2 (Rett syndrome).

Other syndromic causes that may be associated with ID include Neurofibromatosis I (NF1) and mucopolysaccharidoses (MPS). MPS are a group of rare diseases (rare, orphan), with a low prevalence. Treatment is currently transdisciplinary and with enzyme replacement for some forms.

Clinical Semiology of Intellectual Disability

Language. Children with ID usually have difficulties in expressing and articulating language. Mild cases may achieve slightly poorer language than normally developing children. Severe or profound cases are unable to communicate or speak only a few words.

Perception. They are slow to perceive environmental stimuli and to react. Difficulty in distinguishing small differences in shape, size and colour.

Cognition. The ability to analyse, reason, comprehend and calculate, as well as abstract thinking, is impaired. With mild DI they learn to read and achieve a basic grade in mathematics.

Concentration and memory. They have a low and brief capacity. They are slow to recall memories (which are often inaccurate) although there are exceptions (e.g. savants).

Emotions. They are naïve and immature although they may improve with age. With little capacity for self-control and frequent impulsive and aggressive behaviour. Some are shy and withdrawn.

Movement and behaviour. They have poor coordination, clumsiness or excessive movement, inability to sit, and restlessness. In moderate or severe ID, stereotyped or meaningless movements (rocking, cranial self-hitting, tearing of clothes, hair pulling, genital touching,...), or (self-)-aggressive, destructive or violent behaviour are frequent.

Behavioural problems. Lack of concentration, impulsivity, tantrums, irritability and crying. Self-aggressive and aggressive behaviour, sometimes serious.

Concept. Characteristics of the Disorder according to the DSM-5 Domains.

ID involves the impairment of general mental abilities that affect adaptive functioning in three domains or areas that underlie the degree of effectiveness with which the individual copes with everyday tasks:

- *Conceptual mastery.* Includes skills in language, reading, writing, mathematics, reasoning, knowledge and memory.

- *Social domain.* Refers to social judgement, interpersonal communication skills, empathy, and the ability to make and maintain friendships.

- *Practical proficiency.* It focuses on self-management, in areas such as personal care, work responsibilities, money management, leisure and organisation of school and work tasks.

Diagnosis - ICD/DSM-5

The following three requirements are necessary:

- Intellectual abilities, below the population average (IQ <70), e.g. by WISC-V.
- Difficulties in adaptive skills (e.g. through Vineland - II)
- Onset in the developmental period: before the age of 18.

The numerical CIT score is excluded as the sole diagnostic criterion, although it should be included as a description of ID. Although Intellectual Disability does not include a specific age requirement, symptoms must begin during the developmental period and are diagnosed on the basis of the severity of deficits in adaptive functions. It is a chronic disorder, usually comorbid with others such as depression, Attention Deficit Hyperactivity Disorder and Autistic Spectrum Disorder.

Overall assessment

To diagnose ID, the DSM-5 emphasises the need for a full clinical assessment and standardised intelligence tests, together with an assessment of the severity of the deficit on the basis of adaptive functioning, rather than using the IQ number alone.

According to the DSM and ICD, ID involves deficits or impairments in adaptive functioning in at least two of the following areas: communication, self-care, home living, social/interpersonal skills, use of community resources, self-direction, functional academic skills, work, leisure, health and safety. When only one area is affected, it is diagnosed as a Specific Disorder (e.g. Language, or SLD).

Often, children with ID are referred for specialised care because of behavioural problems rather than low intelligence. Moderate and severe ID are identified early because of significant delays in Developmental Milestones. Often the milder forms do not become palpable until the beginning of primary schooling when academic difficulties become evident, or even later, during puberty/adolescence, by the time they reach Compulsory Secondary Education (ESO). It is not adequately defined to what extent the early onset of a delay implies its persistence or how it may progress to other disorders.

Pervasive Developmental Delay (PDD).

RGD is one of the Neurodevelopmental Disorders already listed in DSM-IV as "Mental Retardation of Unspecified Severity". RGD is the diagnosis that applies to <5 years of age and when other diagnoses (e.g, Intellectual Disability, Autism Spectrum Disorder, Attention Deficit Disorder, Specific Language Disorder, Motor Coordination Disorder, Specific Learning Disorders, etc.) still do not meet criteria.) do not yet meet diagnostic criteria or cannot be confirmed, because the child with RGD is unable to participate in formal, standardized assessments surrounding language, learning, and motor functioning, even though he/she has not reached age-appropriate developmental milestones in several areas (more than one). RGD indicates a significant delay in the acquisition of developmental milestones, namely: motor, speech and language; cognition; social functioning; and activities of daily living.

A high number of children with MDD will meet the diagnostic criteria for ID once they reach school age. Approximately 5-10% of the paediatric population suffers from a Developmental Disorder, an estimate that is affected by multiple factors such as age and socio-economic status; therefore, with higher prevalence in the developing world compared to westernised countries. The prevalence of MDD is as high as 15% in children under 5 years of age.

In RGD the aetiologies are also classified as pre-, peri- and postnatal. They range from smdromes and various genetic anomaKas to hypoxic-ischemic (sequelae) encephalopathy and infections of the central nervous system. RGD carries a high risk of later cognitive, behavioural or academic problems. Speech and language delays are linked with later problems in reading, writing, attention and socialisation. Diagnosis of the primary aetiology is a vital step in the treatment protocol for RGD.

In the face of possible RGD, although with the disadvantage that some will be diagnosed with multiple mental disorders, early assessment is very important in order to have an intervention protocol designed before school age. Few cases will be able to receive specific treatment. Typical treatments include psychomotor, language and occupational therapy, and if necessary, physiotherapy and parental support. Delayed language acquisition is the best predictor of RGD and future ID.

Children diagnosed as RGD adopted from developing countries and lacking adequate individual attention resulting in poor skills (motor, language, social and cognitive), when raised in a nurturing environment, often overcome their deficits before starting school.

In summary, early diagnosis of RGD is crucial for early intervention, especially in children with more severe delays. It also helps to avoid future socio-behavioural problems (e.g. social anxiety, bipolar affective disorder, depressive psychosis). Early diagnosis and intervention is demonstrably effective in reducing the risk of developing Attention Deficit Hyperactivity Disorder (ADHD).

Diagnosis

Neonatal screening for metabolic diseases, previously known as the heel prick test, on a dried blood sample on paper, is performed using dual tandem mass technology (GC-MS/MS) and allows the detection of 30 pathologies, extended in our Andalusian Community since 2016 with the detection of Cystic Fibrosis.

A full diagnostic assessment includes:

• Detailed anamnesis about parental and family history (with pedigree and review of medical records): genetic disorders, infections during pregnancy, prenatal exposure to toxins, perinatal injury, prematurity and metabolic disorders. DI of prenatal origin is more frequent than perinatal and postnatal origin combined, and the aetiology can be established in 40-60% of patients with DI (2/3 of severe DI and 50% of mild DI). An anamnesis (followed by a thorough physical examination) may suggest the time of damage (perinatal, postnatal and especially prenatal) even if it is not possible to determine the specific aetiology. Family history may provide unspecific indications of a hereditary disorder (recurrent miscarriages, unexplained early deaths and developmental, sensory, psychiatric, learning disabilities with DI.

• Psychomotor and intellectual development: motor and language skills, socialisation, comprehension and mathematical calculation. And behavioural assessment. Some behavioural traits allow to point out a characteristic "behavioural phenotype". For example, the continuous expression of joy together with easy and excessive laughter in Angelman syndrome; hyperexcitability and bulimia in Prader-Willi syndrome; hypersocial and familiar contact in Williams-Beuren syndrome, together with a loquacious and fluent language in contrast to the mental deficiency and the global visuospatial difficulties they present.

• Environment in which the child grows up: education, resources and family environment.

• Physical and neurological examination. Focusing on the description of possible even minor malformations, and on facial features. The head circumference should always be measured, possible ocular anomaKas or deafness should be recorded, and skin patches and dermatoglyphs should be assessed. There are a number of clinical signs and symptoms such as ID, short stature or microcephaly; and dysmorphic features (facial, distal parts of limbs and genitalia) that point to the possibility of chromosomopaphy. In some pathologies, using quantitative scales with data from the clinical history and clinical signs and symptoms, candidates for a particular genetic study can be selected.

Upon suspicion of a developmental disorder, in addition to medical tests, a complete psychological assessment with age-appropriate tests is mandatory.

• Brunet-Lezine Test: Applicable from 1 month to 6 years; assesses posture, oculo-motor coordination, sociability and language.

• Weschler Test for Preschool and Primary School (WPPSI, administered for ages 4 to 6 years. It assesses general, verbal and manipulative intelligence.

• WISC-V (Weschler for schoolchildren), at school age and includes different Factors and several sub-tests for each factor: Verbal Comprehension (VC), Perceptual Reasoning (PR), Working Memory (WM) and Processing Speed (PS).

• Vineland Adaptive Behaviour Scale. It allows comparison of the child's functional abilities with those of others of similar age and education. Not forgetting an appropriate clinical judgement to put the disorder in context.

Laboratory examinations

• 2^ Line: Haemogram Ferritin, Array CGH, Fragile X, CK, Plumbemia, Thyroid function, uric acid, Biotinidase. 2^ Line: Metabolic study; Neuroimaging, EEG, other Genetic studies.

In order to increase the diagnostic yield of the genetic tests, several requirements were defined in the application report for these tests: Absence of sequelae syndrome (PCI of proven perinatal cause); Degree of intellectual disability (moderate or severe); Presence of dysmorphic/malformational features; Family history (+).

Genomic microarrays (array CGH) have displaced G-banded karyotyping as a first level test because they allow genomic detection of copy number variations (CNVs) with higher resolution than optical microscopy. Overall, as of 2016, more than 812 genes associated with linked ID have been identified, more than 141 of them X-linked. Current cytogenetic studies have revealed several microdeletions and autosomal recurrent duplications that explain clinically differentiated ID smdromes, such as Prader-Willi, Angelman, Williams, Smith-Magenis, Miller-Dieker and DiGeorge smdromes.

In 2010, the ACMG (American College of Medical Genetics and Genomics) established genomic microarray studies (array CGH) as a 1^ line genetic test in the genetic diagnosis of children with congenital malformations / RGD / Intellectual disability. A common alternative to performing an exome is a "gene panel" for a specific phenotype. These panels can be performed on an exome or genome platform with reporting limited to the genes/phenotype indicated. In 2021, the same ACMG strongly recommends that exome or genome sequencing (NGS) be considered as the first or second level genetic test for patients with congenital malformations / RGD / Intellectual disability. In different neurodevelopmental disorders, array-CGH may be requested in unresolved cases or in some cases to precisely delineate the genomic region of a large CNV identified by NGS, and only test for Fragile X in highly suspicious cases (phenotype and/or family history).

X-linked intellectual disability (XLMR) is a common disease, with complex clinical and genetic heterogeneity, due to multiple mutations on the X chromosome. It affects between 1/600-1/1000 males and a considerable number of females. Among them, Fragile X syndrome is the most frequent cause of hereditary ID, with 35% of female carriers going on to have some degree of ID. In current practice, the trend is to screen for fragile X in all cases of ID of unknown cause, always in conjunction with Array CGH or high-resolution karyotyping.

Differential diagnosis

Medical. It aims to rule out sensorineural pathology as well as treatable and potentially reversible pathologies by means of a detailed family history (e.g., consanguinity) and clinical examination. Sometimes there are undetected or undertreated pathologies. It is very important to remember that the occurrence of regression (loss of previously acquired skills) is a medical emergency, because it implies the presence of a progressive encephalopathy, as opposed to a static encephalopathy (e.g. infantile cerebral palsy; ICP). In infantile cerebral palsy the symptomatic expressivity changes or becomes more apparent depending on the stage of development, but the change is very slow and does not lead to an increase in impairment.

Psychiatric. Severe stimulation deficits in the early stages of neurodevelopment are a cause of ID. Child abuse and maltreatment are often associated with lack of affection. In this broad conceptual framework, it should be remembered that for the WHO, the main predictor of ID is the presence of ID in the mother. ASD [and also the developmental disorders of reading, writing, mathematics,...] have their own criteria for diagnosis, complementary examinations and treatment. Psychiatric co-morbidity is common in ID, e.g. Anxiety Disorder (~50%), Oppositional Defiant Behaviour Disorders, ASD itself, ADHD (symptomatic) and Depressive Disorders. The concept of comorbidity refers to patients who simultaneously meet the clinical diagnostic criteria of two or more pathologies.

Other considerations. When dealing with a patient with ID, it is essential to monitor both the mental health of the parents and their *coping skills*. The presence of depression in the mother is common; as well as the incidence of serious marital conflicts, with situations of abuse/maltreatment in the family environment; and in the school environment with bullying by peers and serious school exclusion. Even more so in the absence of adequate economic resources and/or little support from the family environment, which leads to less environmental stimulation.

Degree of impairment (DSM-5) in Mild Intellectual Disability

The degree of involvement should be separated into three areas:

- *Conceptual area:* Difficulties in skills to meet age-related expectations.
- *Social area:* Immaturity in social interactions compared to his age group due to lack of understanding and management of the cues that direct social relations.
- *Practical area:* has capacity for personal autonomy, needing support only in more complex activities of daily life in relation to peers.

The assessment of intelligence using these three domains (conceptual, social and practical) is intended to ensure that the clinical diagnosis is based on the impact of the deficit on the general mental skills needed for daily living; with particular importance for implementing a treatment plan. CIT measures have less validity at the lower end of the normal range.

The use of neurodevelopmental disorder diagnosis specifiers is intended to enrich the description of the clinical course and current symptomatology. In addition to specifiers such as age of onset or severity of onset, neurodevelopmental disorders may include the specifier "associated with a medical condition (e.g., seizure disorder) or genetic disease (e.g., trisomy 21) or environmental factor (e.g., low birth weight)".

Treatment

It should always include family counselling with the implementation of psycho-pedagogical methods, following individualised assessment of the difficulties. In few cases patients will be subsidised by a specific medical (aetiological) treatment, even with the rapidly increasing availability of metabolic-enzymatic treatments and even gene therapy by genome editing (*cutting out* the mutated area and *pasting* the correct gene sequence synthesised in the laboratory) in the relatively near future (e.g. CRISPeR).

Mild ID accounts for about 80% of cases. Although they have very limited abilities to use abstract concepts, analyse and synthesise, the aim of the treatment is to learn the practice of essential skills to lead a life with no or minimal dependency before reaching adulthood; since they are able to communicate and to achieve reading and basic mathematical skills, to do housework, self-care and to achieve non- or semi-skilled work. To achieve this, they benefit from mainstream schooling. Although they always need some support, the real and always achievable goal of the treatment is individual autonomy in adulthood, making their neurodevelopmental potentialities real. This non-dependence is not achieved in moderate ID (CIT between 35 and 49-54), since they will only be able to communicate and perform self-care with some support.

Prevention.

The effective treatment is Prevention. *Primary*: prenatal, perinatal and postnatal, bearing in mind the time of incidence of the different aetiologies, providing comprehensive health services, introducing measures that have been shown to be effective at the right time. It is considered that 20% of the causes of DI are avoidable. With the objective of Primary Prevention, the diagnostic process begins before pregnancy with the recommendation of folic acid intake supplementation in all women who plan their pregnancy, continuing with the care of pregnancy and childbirth. *Secondary*: with early diagnosis, care and early intervention in the neurodevelopmental stage, which involves maximum neuronal plasticity. *Tertiary*: Family support, Stimulation, Training, Occupational therapy; based on Child Development Care (WHO, UNICEF).

Pharmacotherapy

There is little evidence of its efficacy, although it should be remembered that the absence of evidence does not imply the absence of evidence (of efficacy). Pharmacotherapy should be used after a global assessment and always together with psychosocial treatment/attention. In paediatrics the most commonly used atypical antipsychotic is Risperidone, often together with stimulant drugs (e.g. methylphenidate) because they help in the behavioural control and management of patients, and because it is assumed that they do not increase the risk of incidence of other pathologies, but even decrease it. Several studies in patients with controlled epilepsy [symptomatic, comorbid with disability] show that treatment with stimulants decreases the incidence of new seizures. Non-stimulant drugs (Atomoxetine, Guanfacine) help in the control of emotional symptoms and aggressive/impulsive behaviour, and unlike stimulant drugs their effect is prolonged 24 hours a day.

Bibliograffa

1. Galan-Gomez E et al. Genetic studies in inespeafic mental retardation. An Pediatr Contin 2012;10:7-15

2. Greenspan S. Borderline intellectual functioning: an update. Curr Opin Psychiatry 2017;30:113-122. doi: 10.1097/YCO.0000000000000317.

3. Iwase S et al. Epigenetic Etiology of Intellectual Disability. J Neurosci 2017;37:10773-10782. doi: 10.1523/JNEUROSCI.1840-17.2017.

4.   Mithyantha R et al. Current evidence-based recommendations on investigating children with global developmental delay. Arch Dis Child 2017;102:1071-1076. doi: 10.1136/archdischild-2016-311271.

5.   Moeschler JB, Shevell M. Comprehensive evaluation of the child with intellectual disability or global developmental delay. Pediatrics 2014: e903-e918. doi: 10.1542/peds.2014- 1839.

6.   Schalock RL et al. The renaming of mental retardation: Understanding the change to the term intellectual disability. Intellectual and Developmental Disabilities 2007; 45: 116-124. doi: 10.1352/1934-9556(2007)45[116:TROMRU]2.0.CO;2.

7.   Sullivan P, Knutson J. Maltreatment and disabilities: A population-based epidemiological study. Child Abuse & Neglect 2000;24: 1257-1273.

8.   Thomaidis L et al. Predictors of severity and outcome of global developmental delay without definitive etiologic yield: a prospective observational study. BMC Pediatrics 2014;14: 1471-2431

9.   Vissers L et al. Genetic studies in intellectual disability and related disorders. Nat Rev Genet 2016; 17: 9-18. doi: 10.1038/nrg3999.

10.   Zigler E et al. On the definition and classification of mental retardation. Am J Mental Deficiency 1994; 89: 215-230.

27. Occupational therapy in neonatal units

Dr. Esther Ocete Hita

Child development is a dynamic, highly complex process, based on biological, psychological and social evolution. The first years of life are a particularly critical stage of life, since it is here that the perceptual, motor, cognitive, linguistic and social skills that will enable a balanced interaction with the surrounding world are shaped. At the same time, the negative consequences that the presence of biological risk factors can have on a child's development have been extensively studied.

(congenital diseases, perinatal injuries, etc.), and how this will be enhanced if the child is placed in an environment lacking stimuli and opportunities (economic, socio-cultural, etc.) that prevent him/her from receiving adequate and systematic medical treatment.

An important risk factor today is early birth, as advances in perinatal medicine have increased the survival of very low birth weight preterm infants. The World Health Organisation defines a preterm birth as one born before 37 weeks of pregnancy, which corresponds to 1% of all live births. Within this category, those with a birth weight of 1500 g. or less correspond to the group that needs the most attention, because of the risk of disability later in life.

Over the past two decades, a variety of interventions have been used in preterm infants to compensate for their immaturity and abbreviated intrauterine experience. They attempt to compensate for the process that was abruptly interrupted by early delivery and, according to research, have beneficial effects on short-term growth and weight gain, decrease ventilatory support, reduce hospitalisation days and enhance neonatal development.

Bearing in mind that the aim of early care is to offer children with deficits or at risk of suffering them a set of optimising actions that manage to compensate or facilitate adequate maturation in all areas, two complementary and simultaneous instances of intervention can be highlighted within it. On the one hand, the stimulating intervention of the neonate (Early Intervention itself) and, on the other hand, the management of the environment in the neonatal care unit.

Environmental management and regulation

Due to its peculiar characteristics, the preterm infant has difficulty in assimilating environmental stimuli and reduced internal organisation, manifested by changes in skin colour, increased respiratory effort, poor regulation of body temperature and inability to maintain a state of calm alertness. These signs affect the child's ability to interact with parents and the environment, devoting effort only to self-regulation.

Preterm infants are neurologically immature; consequently, they have difficulty adapting to the invasive environment of the Neonatal Care Unit. This environment is characterised by bright lights, noise and frequent manipulation of the neonate. In this effort to cope with the extra-uterine environment, preterm infants attempt to self-regulate physiologically. They often manifest signs and signals of stress.

Intrauterine environment

The foetus begins its life in an environment that modulates all the stimuli that act on it during its development: the maternal uterus. This intrauterine habitat is characterised as a warm, dark, warm, warm environment that provides containment and comfort, as well as the nutrients and hormones necessary for the normal development of the developing child.

The foetus senses its mother's physiological noises (auditory stimulation), moves when its mother does and spontaneously, from the ninth week of gestational age, has vestibular and kinaesthetic stimulation, and is in direct contact with the walls of the amniotic sac (tactile and proprioceptive stimulation). In addition, other basic functions such as nutrition, thermoregulation and the modulation of the sleep-wake cycle are developed through this matrix, as a means of connection with its mother.

From the postural point of view, the maternal uterus provides the foetus with the global flexion of its body, favours the development in the midline, the containment and, of course, the necessary comfort, positioning it correctly so that nature can act on it.

Children who are born prematurely are dramatically deprived of this pathophysical environment and miss out on the intrauterine stimulation necessary to complete proper development.

Extrauterine environment: Neonatal Care Unit (NICU)

Neonates attempt to cope with the stimulation of bright lights, alarms, loud monitor noises and human voices in the NICU. To protect themselves from the demands of the external environment, they exhibit defensive behaviours that correspond to signs of stress and self-regulation.

Signs of stress

When premature infants in the NICU are overloaded by the continuous stimulation provided by the environment and manipulations related to their care, they often show overt signs of stress. These signs of stimulus overload may correspond to physical signs or physiological changes. They indicate that the neonate does not require additional stimulation.

Signals of stimulus overload include: averting the eyes or turning the head away from the stimulus, frowning, tightly pursed lips, twisting movements of the arms, legs, trunk, etc.

Signs of self-regulation

Although neonates may exhibit behaviours that are indicative of stress, they may also show signs of self-regulation and organisation. These behaviours are intended to calm the newborn and help it recover from stress. This happens when the infant's central nervous system is unable to regulate incoming stimulation. The infant begins to become hyperactive and more alert and shows increasing efforts to organise its motor and physiological systems to achieve a state of calm. These self-regulatory efforts may deplete the neonate's enemas, particularly if he/she has difficulty calming down. Signs of self-regulation include the following: aversion to gaze, intense sucking to calm down, constant movement in search of contact, etc.

General and specific objectives of occupational therapy in neonatal units.

1. To apply global motor and neurosensorial stimulation techniques focused on favouring adequate psychomotor development in children with a history of prematurity.

*   Assess and perform postural monitoring of neonates.

*   To carry out vestibular, kinaesthetic, tactile, auditory, etc., stimulation activities for those children who are able to assimilate these stimuli.

*   To stimulate the organisation and moderation of sensory information received by the child.

*   To monitor children's development up to 24 months of age.

*   Enable the development of strategies that contribute to a better understanding and understanding of the
establishing the link between the newborn and the family during hospitalisation.

2. To regulate and adapt the environment of the neonatal care unit to avoid harmful stimuli to the infant and its development.

*   Assess and monitor harmful environmental pollutants.

*   To reduce the stress of hospitalised neonates.

*   To inform the Neonatal Unit staff on the recognition of neonatal stimulation signs and their management.

Activities

Early intervention and stimulation, by activating sensory systems important for maturation, aims primarily to compensate for the disruption of experiences and to allow the resumption of a process that was suddenly interrupted by premature birth.

Within this, the following interventions can be highlighted:

- Observe the child's level of spontaneous activity and response to environmental stimuli.
- Apply global neurosensory stimulation according to corrected age (visual, tactile, auditory, vestibular, stimulate exploratory and play skills, hand-eye coordination, etc.).
- To give advice to parents on modalities of psychomotor development stimulation and management at home according to the specific needs of the child.
- To reinforce the mother-child bonding and to favour the paternal-filial relationship.

Interventions in neonatology have been guided by two trends or schools of thought. The first argues that, because preterm infants are born early, essential intrauterine experiences necessary for growth and development have been lost. Thus, it is necessary to stimulate the pathophysical aspects of the womb. The other stream of opinion emphasises the differences between preterm and term infants. According to this trend, supplementary sensory stimulation is needed for preterm infants to catch up with term infants.

Consequently, if both tendencies are combined, sensory-motor interventions can be protective as well as stimulating.

The main elements through which intervention can take place are as follows:

1. Positioning and handling of the preterm newborn.

Handling and positioning of the premature infant is one of the first and most important ways for caregivers to intervene in its development.

When the preterm infant becomes disorganised and cries, interaction with the environment may be developmentally inappropriate. Proper handling and positioning of newborns before and after a procedure helps them return to the calm alertness necessary for growth and development. Proper handling and positioning produces a calm and restful state for the neonate.

If repositioning occurs while the neonate is awake or in active sleep, the therapist can proceed to touch and move the neonate slowly and purposefully. This slow and deliberate manipulation is comfortable for the premature infant, who has decreased muscle tone and is therefore inefficient in counteracting the effects that gravity exerts on them during changes of position.

Manipulation and positioning are also involved with tactile stimulation, which provides a kind of stimulation that has important consequences for the development of the preterm infant.

Some important elements to consider for proper positioning are:
- Use nests and coils as support elements to provide containment.
- Minimise the effects of gravity on babies.
- Provide external stability and containment that resembles the intrauterine environment to increase the baby's ability to maintain a flexed posture.
- Stimulate active flexion of limbs and trunk.
- Promote the orientation to the middle Knea of the hands and the hand-mouth activity.
- To reduce cranial deformities due to pressure and rotation of the neck.

2. Environmental Adaptation

The elements that can be modulated in Neonatal Care Units are noise and bright light.

Noise modulation at UCN.

Newborns in Neonatal Care Units are continuously exposed to auditory stimulation for prolonged periods of time. For this reason, it is necessary to establish intervention routines that modify noise levels.

The noise level can be significantly reduced through individual actions, but also through global or systemic changes.

Some unnecessary sounds can be eliminated through the following interventions:

- Decrease the alarm intensity of monitors and telephones.
- Limit conversations close to the newborn.
- Respond quickly to turn off alarms.
- Turn off radios in the unit.
- Locate the most labile patients away from high traffic areas.
- Decrease the child's activity level and reduce stress.
- Intermittent stimulation, such as musical boxes or recordings of parents' voices, may be used only after assessing the infant's ability to tolerate these sounds. If the newborn shows signs of stress or physiological instability, stimulation should be discontinued.

Modulation of brightness at UCN

Neonates are kept in care units that are continuously illuminated.

Research has reached consensus on the effect of the loss of daylight and artificial light cycles on the sleep states of neonates.

It can be concluded that in Neonatal Care Units there is a need to measure the level of light necessary to support and improve the individual biological rhythm of the neonate, and also to allow the medical procedures inherent to their care to be carried out.

Possible interventions include the following:

- Use blankets over incubators.
- Place the most stable patients in areas where it is possible to establish day-night light cycles.
- Install dim light penodos in the unit.
- Use individualised lighting for the execution of therapeutic procedures.
- Use eye protection for premature infants in phototherapy.

More mature and stable infants are able to tolerate more visual stimulation. They may be able to visually explore toys or mobiles located within their visual field. Face-to-face interaction during breastfeeding or the newborn's alertness may be appropriate for visual stimulation.

3. Interaction with parents

The early relationship between parents and their children is the cornerstone of a child's development. These interactions give children confidence and security and allow them to develop healthy emotional bonds that are important for the attachment process.

In recent years, researchers and clinicians have expressed a growing need to strengthen a positive emotional environment for parents and their children at UCN. This reflects an awareness of the need for families and their important role in promoting the well-being of their children. Interventions have been developed to assist families while the newborn is hospitalised in the NICU and during the transition to home.

Interventions that facilitate positive interactions between the preterm infant and parents within the hospital institution include the following:

- Teach parents to recognise the different states of their child.
- Encourage parents to interact with their child when the child's condition and medical conditions permit.
- Help parents recognise signs of stress in children in order to modify stimulation and interaction.
- To assist parents in relation to the expectations of their child's future development.
- Teach comforting manoeuvres for the child.
- Teach parents positioning techniques.
- Keep parents informed of their child's condition.

Bibliography

1. Fernandez MP. Sensorimotor intervention in preterm infants. 2016 [cited 2016 Sep 10, 2022];13(4). Available from: https://www.revistapediatria.cl/volumenes/2004/vol1num1/5.html
2. de Rose ML. Promoting occupational self development from the neonatal period. Tog [Internet]. 2013 [cited 2013 Oct 4, 2022];(18):2-4. Available from: https://dialnet.unirioja.es/servlet/articulo?codigo=4509109
3. AOTA. Occupational Therapy Practice Framework: Domain and Process-fourth edition. Am J Occup Ther [Internet]. 2020 [cited 2022 Apr 4];74(2). Available from: https://research.aota.org/ajot/article-abstract/74/Supplement_2/7412410010p1/8382/OccupationalTherapy-. Practice-Framework-Domain-and?redirectedFrom=fulltext
4. Pinon Formoso A. Benefits provided by the attachment-based care methodology [Internet]. Universidade da Coruna; 2014 [cited 2022 Oct 9, 2022]. Available from: https://ruc.udc.es/dspace/bitstream/handle/2183/13664/TFG Enfermaria Pi%C3%B1%C3%B3n %20Formoso Ariazna.pdf?sequence=2&isAllowed=y1
5. Pallas Alonso CR. Developmental care in neonatal units. Anal dePediatnaContrnuada [Internet]. 2014;12(2):62-7. Available in: https://www.elsevier.es/es-revista-anales-pediatria-continuada-51-pdf-S1696281814701702
6. Espm MP, Caro MJL, Serrano AC, Rodnguez AC, Gonzalez JAM, RodnguezIMR. Developmental care in neonatology units. In: ASUNIVEP, editor. Health and Care during development [Internet]. ASUNIVEP; [cited Sep 24, 2022]. p. 181-6. Available in : https://www.formacionasunivep.com/Vciise/files/libros/LIBRO_5.pdf#page=

28. Occupational therapy for institutionalised children

Dr. Esther Ocete Hita

Childhood is the first opportunity for human beings to get to know the world around them and to develop in the environment in which they live. During the development of the human being there are a series of physical, mental, emotional and social changes. These are manifested as children grow and develop. During the first five years of life, the foundations for future health and happiness are laid, as well as for growth, development and learning in school, family and community.

The family is the first socialising agent, where the child's first interactions take place, and it is in this context that the foundations for affective and social relationships are laid, thus attachment is considered fundamental in the social development of children. Similarly, the family's role is to foster the development of skills in a nurturing environment and to provide stimuli for optimal development. Experiences in childhood will have a positive impact as long as they take place in nurturing, protective and stimulating relationships, but they can also have a negative impact if they take place in environments filled with stress, hostility, insufficient basic care and neglect. For this reason the environment exerts an important influence on the child's development, which can facilitate or hinder it.

Among the factors that hinder a child's development is the social environment that does not provide adequate time and space for play. Through play, feelings, emotions, desires and curiosity can be expressed, which favours the creative process and with this the discovery of abilities and qualities that allow the child to develop skills for an adequate performance, both in daily activities and in social interactions. The family's role is to foster the development of skills in a nurturing environment and to provide stimuli for optimal development, but what happens to children who are not in a favourable socialising context? Certainly, social problems limit the child's opportunity for holistic development and personal growth, affecting social behaviour and impacting on all domains (psychosocial, emotional, neurological, cognitive and physical), influencing the child's ability to relate healthily to society and to be competent. When the child is immersed in a context that is not appropriate for his or her age, the areas and components of performance are affected, and therefore his or her performance in these areas is altered.

Institutionalisation has effects on children such as:

o Deterioration of basic confidence: the child perceives a frustrated and emerging world, making it difficult for him/her to adapt to it.

o Low self-image: it depends on the self-image whether the child will face the world with more or less confidence, with more or less creativity.

o Distortion in interpersonal relationships: mainly in areas such as detachment and instability in affection and indiscriminate relationships.

All of the above effects result in a feeling of frustration which Dollard considers to be the cause for the aggressive reaction.

Marginal Behaviours:

o Difficulties in self-regulation of behaviour: The child learns to depend on routine and external controls and loses autonomy and becomes dependent.

o Lack of initiative: The feeling of hopelessness and the feeling of not having much control over events, plus the lack of varied experiences, makes them face situations with their own limitations. They move as far as they are taught, do what is allowed, repeat more and try less.

o Survival Behaviours: Fighting for space; kicking for attention; self-stimulatory movements for gratification in an unrewarding environment and to avoid dissatisfaction; limited use of objects; children restrict and impoverish their actions due to lack of opportunities and role models. They accumulate objects, which has a background in the need to contain something that is their own and in relation to the general need they feel. Occupational therapy in paediatrics specialises in the prevention, functional diagnosis, treatment and research of daily occupations in different areas: Prevention, functional diagnosis, treatment and investigation of daily occupations in different areas to increase independent functioning and improve the development of children who present difficulties in their daily performance. It also includes the adaptation of tasks or the environment to achieve maximum independence and improve quality of life. So that the intervention of the discipline provides an integral treatment for the benefit of the quality of life of institutionalised children, thus facilitating their occupational performance and their relationship with their environment.

UNICEF (2015), mentions that, during childhood, children should participate in recreational and educational activities, so that they develop strong and self-confident, receiving love and encouragement from the adults around them. In this period of their life children should be protected from abuse, exploitation and violence in the physical, social and family environment. From the physical environment the person receives consistent feedback, whereas from the social environment the responses are more variable.

The environment for play to emerge must offer safety; variety of objects, materials, people or activities with which to interact; freedom to choose whether or not to play; times when the child is not tired, hungry or stressed; and environmental cues (human or object) that communicate that this is "play".

The institutionalised environment is characterised not only by maternal deprivation, but also by reduced handling, reduced opportunities for interaction and reduced stimulation. The lack of interaction of the child with a mother figure and a nurturing environment in the institutionalised infant constitutes a negative impact on intellectual, physical, emotional, social and language development. This is associated with the decreased play time that the caregiver(s) spend with the children at play, coupled with the existence of children who are "favoured" by the caregiver(s), who have greater advantages in play than those who are not and who have a stronger relationship with the caregiver(s). In addition, the varied number of caregivers present, who fulfil various roles within the institution, has a negative impact on the infant in relation to the development of the self and their interaction with their environment. In addition, children in an institutionalised environment tend to be more passive in feeding and play. In summary, it is worth mentioning that "play in childhood provides a unique window to assess and understand the effects of deprivation and to provide intervention for children who have experienced such conditions.

The importance of the early years

Childhood is a period during which many milestones are reached. However, it is important to remember that human development has a number of characteristics: it is lifelong, it depends on environments and contexts, it is multidimensional and multidirectional, and it is flexible and plastic. In this way, environment and context are two determining aspects for the occupational development of the child in particular, and of the human being in general.

The American Occupational Therapy Association defines environments (physical and social) as the settings in which occupations are performed, while contexts (cultural, personal, temporal and virtual) are a set of conditions that influence occupational performance. An impoverished or unstimulating environment can influence both child development and quality. Also of vital importance are the children's relationships, care and/or links with their family/primary caregivers, which must be sufficiently good to avoid developmental problems. Thus, both the place and the relationships that occur in the early years can condition the child's development, as this will be the result of the interaction between his or her potential capacities and his or her environment. In this way, a maturing brain presents a greater vulnerability to adverse environmental conditions and a developmental disorder can be produced by unfavourable social circumstances, including situations of neglect, mistreatment or abuse or institutionalisation.

It should be remembered that many of the children who spend part of their lives in residential centres under state care have gone through serious social situations that have had an impact on their development and health.

Life in an orphanage is characterised by the fact that there are multiple caregivers who take turns to care for the children, so there is a high child to caregiver ratio and the environment may be set up in such a way that they may have less opportunity for movement and play.

Different diseases and/or pathologies have been observed in orphaned, institutionalised and adopted children: nutritional disorders, rickets, iron deficiency anaemia, difficulties in psychomotor development, communication and language disorders, behavioural disorders, attention deficit and hyperactivity disorder, emotional problems and psychological and psychiatric disorders.

Teona de Integration Sensorial

Sensory Integration (SI) is a neurobiological process that consists of the adequate organisation of sensations coming from the senses in the Central Nervous System for the elaboration of adaptive responses in daily life. Thus, a sensory processing disorder results from a problem related to an inadequate integration of sensations in the brain, which can lead to problems in modulation, discrimination or sensory-based motor difficulties.

The repercussions can lead to difficulties in daily life and participation, including learning, behavioural, social, emotional (self-esteem and self-control), motor coordination and attention problems. For all these reasons, early detection of this situation is essential to prevent future occupational dysfunctions. It is suggested that some of these occupational dysfunctions shown by orphaned, institutionalised and adopted children could be due to difficulties in SI.

Among the objectives of the intervention by the institutions are to promote a set of practices aimed at ensuring the reintegration of the child into his/her family environment, the preparation for autonomous life, as well as the generation of conditions that prepare him/her, and facilitate the construction of a life project for social inclusion, avoiding isolation and maladjustment. A stable, active and reliable personal social network protects children and adolescents from various risk factors and acts as a helping agent. The support network fulfils the following functions: social interaction, which refers to the carrying out of joint activities; emotional support, which consists of exchanges that provide support, encouragement, understanding and security; social regulation, which seeks to promote functional and normative adaptation to the environment; cognitive gwa and exchange of knowledge, which provides role models and social interactions; access to new contacts, which facilitates openness for connection to other networks.

It is found that the most applied programmes for intervention and promotion of mental health in the institutionalised population are the systemic perspectives and the cognitive and behavioural approaches. The relevance of the systemic approach is more applicable to family care, followed by cognitive and behavioural approaches. Nowadays, it is important that the different approaches seek to strengthen support networks, to improve parenting patterns and to strengthen parental roles. In the intervention processes with children and adolescents, the cognitive and behavioural approach is used to strengthen social skills and promote the assertive expression of emotions and overcoming the experiences of vulnerability that preceded their entry into protection. It is recommended to emphasise prevention rather than treatment; to recognise the strengths and competencies of individuals; to work from an ecological perspective; to promote collaboration between different disciplines; to promote a sense of community, respect for difference and the generation of community mental health services through intrasectoral and intersectoral collaboration.

The functions of the occupational therapist in institutionalised children will be aimed at:

- Global evaluation and assessment of the person, his/her abilities and limitations.
- Elaboration of treatment programmes according to individualised objectives in accordance with the abilities, needs and interests of the person.
- Training and re-education in basic and instrumental activities of daily living (hygiene, eating, use of public transport, use of money, etc.).
- Assessment, design, prescription and training of orthoses, prostheses and support products.
- Adaptation and transformation of the environment by eliminating physical and/or social barriers that hinder the participation of people in their occupations.
- Sensory stimulation and integration.
- Advice on leisure and free time.
- Guidance/job counselling to increase employability and employability opportunities.
- Collaboration with public and/or private institutions for the development of

programmes aimed at the promotion of health and social participation of the population with or without disabilities.

The therapeutic objectives for institutionalised children are as follows:

Specific objectives

A.   In relation to the need to favour the socio-emotional development of children while they remain in the alternative care system:

1.   To offer the child a space of therapeutic containment that promotes their emotional security.

2.   To identify the characteristics, relational functioning and needs of each child admitted in order to plan the therapeutic intervention.

3.   To sensitise and integrate in the therapeutic process the significant caregivers of the children assisted, promoting a protective environment, which facilitates their bonding and capacity for emotional regulation.

4.   Therapeutically accompanying the child in his or her developmental trajectory, in order to integrate in a basic way the violations of rights experienced, including the process of declaration of adoptability.

B.   In relation to the need to facilitate the bonding of the child with his future adoptive family

5.   To collaborate from the child's perspective in the process of searching for an adoptive family, participating in the decision making about the pre-selected families.

6.   To prepare the child for his/her insertion in an alternative family to the family of origin.

7.   To prepare the alternative family to the family of origin to take on the child, in the exercise of positive parenthood.

C.   In relation to the need to support parental figures in order to adequately exercise adoptive parenthood:

8.   To support families in the stage of family integration, fostering their bonding and child care skills.

9.   To provide specialised therapeutic intervention for adoptive families with adoption-related difficulties, supporting their family development trajectory.

Bibliograffa

1.   Hers, B. Popovici, E., Apetrei, R., Zolotusca, L., Beldescu, N., Calomfiescu, A. & Col. Acquired immunodeficiency syndrome in Romania. Lancet, 338,   645-649. https://doi.org/10.1016/0140-6736(91)91230-R.

2.   Gonzalez, C, Ampudia, A., & Guevara, Y.. Intervention program for the development of social skills in institutionalized children. Acta colombiana de Psicolog^a, 15(2), 43-52.2012, http://www.redalyc.org/articulo.oa?id=79825836008

3.   Martin, E. Perceived social support in children and adolescents in residential care. International journal of psychology and psychological therapy, 2011, 11(1), 107-120. http://www.ijpsy.com/volumen11/num1/285/apoyo-socialpercibido-en-nios-y-adolescentes- EN.pdf.

4.   UNICEF.2015 La situación de niños, ninas y adolescentes en las instituciones de

protección y cuidado de América Latina y el Caribe. United Nations Children's Fund.

5. Manrique, A. M., & Henny, E. (2017). Factors and components of occupational performance in boys and girls, at social risk and institutionalized in early childhood. Revista Chilena De Terapia Ocupacional, 17(1), 141-154. https://doi.org/10.5354/0719-5346.2017.46387

29. Epilepsy in Paediatrics

Dr. Antonio Molina-Carballo

Introduction

Epilepsy is the most common and severe neurological pathology, affecting an estimated 50 million people worldwide. There are more than 40 different types of epilepsy, with at least 29 syndromes and about 12 clinical pictures defined by a specific or underlying cause. Epilepsy can manifest itself with up to 63 different types of seizures and each patient may have one or several different types. Many people with epilepsy also suffer from difficulties with intellectual functioning, behaviour and social communication.

Definition

Epilepsy as a brain disorder characterised by an ongoing predisposition to seizures is defined clinically as the occurrence of two or more unprovoked (or reflex) seizures. Diagnosis after a single seizure and a probability of recurrence >60% or the diagnosis of an epileptic syndrome is currently accepted. The probability of recurrence can be calculated by taking into account factors such as anomaKas in the electroencephalogram (EEG) or in imaging tests (structural magnetic resonance imaging, MRI), and a family history of epilepsy. The concept of "unprovoked seizure" refers to the absence of disease or brain damage in close relation to the seizure.

Epidemiolog^a

Incidence. It is maximal at both ends of life. 1er year: 120 / 105. 1-10 years: 40-50 / 105, Adolescence: 20 / 105, >1 seizure: 1% (<15 years), Epilepsy: 0.4-0.8% at 11 years. *Prevalence.* Active epilepsy (in treatment or with seizures in the last 5 years): 4.3-9.3 / 1000.

Diagnosis

It is almost exclusively clinical. It begins with a description of the seizure and an EEG, if possible within the first 24 hours after the seizure. Subsequently, if anomaKas are found that reinforce the clinical suspicion of a seizure, a prolonged EEG recording (including sleep recording) in sleep deprivation is recommended to adequately characterise the anomaKas.

Description of crises

The seizure should be defined on the basis of the predominant and earliest onset clinical feature, as focal, generalised or "unknown". The alertness/consciousness may be focal conscious or focal with altered consciousness, if this occurs at any time during the seizure, indicating also whether there is arrest of activity.

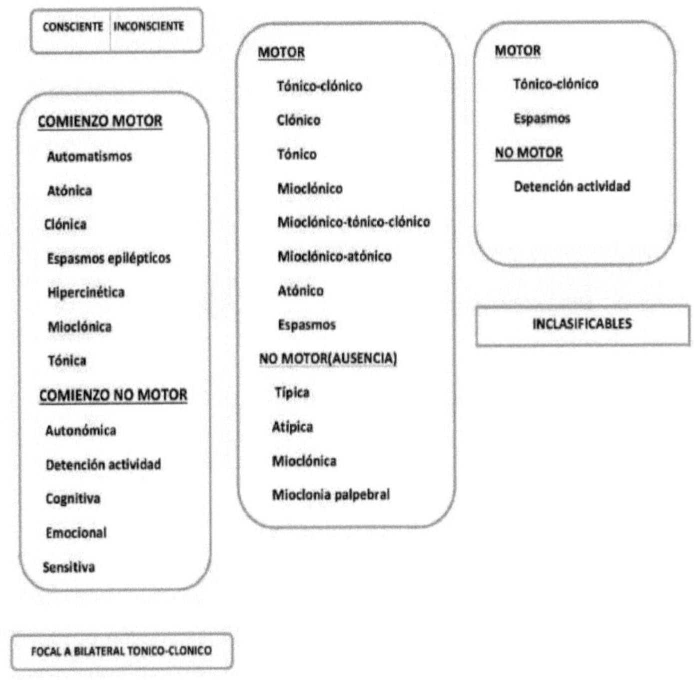

Figure 29.1. *Classification of seizure types; ILAE (2017).*

Non-epileptic seizures

Onset is much more common in adulthood, episodes are of variable character, associated with prolonged sitting or standing, previous sweating or dizziness during the episode, bizarre eyewitness descriptions, stress-induced, dramatic events, recurrent hospitalisation of the patient, and lack of response or even worsening with antiepileptic treatment. In these patients there is often *evidence of behavioural disturbance*, together with a past history of unexplained physical symptoms or a past psychiatric history, especially of self-abuse. They are more common in females, in paramedical professions, and in the presence of traumatic childhood or major life stressors. The classification of seizure types is given in Figure 29.1.

EEG

Although the diagnosis of epilepsy is clinical and EEG, the EEG does not make the diagnosis, as it must be interpreted in the clinical context, except with the recording of a seizure.

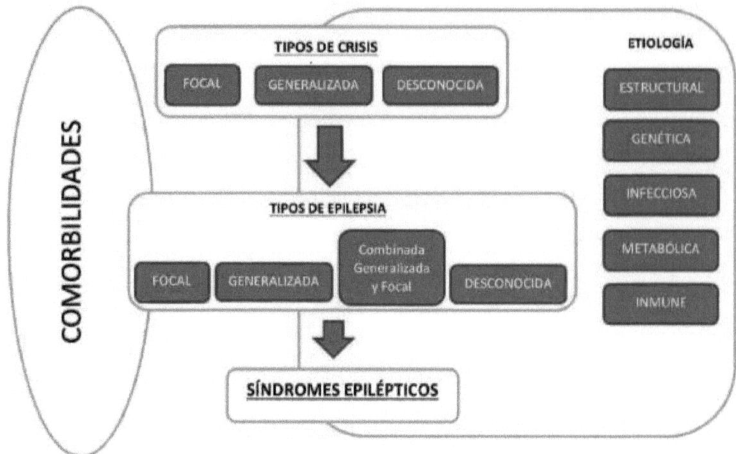

Figure 29.2. Classification of epilepsies, ILAE, 2017.

Diagnostic imaging

Structural MRI has a high sensitivity for detecting subtle epileptogenic lesions, such as hippocampal sclerosis and focal cortical dysplasia. Early identification of focal lesions improves the likelihood that a patient will be a good candidate for epilepsy surgery.

Classification of epilepsies.

It is shown in Figure 29.2.

Forecast

The probability of recurrence after a first attack is 40%, doubling (80%) after the second attack. The first recurrence usually occurs within 6 months of onset in 75% of cases. Epilepsy is considered to be resolved in subjects who have an age-dependent epileptic syndrome and have passed the corresponding age, and in those who have remained seizure-free for the last 10 years without having taken anti-epileptic medication for at least 5 years.

Epileptic syndromes.

Smdromes can be subdivided into those with:

1. Generalised onset seizures,
2. Focal onset seizures, generalised focal onset seizures, and
3. Developmental and/or epileptic encephalopathy or progressive neurological deterioration

Each of them has an age-dependent crisis onset. Another group of smdromes may have a variable age onset.

Generalised vs. focal epilepsies.

Types of focal epilepsies

*   *Focal with intact vs. altered consciousness*. Focal seizures with altered consciousness:

lesions in temporal or frontal lobes. Difficult to distinguish in children, due to poor regional specialisation in the immature brain.

• *Non-lesional vs. lesional.* A lesion that is evident on neuroimaging should be examined in an Epilepsy Surgery Unit: If it can be removed, it can probably lead to cure.

Types of Epilepsy by age

• *Paediatric age:* probable "primary" aetiology: genetic, non-structural, with generalised seizures. The exception that breaks the rule: focal rolandic or occipital seizures, which, despite being focal, are "benign" because they are self-limited at paediatric age and do not cause cognitive impairment.

• *Adults:* epilepsy is assumed to be of secondary aetiology (structural lesion), until proven otherwise.

Epileptic syndromes and atypical seizures in neonates and infants

In early stages, seizures are usually symptomatic of brain dysfunction and are difficult to diagnose. Their typology does not indicate the pattern of later seizures.

Aetiology

Includes perinatal hypoxic-ischemic encephalopathy (infarction, haemorrhage, brain trauma and brain malformations) and other hypoxic events in the neonatal period.

Typology

They are subtle seizures, very difficult to recognise and to differentiate from non-epileptic events. Rarely associated with EEG changes. They are habitual and involuntary but repetitive and stereotyped movements, e.g. eye rolling, pedal movements, mouth movements, apnoeas. There is usually a clmic-EEG dissociation (no EEG changes).

Classification

1. Self-limiting epilepsies
a. Neonatal.
b. Neonatal infant family.
c. Genetic epilepsy with febrile seizures plus.
d. Myoclonus of infancy.
2. Epileptic and developmental encephalopathies.
a. Precocious.
b. Of the infant with migratory focal crises.
c. Infantile Spasms Syndrome.
d. Dravet syndrome.
3. Smdromes with spetffic aetiology.

Neonatal self-limited epilepsy

With focal, multifocal clomas (4-6 days of life). With normal intercrisis physical examination. Of unknown aetiology, they have a good prognosis. There are sporadic forms and another familial syndrome.

Neonatal epileptic encephalopathies

These are severe neonatal epileptic encephalopathies, which share the presence in the EEG of paroxysms followed by suppression of the tracing, with neurological involvement that persists between episodes. And poor prognosis.

Epileptic Spasms Syndrome of the Infant

The peak incidence of infantile spasms occurs between 3-8 months, expressed as sudden, sudden, momentary, single or clustered flexions or extensions involving trunk and limbs. Accompanied by crying, grimacing or eye movements. Usually on waking. It is the most frequent epileptic syndrome in infancy. If characterised by the presence of: a) epileptic spasms, b) hypsarrhythmia ["chaotic rhythm" (absence of baseline rhythm)] on the EEG, and c) arrest or regression of neurodevelopment, it is known as West syndrome. Without the presence of hypsarrhythmia on the EEG, the diagnosis is infantile spasm syndrome, not West syndrome.

Forecast

Although it depends on the aetiology, it is usually poor. In West's syndrome, normal cognitive development, < 50% in those of genetic or unknown cause (a minone), does not reach 10% in symptomatic cases. Along with cognitive impairment, there is a high risk of autistic spectrum disorder and chronic epilepsy (60%), including Lennox-Gastaut syndrome.

Febrile Seizures

Febrile seizures are the most frequent type of seizures in the first 2 years of life (3% of all children). They are seizures accompanied by fever, without infection of the central nervous system. They are usually benign with a normal cognitive prognosis. They rarely require complementary examinations or preventive treatment.

Febrile ^pic (and therefore benign) seizures account for 80-85% of the total. The first febrile seizure occurs within an age range of 6 months to 5 years, with high or moderate fever (> 38.5°C), at the onset of fever, and lasts less than 5 minutes. By definition, they are generalised seizures, usually tonic-clonic, without a post-clonic period and usually single [risk of recurrence of the first seizure 33% (50% after the second seizure), with a risk of subsequent epilepsy of 2-3%]. With no personal history of interest, there is usually a family history of febrile seizures alone in up to 20-25% of patients.

If the above requirements are not met, the febrile seizure is diagnosed as atypical, and may also have a focal onset, usually paroxysmal EEG abnormalities, a personal neurological history (pervasive developmental delay, cerebral palsy), first-degree relatives with epilepsy, and a high risk of recurrence and subsequent epilepsy.

Treatment

Benzodiazepines are administered for the treatment of seizures: diazepam intravenous or rectal; midazolam: IV, intramuscular, buccal or intranasal. Prophylactic drug treatment is not recommended.

Generalised epilepsy with Febrile Seizures Plus

It is a syndrome that can be associated with multiple types of crises, basically febrile crises that last beyond the age of 5 years. It can also be associated with cognitive impairment.

Dravet Syndrome

It is a rare and severe epileptic encephalopathy mainly due to loss-of-function mutations in the SCN1A gene (>80% of cases). It begins in young infants and preschoolers, typically between only one month and 18 months of age. Hyperthermia, which may be associated with vaccination, triggers prolonged seizures in most patients. Subsequently, the presence of recurrent generalised tonic-clonic or haemiconvulsive seizures, without fever, usually prolonged, is a prerequisite for diagnosis. Also myoclonic seizures. Obtunded state, focal discognitive seizures and atypical absences are common. In addition to fever, other seizure triggers may include flashing lights, visual patterns, bathing, feeding and overexertion. Neurological and cognitive deterioration develops, with risk of epilepsy-related sudden death (the affected gene is also expressed at the cardiac level). Seizures are difficult to control in Dravet syndrome.

Preschool-onset epilepsies

Myoclonus-atonic epilepsy

Formerly called Doose syndrome, it is of genetic aetiology and owes its present name to the characteristic initial myoclonic component which is followed by a drop or near-fall due to loss of muscle tone. The patient also suffers from other types of seizures, including absence and tonic-clonic seizures, as well as status myoclonus or non-convulsive status epilepticus. Tonic seizures are not typical. Seizure onset is between 18 months-5 years, with a clear predominance in males. Prognosis is variable, with long-term remission in most, and with 1/3 of patients developing intractable epilepsy with associated intellectual disability. Persistence of EEGraphic anomaKas despite treatment is often associated with poor prognosis.

Epileptic Encephalopathies (EED/EE) with Epileptic Wave-Point Slow Sleep Activation (APOSL)

They are a spectrum of epileptic encephalopathies (EE) and/or developmental encephalopathies (EED) with the presence in the EEG of slow spike-wave discharges; a tracing that undergoes a marked activation during slow wave sleep (NREM sleep) that may become continuous. They account for 0.5% of paediatric epilepsies. They are characterised by the occurrence of a fluctuation/regression in cognition, behaviour, motor skills or autistic traits; appearing or worsening after the onset of epilepsy, together with the presence of abundant focal interictal epileptiform activity in the waking state that tends to diffuse and become almost continuous [Status epilepticus electrically] during NREM sleep. In their spectrum, which share behavioural phenotype and endophenotype with presence of centro-temporal spikes, different epilepsies are included:

- Benign atypical focal (partial) epilepsy of childhood.
- Encephalopathies with peak-wave activation during NREM sleep: Encephalopathy Epilepsy and Developmental Disorders (EED-APOSL), and Epileptic Encephalopathy (EE-APOSL).
- Landau-Kleffner syndrome.

Developmental autistic regression occurs in approximately 30% of children with Autism Spectrum Disorder (ASD) and is associated with an epileptiform EEG in 20% of them.

APOSL Syndromes (APOSL (Apophysial Wave-Point Activation during Slow Sleep)

Due to the significant epileptic activation during slow sleep, patients with this syndrome are unable to consolidate during the night the learning achieved during the day. By analogy with the Greek mythological character Penelope [she unravels during the night the clothes she wove during the day for her husband Ulysses while waiting for his return], it has been called Penelope syndrome. It appears from the 2nd year of life. The diagnosis is made (by prolonged v^deo-EEG recording in sleep) in the context of severe epilepsy with cognitive impairment. Early and aggressive treatment (anti-epileptic polytherapy) is essential. The prognosis is generally severe due to cognitive impairment, with good seizure control or resolution, and seems to be associated with non-resolution of the electrical status in the first 6 months of treatment.

Landau-Kleffner acquired epileptic aphasia (SLK)

It is a specific presentation of POCSL where acquired aphasia is the primary symptom. In older preschoolers or school children. When present (2/3), seizures are usually focal, but may have tonic-clonic seizures and atypical absences with striking facial and perioral myoclonus. Clonic seizures occur most frequently during sleep. Cognitive-behavioural disturbances are always part of the clinical picture. As the symptomatology always includes language impairment, this syndrome and, in general, epileptic syndromes with continuous spike-wave during sleep, are the reason for always indicating EEG in the presence of delayed language acquisition, with an even higher degree of indication if language arrest or regression is involved. Epileptic pathology has a good response to treatment, both clinically and electroencephalographically, with resolution of POCSL. Aphasia recovers with speech rehabilitation treatment, but persistence of cognitive repercussions is common until mild-moderate intellectual disability and, sometimes, persistence of associated behavioural disorders.

Focal apical epilepsy of infancy

It is considered a mild form of epileptic encephalopathy with APOSL or a more severe form of self-limited focal epilepsy with central temporal spikes (formerly rolandic epilepsy). The reason for this aggravation of rolandic epilepsy is unknown. Intense epileptic activity in the dominant temporal lobe affects ling^stic abilities as in Landau-Kleffner syndrome. In contrast, the mainly frontal localisation of POCSLL affects mainly executive and higher cognitive functions.

Treatment of EED/EE with Point-Wave Activation in Slow Sleep (APOSL)

The aim is to make APOSL disappear or at least improve the EEG tracing. To achieve this, initial triple anticonvulsant therapy (valproate + levetiracetam + clobazam, at usual doses) is proposed for at least 3-6 months, with subsequent prolonged monotherapy. If no response, corticosteroids are prescribed. Epilepsy surgery is indicated if the patient has a resectable lesion. Seizures are usually self-limited and usually disappear during adolescence, but neurocognitive sequelae (even moderate or severe) persist.

Lennox-Gastaut syndrome

It is an age-dependent epileptic encephalopathy, severe, although currently very rare, with onset between 2-8 years of age. Multiple aetiology (hypoxic-ischemic encephalopathy, meningoencephalitis, cortical malformations / neurocutaneous disorders, metabolic disorders or tumours) and in other cases unknown, probably genetic.

Clinical. Onset is usually between 2-7 years, with frequent previous history of West syndrome, and debut with status epilepticus in one third of patients. All types of epileptic seizures may occur throughout the course of the disease. The classic classic triad includes intellectual disability, atypical absences and tonic seizures (very typical of the disorder and required for diagnosis). There is persistence of seizures despite anticonvulsant polytherapy in 80% of patients. Intellectual disability is present in 80-90% of cases, and is usually severe (CIT: 20-34).

Self-limiting paediatric focal epilepsies

Self-limited to the paediatric age [they remit - even without treatment - by the end of adolescence]; two groups of smdromes are described, depending on the long-term prognosis:

Group 1:

1. Self-limited Focal Epilepsy with Central-Temporal Spikes.

2. Self-limited focal epilepsy with autonomic seizures.

Group 2:

1.   Childhood Focal Occipital Visual Epilepsy (EFOVI / COVE).

2.   Focal Occipital Photosensitive Focal Epilepsy (EFOF / POLE)

In Group 1, remission is achieved in all cases. In Group 2, onset may be at a variable age, and remission is highly probable; however, some patients may have persistent seizures after adolescence.

Self-limited Focal Epilepsy with Central-Temporal Spikes (EFA-PCT / SeLECTS)

It is a <u>non-lesional </u>focal epilepsy of childhood with **centrotemporal** spikes (rolandic, sylvian; SeLECTS). With familial incidence. It is the prototypical genetic focal epilepsy of childhood defined by age-related onset, normal psychomotor development/intellectual capacity, special features [clinical and EEG, including sleep activation (increased presence of interictal epileptiform discharges)]. The long-term prognosis of EFA-PCT is excellent, with remission during adolescence. It accounts for 14-16% of all childhood epilepsies. Onset is between 4-12 years, (mean 9.9) and predominantly male: 55-69%.

Seizure types. Spastic orophanngeal seizures without alteration of consciousness (cessation of speech, profuse salivation, guttural sounds). They may also be hemifacial motor seizures, characteristic, which may be preceded by numbness, paraesthesia, or a sensation of numbness around the mouth, cheeks, or nose. Much more frequent in sleep (onset and/or awakening). They are usually brief (usually < 2'), if prolonged they may progress from focal to bilateral tonic-clonic seizures.

Self-limited Focal Epilepsy with Autonomic Seizures (EFA-CA / SeLEAS)

Of the benign childhood occipital epilepsies, the most common form is the early-onset type (*pr.* Panayiotopoulos syndrome). Onset is usually between 3 and 6 years of age [range: 1 - 14 years]. The most prominent feature is an autonomic component (*autonomic seizures),* classically a seizure with recurrent vomiting with onset during sleep (*ictal vomiting*). Seizures may be prolonged (from at least 5 minutes and sometimes even hours), with nausea, vomiting and ocular deviation with preserved consciousness.

Focal Occipital Visual Epilepsy in Children (EFOVI / COVE)

Of ta^a infantile onset (*pr.,* Gastaut type), it reaches its highest incidence between 811 years of age. Symptomatology is more classically occipital (visual cortex) than Panayiotopoulos, as symptoms begin with transient amaurosis, phosphenes and tend to be complex visual illusions, visual hallucinations, ocular deviation, nystagmus, transient loss of vision, ocular pain. Postictal headache is common and striking. Often with posterior headache (migrainous features) in older children.

Another subgroup, later onset, variable, more persistent, and rare in children, is Photosensitive Occipital Lobular Epilepsy (POLE).

Focal epilepsies of variable age onset.

•   Infantile occipital visual epilepsy (COVE), and 2. Photosensitive occipital lobe epilepsy (POLE).

•   *Focal epilepsy syndromes with genetic, structural or genetic-structural aetiologies*: 1. sleep-related hypermotor epilepsy; 2. familial mesial temporal lobe epilepsy; 3. familial focal epilepsy with variable foci; and 4. auditory epilepsy.

•   *Epilepsy syndromes with developmental encephalopathy (DE), epileptic encephalopathy (EE), or both, and epilepsy syndromes with progressive neurological deterioration*: 1. Progressive Myoclonic Epilepsies; and 2.

In addition, there are smdromes with focal epilepsy combined with generalised epilepsy, such as epilepsy with reading-induced seizures. The EGGs described below may also begin at a variable age.

Generalised epilepsies

Genetic Generalised Epilepsy Syndromes (GES)

Benign myoclonic epilepsy of infancy; 2 and 3. Absence epilepsy in its infantile and juvenile forms; 4. They appear in healthy individuals with normal development, neurological examination and structural neuroimaging. They are probably related to the same dysfunctional process of brain maturation that is usually mild and reversible, and have a genetic predisposition.

Myoclonic epilepsy of the infant

It is a well-defined epileptic syndrome with a probable genetic origin, characterised by myoclonic seizures with no other seizure types, except rarely typical febrile seizures. Myoclomas predominate in the head and upper extremities, and are usually very brief (1-3 s). It is a self-limited syndrome within the first three years of life and shows a good final prognosis.

Epilepsy-Childhood/juvenile absence

In childhood absence epilepsy, seizures begin between 3-8 years of age, have a high daily frequency (even hundreds in 1 day) and cannot be induced by sensory stimuli, but are instead sensitive to hyperventilation. There is often spontaneous resolution around adolescence.

Absences

Clonic absences: Impairment of consciousness with sudden cessation of all activity, preserving postural tone, with fixed gaze and, usually in < 10 seconds (range 3-20 seconds), return to previous activity without recalling the episode. In 90% of disconnection episodes with some type of motor automatism. *Typical EEG absence.*

Generalised, synchronous, symmetrical and bilateral spike-wave discharges at 3 - 3.5 Hz (cycles per second). Abrupt onset and abrupt termination in the EEG recording, coincident with the disconnection clinic.

Prognosis. Good, in general, with withdrawal of treatment in about 2 years, and no relapse in 80% of cases. 40% of patients are associated with CTCG.

Juvenile Myoclonic Epilepsy (JME)

Juvenile myoclonic epilepsy accounts for 5-10% of all cases of epilepsy and 18% of all cases with generalised genetic epilepsies. Characteristics. Typical features of JME include: 1) age at onset between 10 - 25 years, in otherwise healthy patients, with good intellectual performance; 2) seizure triad: myoclonus, generalised tonic-clonic seizures and/or absence seizures, of which only myoclonus is a mandatory criterion; 3) cognitive dysfunction that may impact interpersonal relationships and social outcome; 4) possibility of seizure control in up to 80% of patients; 5) tendency to persist for life, with a morning preponderance; 6) after decades from clinical onset, only one third of patients will be untreated; and 7) prognostic factors for persistence [long duration of illness; combination of all three seizure types; non-classical clinical presentations (absence epilepsy progressing to JME; focal EEG abnormalities; psychiatric comorbidities; expression of reflex features; and different genetic variants].

Precipitating factors for seizures are described as lack of sleep, excessive alcohol intake, sudden awakening, extreme fatigue and/or stress in 50% of cases. There is a family history of epilepsy in up to 50% of cases.

Prognosis. Rare spontaneous resolution; although 2/3 of patients are seizure-free, more than half require lifelong treatment. Not associated with intellectual impairment.

Genetic Generalised Epilepsy with tonic-clonic seizures only (CGTC)

Isolated GTC seizures (CGTCA) are the "classic" type of seizure, already described in the Bible. They start with rigidity (tonic phase) followed by repetitive clonic activity of all 4 limbs. Usually with ocular retrovulsion (eyes open), sometimes with foaming at the mouth, difficult and noisy breathing, cyanosis and urinary incontinence. It may be generalised from onset, or focal to bilateral tonic-clonic. There may be a personal history of previous febrile seizures. Generalised tonic-clonic seizures may occur at any age except neonates (due to immaturity: absence of epileptogenic network). In the paediatric age group, they are the most frequent type of epileptic seizure.

Epilepsy with CTCGA starts in the age range 5 - 41 years, although it is more frequent in adolescents and young adults, and during adolescence it is included in the group of IGE with variable phenotypes. There are paediatric patients with CGTCA with age-dependent onset, similar electro-clinical features and good response to AEDs allowing discontinuation of treatment. In contrast, adolescent-onset EGI-CGTCA, although a separable, relatively benign syndrome with complete remission in 75%, is associated with a high rate of learning disabilities and unsatisfactory social outcome.

Behaviour to follow in the event of a seizure

It can be summed up in 6 points: 1. 2. Place the patient on their side with their head resting on a pillow, removing objects with which they can hit themselves. Measure the duration of the seizure/record the episode. 4. Wait for the seizure to subside spontaneously. If it lasts longer than two minutes, administer diacepam rectally or midazolam orally, or call the emergency department. 5. Do not restrain the child, do not put anything in the child's mouth, do not give the child anything to eat or drink, and do not bathe the child. And 6. Go to the emergency room if it is the first time it has happened or if the child has suffered any damage. And if the crisis has been prolonged.

Emergency/Emergency Pharmacological Treatment in the event of a Crisis

Diazepam. Administered rectally or by I.V. it has an immediate effect, in 1-3', with a very short duration of effect (5-15'). The initial dose is 0.25-0.4 mg/kg (maximum 20 mg) and can be repeated in 10-15', up to a maximum of 40 mg in 24 h. May cause decreased consciousness, and respiratory depression (especially if IV administration is rapid).

Midazolam. V^a orobuccal (cheek) / IV / IM, effect is obtained in 1.5-5', with short action (between 1-5 h). Initial dose is 0.05-0.2 mg/kg (maximum 5 mg). Similar side effects to diazepam. As an advantage over diazepam it can be administered IM.

Epilepsy prevention

For the WHO, epilepsy is a public health imperative, requiring urgent priority action. The main gaps are in awareness, diagnosis, treatment and health policies. With around 50 million people affected worldwide, epilepsy is one of the most common and serious brain disorders. Nearly 80% of people with epilepsy live in low- and middle-income countries. A quarter of all epilepsy episodes are preventable.

Measures should be aimed at minimising the main factors that can trigger seizures (perinatal infarction, CNS infections, traumatic brain injury and stroke), which are crucial for primary prevention. Interventions as part of public health programmes for maternal and neonatal care, communicable disease control, injury prevention and cardiovascular disease can also reduce these risk factors. For secondary prevention, treatments initiated early after an injury aim to limit its extent or to interrupt epileptogenesis, although the latter intervention requires a much better understanding of its complex mechanisms.

Comorbidities and Complications of Epilepsy in Children and Adolescents

Adolescents

Psychological stress associated with epilepsy may be the main problem faced by the child or family. Health-related quality of life may be affected even after a single seizure, but in general, deficits in quality of life are related to the frequency and severity of seizures, as well as to the socio-economic/cultural status of the family. The child may have difficulties in school due to being seen as different by peers, with poor academic performance as a result of limited cognitive functioning, low self-esteem and/or depressive symptoms. Secondary" ADHD (a consequence of the epilepsy itself) is common, with a predominantly inattentive presentation, although different drugs may worsen the attention deficit. With controlled epilepsy, concomitant pharmacological treatment of epilepsy and ADHD reduces the number of relapses.

Bibliography.

1. Beghi E et al. The natural history and prognosis of epilepsy. Epileptic Disord 2015; 17:

243-53. doi:10.1684/epd.2015.0751

2.   Beghi E. The Epidemiology of Epilepsy. Neuroepidemiology 2019; 1-7. doi: 10.1159/000503831

3.   Camfield P, Camfield C. Incidence, prevalence and aetiology of seizures and epilepsy in children. Epileptic Disord 2015; 17: 117-123. doi:10.1684/epd.2015.0736

4.   Hirsch E, French J, Scheffer IE, et al. ILAE definition of the Idiopathic Generalized Epilepsy Syndromes: Position statement by the ILAE Task Force on Nosology and Definitions. Epilepsia 2022;63:1475-1499. Doi: 10.1111/epi.17236

5.   Riney K, Bogacz A, Somerville E et al. ILAE classification and definition of epilepsy syndromes with onset at a variable age: position statement by the ILAE Task Force on Nosology and Definitions. Epilepsia 2022;63:1443-1474. Doi: 10.1111/epi.17240.

6.   Specchio N, Wirrell EC, Scheffer IE, et al. ILAE classification and definition of epilepsy syndromes with onset in childhood: Position paper by the ILAE Task Force on Nosology and Definitions. Epilepsia 2022;63:1398-1442. Doi: 10.1111/epi.17241

7.   Wirrell EC, Nabbout R, Scheffer IE, et al. Methodology for classification and definition of epilepsy syndromes with list of syndromes: Report of the ILAE Task Force on Nosology and Definitions. Epilepsia. 2022;63:1333-1348. Doi: 10.1111/epi.17237.

8.   Zuberi SM, Wirrell E, Yozawitz E, et al. ILAE classification and definition of epilepsy syndromes with onset in neonates and infants: Position statement by the ILAE Task Force on Nosology and Definitions. Epilepsia 2022;63:1349-1397. Doi: 10.1111/epi.17239.

PART IV

30. Neuromuscular Pathology

Dr. Antonio Molina-Carballo

In the first months of life a frequent reason for consultation is delay in the acquisition of developmental motor milestones, which is often accompanied in the following months by concern about neurodevelopment as a whole. In the first year of life, in the presence of a hypotonic infant, the clinical picture is much more likely to be due to a combined Hypotoma with both central and peripheral involvement, or to one of the congenital Myopathies, than to a Duchenne Muscular Dystrophy.

Anatomo-physiological recall

The anatomical pathways involved in the regulation of muscle tone are initiated in the motor cortex, where the upper motor neuron is located, and in the medullary anterior horn, which is the location of the lower motor unit. The state of muscle contraction at rest is determined by the alpha motor neuron, and modified by afferent input from the muscle spindle via the dorsal ganglion cell and by supraspinal pathways from the motor cortex, reticular formation and vestibular nucleus, cerebellum and basal ganglia.

Classification / Aetiologies

Therefore, the pathologies causing hypotoma may anatomically affect one or more of these locations. Consequently, they may be:

a) For general (secondary) pathologies;

b) For central neurogenic conditions; and

c) By peripheral alteration:

- of the neuromotor plate
- Muscle involvement

Diagnosis

The diagnostic process is initiated by a clinical history with detailed anamnesis of pregnancy and childbirth, family medical history and three generations of family history, and usually allows a diagnosis of suspicion to be reached. Central causes (60-80%) of hypotoma are more frequent than peripheral causes (15-30%).

Physical exploration

The first objective of the physical examination is to establish whether the hypotome is due to a disorder of the central nervous system, the peripheral neuromuscular system or a combination of both. The presence of significant muscle weakness is a reliable indicator of a lesion affecting the lower motor unit (lesions affecting the anterior medullary horn cells, peripheral nerve, neuromuscular junction or muscle). Conversely, newborns with hypotoma, but without significant muscle weakness (retaining anti-gravitational movements) are likely to have an upper motor unit lesion, a metabolic cause or a syndromic cause.

Inspection of the infant. Normal muscle tone is necessary to reach the milestones of psychomotor development during the first year of life (e.g. head support, turning, crawling, sitting, standing). Hypotomia leads to decreased postural control with increased range of motion of the joints. Muscle tone is examined by observing the infant's posture in: 1. supine position, 2. in ventral and upright suspensions, and 3. in anterior traction. In supine, hypotonic infants adopt a 'frog posture' with full abduction and external rotation of the legs, with arms in flaccid extension, weak Moro reflex, weak sucking and little or no voluntary movement. In the traction of both arms seeking sedation, they do not actively bring forward their head, which on the contrary lags behind; with the sensation of slipping between our hands in vertical suspension, and they adopt an inverted 'U' position in ventral suspension.

Other clinical features that help distinguish between central and peripheral aetiologies of hypotoma include:

1. Alertness/awareness: children with neuromuscular diseases maintain alertness with good visual connection, whereas in CNS involvement they may have a depressed level of awareness with poor facial expressivity and difficulty in gaze. In central hypotoma, there is significant axial weakness (trunk axis), with preserved limb strength and with heightened-vivid reflexes, feeding difficulties and preserved neonatal reflexes. In contrast, in neuromuscular disorders there is muscle weakness with little or no anti-gravitational movements and areflexia. Fasciculations suggest a peripheral origin of the hypotoma.

2. The pattern of weakness: in peripheral hypotomas, weakness of distal muscles predominates. In generalised hypotomas there is usually a greater proximal involvement of the limbs, with respect to the diaphragm and facial muscles. A precise distinction is not always possible and features may overlap in pathologies with combined CNS and lower motor unit involvement.

3. Dysmorphic features (major or minor malformations). Their description helps to suspect a syndromic diagnosis.

In myasthenic smdromes, the oculomotor and bulbar muscles are most affected, with eyelid ptosis and fluctuation in muscle strength. The "myopathic facies" may be present in: 1) congenital muscular dystrophy, 2) myotonic dystrophy and 3) myasthenic smdromes.

After examining the infant, and assessing the family history for a history of Charcot-Marie-Tooth disease, spinal muscular atrophy, or one of the known congenital myopathies, physical examination of the mother is important:

- Stiffness of the hands after repeated and rapid opening/closing of the punctum, or presence of myotome on percussion of the muscle, with facial weakness, in myotonic dystrophy congenita.

- Mild facial weakness in the mother of a male with X-linked myotubular myopathy.

- Fatigability and palpebral ptosis in the mother with myasthenia gravis.

Electroneuromyography (EMG) locates the site of involvement within the lower motor unit, for subsequent molecular studies of the genes involved in the disorder. In peripheral neuropathy there is a slower conduction velocity if the pattern is demyelinating, or reduced combined muscle action potentials if axonal.

Cerebral hypotonphus

We often see otherwise healthy infants with congenital hypotomia, who gradually, but very late, reach normal motor skills: benign, transient hypotomia. A second group of patients are carriers of various chromosomopathies, deletion syndromes and genopathies. And the third group of patients with hypotoma corresponds to metabolic disorders (peroxisomal diseases; Zellweger's syndrome. Neonatal adrenoleukodystrophy, among others).

The presence of encephalopathy (altered consciousness/seizures) or Pervasive Developmental Delay in the absence of muscle weakness suggests central hypotoma. In these cases there is hypotoma without weakness together with anomaKas of other brain functions and, frequently, dysmorphic features associated or not with organ malformations; with abnormal sensorium and feeding difficulties. On examination it is possible to observe abnormal hand position, presence of concomitant movements with postural reflexes, with normal or exaggerated stretch reflexes, and in vertical suspension there is a crossing of the legs. The presence of fasciculations (e.g. lingual, such as irregular tremor of the tongue) suggests a peripheral origin of the hypotoma. Some etiologies of central hypotoma are hypoxic-ischemic encephalopathy, intracranial haemorrhage, cerebral malformations, inborn errors of metabolism (IEM), infections of the TORCH complex (toxoplasma, rubella, cytomegalovirus, hepatitis), acquired infections and chromosomal anomata (trisomy 21, Prader-Will syndrome)...).

Genetics

Since 2021, it is recommended to request the complete Exome (or Genome) sequencing in the investigation of hypotonic infants with associated dysmorphias and/or Global Developmental Delay. Array CGH, which in the previous ten years had displaced karyotyping and FISH, is indicated for molecular confirmation of a specific clinical diagnosis.

Neuroimaging

Cranial MRI can show e.g. structural malformations of the CNS, alterations of neuronal migration, anomaKas of the cerebellum or agenesis of the corpus callosum. Computed tomography (CT) may show intracranial calcifications in Aicardi-Goutieres syndrome (AGS) and in congenital infections (e.g. CMV).

Functional neuroimaging

Magnetic resonance spectroscopy (MRS) can reveal distinct patterns of signal alterations in some mitochondrial and white matter disorders.

Combined central and peripheral hypotoma

In addition to being present in multiple genetic and metabolic disorders, a picture of combined hypotoma may be due to hypoxic-ischemic encephalomyopathy; not to mention that perinatal asphyxia may be secondary to motor neuron disease, due to the low respiratory effort. E.g. in Pompe disease (with cardiomegaly), congenital disorders of glycation (CDG; with atrophy) and mitochondrial encephalomyopathies (due to dysfunction of the respiratory chain, which is responsible for ATP production).

peripheral hypotonia (motor unit disturbance)

Absent or diminished anti-gravitational movements with delayed motor acquisitions, together with absent or severely depressed stretch reflexes, absent movements associated with postural reflexes, fasciculations, signs of muscle atrophy and absence of anomaKas of other organs, are highly suggestive of lower motor neuron dysfunction.

Spinal muscular atrophies (SMAs)

SMA is a group of disorders, usually autosomal recessively inherited, that cause degeneration of anterior horn cells in the spinal cord and brainstem. It is the most common cause of hypotoma due to lower motor unit involvement and is diagnosed with molecular genetic testing, usually an MPLA that detects copy number alteration of genes associated with the disorder. In the different SMAs, the time of onset of symptomatology varies.

Werdnig-Hoffman disease

SMA type I begins before 6 months of age with intense hypotoma of proximal predominance, preserving some distal movement, absence of muscle stretch reflexes, alert facial expression, tongue twitching, swallowing problems, diaphragmatic involvement leading to abdominal breathing, and significant intercostal muscle weakness. SMA type II begins between 6 and 12 months of age, with proximal weakness, tremor of the fingers and difficulty in maintaining sedation. SMA III usually presents after one year of life, when the child has reached ambulation but has proximal weakness.

Diagnosis. In the presence of compatible clinical manifestations due to hypotoma without ocular muscle involvement, genetic testing (by MLPA technique) is indicated. EMG (showing fibrillation potentials, with rare presence of fasciculations) and muscle biopsy (showing pan-fascicular atrophy with hypertrophy of type I fibres) are not necessary for diagnosis.

Treatment. The first approved drug was Nusinersen (Spinraza®), a gene therapy based on modified antisense oligonucleotides that bind to a specific sequence in the pre-messenger RNA of the SMN2 gene, modifying its assembly and promoting the expression of the complete SMN protein. It is administered intrathecally, and its efficacy reaches a grade I level of evidence. Other forms of gene therapy are available for intravenous and even oral administration.

Congenital myopathies

They are a group of muscle diseases characterised by characteristic structural abnormalities on muscle biopsy. They typically present with hypotome, respiratory compromise, facial muscle weakness with expressionless face, arched palate and feeding difficulties, with skeletal muscle weakness and delayed acquisition of developmental motor milestones. Since these disorders are clinically and genetically heterogeneous, the specific diagnosis is based on the structural features of the muscle biopsy. Although multiple genes can cause a similar clinical phenotype and muscle pathology, recent advances in molecular genetics have greatly aided in their classification and understanding.

Congenital muscular dystrophies (CMDs). They are a subgroup of congenital myopathies, characterised by muscle weakness at birth or in infancy, with biopsy evidence of dystrophic muscle (signs of necrosis and regeneration, with muscle replacement by fatty and connective tissue), with increased serum creatine kinase.

Myotonic dystrophy type I. It is a multisystem disease of autosomal dominant inheritance, with variable penetrance, due to a CTG triplet expansion mutation in the non-coding region of the Myotonic Dystrophy Protein Kinase gene (DMPK gene) located at 19q13.3. CTG repeats are considered normal between 5-34, premutated asymptomatic between 35-49, and associated with pathology >50.

Myotonic dystrophy can occur at any age. It has a prevalence of 1 in 8,000. Several diagnostic classifications have been proposed based on age of onset and severity of symptoms; with congenital, paediatric, juvenile, adult and asymptomatic adult forms. DM1 probably represents a continuum (spectrum) of symptomatic severity. DM1 is the most common form of adult muscular dystrophy, with symptoms of progressive muscle weakness and myotome, with daytime sleepiness, fatigue, cataracts, endocrine disruption and cardiac arrhythmias as commonly associated symptoms.

Paediatric DM1 becomes clinically evident between 1 and 10 years of age and is often associated with lack of thrift accompanied by abdominal symptoms, muscle hypotoma, variable degrees of cognitive impairment, psychosocial problems, dysarthria and excessive somnolence. Myotonic crises (>2 years of life), cataracts and hypogonadism (testicular atrophy) may occur, along with mild intellectual disability. Muscular atrophy is usually not present until the 3rd decade of life. Many of the characteristic symptoms of adult DM1 are different from those seen in the congenital and paediatric forms, probably related to the relatively more severe phenotype of the early-onset DM1 forms.

Myotonic dystrophy congenita. Congenital MD should be suspected in any newborn with muscle weakness and respiratory distress. It is confirmed by transmission (usually via maternal transmission) of an allele with more than 200 CTG repeats. In the neonatal period, in addition to hypotome (weak cry and sucking) and respiratory distress with/without apnoea, there may be associated facial weakness with raised and arched upper lip (like "carp mouth"), ogival palate and micrognathia; with swallowing difficulties, diaphragmatic paresis, delayed gastric emptying and reflux; with talo-valgus feet. With a probable history of prematurity, decreased foetal movements and polyhydramnios. There is no myotome in the neonate but examination of the mother may reveal hand stiffness on forceful squeezing or myotome to percussion, together with facial weakness, with poor facial expressiveness and carp mouth. Cerebral ventriculomegaly, hypoplasia of the corpus callosum, and/or cerebellar hypoplasia are usually seen on magnetic resonance imaging.

Pronounced micrognathia requires assessment by a multidisciplinary airway team because it contributes to obstructive apnoea and swallowing difficulties, necessitating surgery with implantation of mandibular distractors to control apnoea, although supplementary oxygen supply is necessary. Although, with respect to prognosis, congenital MD has a 'biphasic' course with progressive improvement of the initial manifestations of severe hypotoma, respiratory failure and feeding difficulties, various health problems remain relevant throughout life and more severe than in the paediatric form, such as intellectual disability, and the presence of features of Autistic Spectrum Disorder. Treatment is currently symptomatic.

Myasthenia paediatrica

Myasthenia is a disorder of neuromuscular transmission that causes skeletal muscle fatigue and fluctuating weakness. Paediatric myasthenia is classified into 3 types: congenital myasthenia myasthenia, transient neonatal myasthenia and juvenile myasthenia gravis. It can involve the respiratory muscles leading to respiratory failure requiring ventilatory support.

Congenital myasthenic syndrome. They are a group of diseases (mostly of RA inheritance) with fatiguable weakness (worsening with activity and improving with rest) of limbs, ocular and bulbar musculature, with poor sucking, weak cry, facial weakness and ptosis. With probable arthrogryposis and early respiratory failure with apnoeas. These are not autoimmune diseases, but a group of disorders due to primary ACh deficiency or due to alterations in the structure or function of proteins in the neuromuscular junction.

Transient neonatal myasthenia. It is due to passive transfer of antibodies (measurable in mother and neonate) against the acetylcholine (ACh) receptor. With fatiguable weakness in 10% of neonates born to mothers with myasthenia gravis. Resolves spontaneously, although tube feeding and respiratory support may be required.

Juvenile myasthenia gravis. Juvenile myasthenia gravis is an autoimmune disease, with a prevalence of 5/100,000, mediated by IgG antibodies against nicotinic acetylcholine receptors of the postsynaptic membrane. Juvenile MG tends to affect the extraocular muscles, but can also affect skeletal muscles leading to generalised weakness and fatigue. Suspected diagnosis is based on pharmacological testing (edrophonium), neurophysiological study with repetitive nerve stimulation, electromyography and quantification of antibodies to acetylcholine receptors. Treatment of juvenile MG includes acetylcholinesterase inhibitors, immunosuppressants, plasmapheresis, intravenous immunoglobulins and thymectomy. Children with myasthenia gravis require ophthalmologic supervision to prevent the development of amblyopia due to ptosis or strabismus.

Infant botulism

In neuromuscular transmission, acetylcholine (ACh)-containing vesicles bind to the presynaptic membrane of the nerve terminal with release of ACh into the synaptic cleft. The ACh molecules bind to receptors on the muscle cell, allowing muscle contraction. Binding of botulinum neurotoxin (NTBo) to receptors on the presynaptic terminal causes endocytosis of the receptor, disrupting the protein mechanism underlying ACh fusion and release, with blockade of neurotransmission due to the absence of ACh in the synaptic space.

Infant botulism [under 1 year] occurs in a small population of infants following *Clostridium botulinum* colonisation of their gastrointestinal tract. In 20% of cases by ingestion of contaminated honey. The clinical spectrum ranges from asymptomatic carriers, infants with mild hypotoma and failure to thrive, to severe, progressive, potentially lethal paralysis. Botulinum antitoxin therapy and antibiotics do not modify the clinical course. Some patients require ventilatory support.

Muscle weakness in children

The causes can be manifold. From a spinal pathology in cases of acute or subacute presentation, mainly forms of juvenile spinal muscular atrophy, to deposit diseases such as GM2 gangliosidosis. We are going to focus on myopathies, mainly Duchenne/Becker muscular dystrophy, without going into much more infrequent (and much more benign) forms, and of AR inheritance, such as facioscapulohumeral smdromes and limb girdle dystrophies (scapular and/or pelvic).

Muscular dystrophies. Duchenne disease (DMD)/Becker's disease (BDD).

The distribution pattern of muscle weakness is specific to most muscular dystrophies. The inheritance pattern is X-linked recessive in Duchenne/Becker disease, and autosomal recessive in most muscular dystrophies (which are much less common). Muscle atrophy is progressive, proximal predominant, with loss of muscle stretch reflexes.

Inheritance. Prevalence. DMD/B is a fatal neuromuscular pathology caused by mutations in the dystrophin gene, which is absent (DMD) or functionally deficient (DMB). Dystrophin is a cytoskeletal protein that enables the strength, stability and functionality of myofibrils. The prevalence of DMD is 1.5-2 cases per 10,000 live male neonates. 70% of people with DMD/B have a deletion or duplication in one or more exons in the dystrophin gene.

Clinical / Physical examination. After a usually slow development of motor functions, a progressive muscular weakness appears, which is eventually associated with joint contractures and skeletal deformities. Initially, they have difficulty in raising their arms, climbing stairs, grasping the hand and getting up from the ground. They develop an abnormal gait or "waddling gait" due to weakness of the proximal muscles of the pelvis; they perform a hip circumduction movement to bring the limb forward to compensate for the weakness of the buttocks which prevents them from lifting the limb. This type of gait is associated with significant fatigue, with frequent falls. They associate a neuropathic gait, due to the presence of foot drop due to loss of dorsiflexion of the foot, which makes it necessary to lift the leg more than usual in order to walk; with a tiptoe gait, due to progressive contracture.

On observation, both muscle atrophy and hypertrophy (or rather, pseudohypertrophy, because this is due to fatty substitution of muscle fibres) are observed, with the presence of fasciculations and poor functional ability. Palpation shows increased muscle texture as a sensation of increased muscle tension. Examination shows myotome (slow muscle relaxation after contraction), with poor muscle strength. Most patients have intellectual ability in the mid-low range, although some fall into the mild disability range, due to failure of CNS functions attributed to dystrophin isoforms.

Diagnosis. In the absence of a family history (50% of cases), the very significant increase in the creatinkinase (CK) enzyme (between >10 and >100 times; the only pathology with such a sustained increase) often goes unnoticed and patients are usually referred to the paediatric gastroenterology department for the presence of a persistent slight increase in other transaminases (x5 times). The genetic study (immediately afterwards) by MLPA technique allows the detection of the deletion or duplication of one or more of the 79 exons of the dystrophin gene. Genetic testing should also be performed in women from at-risk families. In addition to genetic counselling (with the possibility of prenatal genetic testing or preimplantation genetic diagnosis). Up to 10% of carriers may develop dilated cardiomyopathy (cardiac screening of carriers is advised when they reach the age of majority).

The severe clinical phenotype (complete absence of dystrophin) is Duchenne disease. The first symptoms appear from the first year of life (e.g. delayed acquisition of gait), and progress to loss of autonomous gait at the beginning of the second decade. The mild clinical phenotype is Becker muscular dystrophy (with molecular alteration allowing the presence - still very scarce and dysfunctional - of dystrophin [the mutation preserves the reading frame], whose first symptoms of muscle weakness usually appear in adolescence. Based on the molecular alteration, it is sometimes difficult to predict whether the clinical phenotype corresponds to a severe form (with 100% heart failure - dilated cardiomyopathy - at 18 years of age, and exitus in the 3rd-4th decade of life); or a mild form, with no shortened vital interval despite muscle weakness that usually requires a wheelchair.

Treatment. The different (and multiple) therapeutic approaches, whether palliative or curative, are aimed at counteracting the pathophysiological consequences of dystrophin deficiency. The absence or loss of dystrophin and the consequent loss of the dystrophin-associated protein complex (DAPC) increases susceptibility to contraction-induced damage.

The palliative treatment indicated with grade I evidence is daily administration of Prednisone at 0.75 mg/kg/d, although drugs such as Deflazacort have demonstrated efficacy; and other treatment regimens may be useful. Corticosteroids delay the onset of scoliosis and improve respiratory and cardiac function. Various drugs are used to decrease oxidative stress (e.g. melatonin, which also has anti-inflammatory properties) or delay the onset of heart failure (e.g. perindropyl). Orthopaedic support from the early stages, and respiratory support (i.e. BIPAP) is essential. And monitoring / treatment of side effects of corticosteroids. Gene therapy, hampered by the impossibility of introducing the Dystrophin gene into the cell nucleus (because it is the largest gene in the economy) also employs different strategies. In recent years, the possibility of gene therapy for any of the molecular diseases has experienced an enormous boom with the introduction of the CRISPeR technique for cut-and-paste genome editing (known as Genome Word); with "promising" efficacy data in DMD.

Palliative treatments to reduce inflammation, membrane fragility, muscle weakness or atrophy, also aim to preserve muscle tissue to increase the efficiency of gene (e.g. exon skipping; CRISPeR; mini- and microdystrophins) and cell therapies (e.g. myoblast transplantation).

Summary

Central hypotome is more common than peripheral hypotome. Absent or weak anti-gravitational movements associated with hypotome is the most sensitive clinical marker of a combined neuromuscular disorder. A detailed medical history, physical examination, brain imaging techniques, together with biochemical and genetic testing lead to an aetiological diagnosis in more than 2/3 of hypotonic children. Genetic disorders and metabolic diseases account for more than half of the cases of hypotonia in infants. Assessment should be multidisciplinary, involving neuro-paediatricians and paediatricians with expertise in metabolic disorders, geneticists and neuro-radiologists.

Treatment is usually symptomatic and supportive. Early diagnosis of inborn errors of metabolism may allow dietary manipulations and use of specific drugs. In all children, treatment is also multidisciplinary, including orthopaedic assessment, physiotherapy, occupational therapy, speech and language therapy, vision and hearing care, as well as psychosocial support for families.

Bibliograffa

1.   Birnkrant DJ et al. Diagnosis and management of Duchenne muscular dystrophy, parts 1, 2 and 3: Lancet Neurol 2018; 17: 251-67; 347-61; 445-55.
2.   Bodensteiner JB. The Evaluation of the Hypotonic Infant. Semin Pediatr Neurol 2008; 15:10-20.
3.   Darras BT, Markowitz JA, Monani UR, De Vivo DC. Spinal muscular atrophies. In: Darras BT, Jones HR Jr, Ryan MM, De Vivo DC, eds. Neuromuscular Disorders of Infancy, Childhood and Adolescence: A Clinician's Approach. 2nd ed. San Diego: Academic Press; 2015: 8, 117-145.
4.   Hartley L, Ranjan R. Evaluation of the floppy infant. Paediat & Child Health 2015; 25: 498-504.
5.   Ho G, Carey KA, Cardamone M, Farrar MA. Myotonic dystrophy type 1: clinical manifestations in children and adolescents Arch Dis Child 2018;:1-5. doi:10.1136/archdischild- 2018-314837.
6.   Parente V, Corti S. Advances in spinal muscular atrophy therapeutics. Ther Adv Neurol Disord 2018; 11: 1-13.
7.   Peragallo JH. Pediatric Myasthenia Gravis. Semin Pediatr Neurol 2017;24:116-121. doi: 10.1016/j.spen.2017.04.003.

31. Orthopaedic disorders in childhood

Dr. Jose Uberos Fernandez

Torsional and angular deformities

In infants and children, deformities such as inward or outward deviation of the foot, genu varum and genu valgum are frequently observed. Torsional or angular malalignment is the most common musculoskeletal problem in infancy.

Torsional disturbances

Rotational malalignment can arise at any level between the hips and the feet. Foot deviation > 10° inward or >30° outward is considered abnormal. Outward or inward deviation of the feet is assessed by the angle of podalic progression, which is the angle between the longitudinal axis of the foot and the Knee of gait progression.

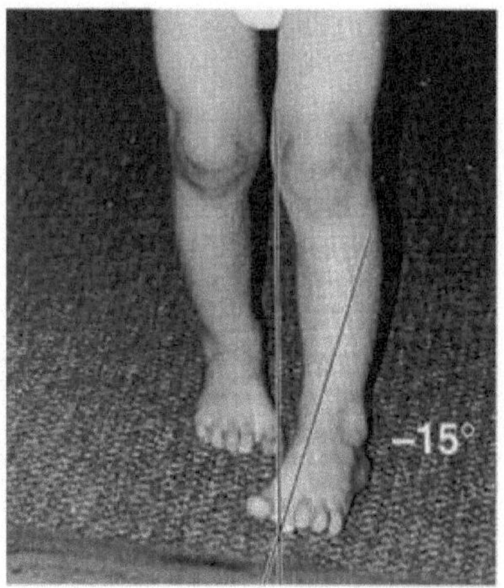

Figure 31.1. Angle of foot progression, determined by the line of gait progression and the longitudinal axis of the foot.

The rotation of the hips is best measured in ventral decubitus with the knees in 90° flexion, this manoeuvre allows maximum inward and outward rotation of the leg.

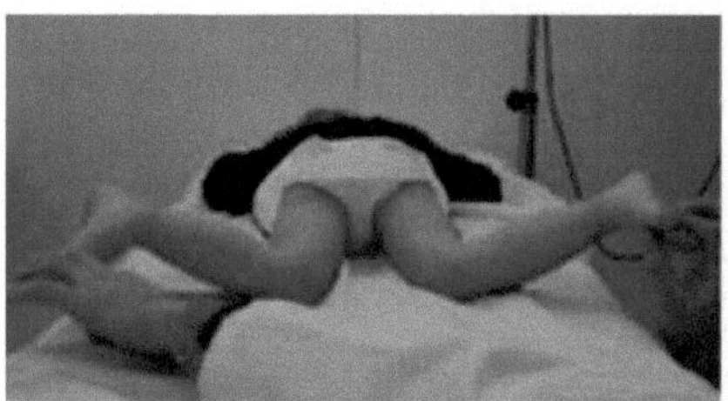 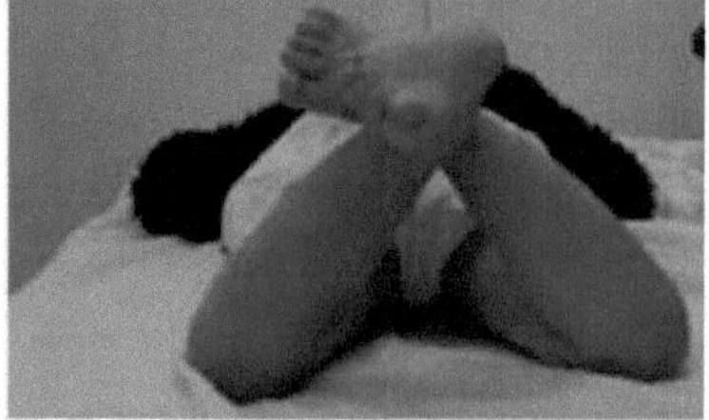

Figure 31.2. Medial rotation of the hip and corresponding lateral rotation.

Tibial rotation is reflected by the thigh-foot angle, formed between the axis of the thigh and the longitudinal axis of the foot, and is explored in the ventral decubitus position with the knees in 90° flexion. The feet should then be checked for the possibility of metatarsus adductus.

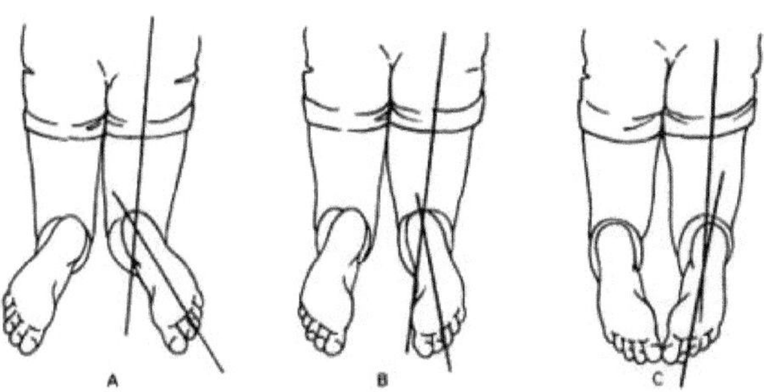

Figure 31.3. Tibial rotation. Assessment of the tibial version. A) 40 degrees external tibial torsion (increased). B) 20 degrees external tibial torsion (normal). C) 10 degrees internal tibial torsion (decreased).

Defective angular alignment.

The neonate presents a physiological genu varum of 15 degrees which progressively decreases to 0 degrees by the age of two years. A progressive genu valgum appears up to 11 degrees at three and a half years of age, then decreases and stabilises at about 7 degrees by 7 years of age. It is therefore normal to find a genu varum until the age of two years and a genu valgum thereafter, being pronounced at around 3-4 years of age. Children with a high degree of elasticity, in the standing position, show a greater genu valgum than in the supine decubitus position. This elasticity tends to decrease with age.

The physical examination is carried out in the supine decubitus position (unloaded assessment) and then with the child in the standing position (loaded assessment). In this way we can observe an increase in genu valgum due to the effect of elasticity at knee level. If a deformity is observed, a complete X-ray of the lower limbs (telemetry under load) should be carried out in order to measure the degree of valgus or varus and to determine whether it is a local or global deformity of the limb.

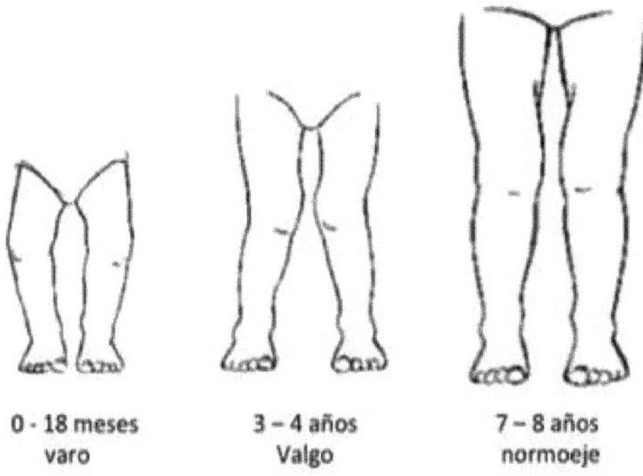

Figure 31.4. Temporal evolution from physiological varus to valgus.

When assessing the frontal plane of a child's lower limbs, the rotational profile should also be explored because alterations in both planes can coexist. An internal tibial rotation causes the appearance of genu varum because in order to align the angle of progression

257

of the foot with the angle of progression of the gait, it causes an external femoral rotation and the knees are facing outwards. Conversely, external tibial rotation can cause the appearance of genu valgum.

Foot and hip malformations

Clubfoot

Also known as congenital clubfoot, it is a congenital malformation that occurs in 1% to 2% of live newborns. It may be bilateral in up to 50% of cases and somewhat more frequent in males. It is usually associated with other pathologies such as spina bifida, congenital hip dysplasia, myotonic dystrophy or arthrogryposis.

Depending on the degree of stiffness, 2 types can be distinguished:

- Type A (mild, flexible form).
- Type B (severe, rigid form): deformity with significant stiffness and marked fibrosis.

Treatment must be started early. Currently, the most commonly used treatment method is the *Ponseti method*, which aims to progressively correct the different deformities by placing serial casts that are changed weekly. Usually, between 5 and 7 casts are necessary, although this will depend on the degree of rigidity and initial deformity. Equinismus is the last deformity to be corrected, but exclusively surgically, by means of a percutaneous tenotomy of the Achilles tendon, which consists of making two incisions in the Achilles tendon without damaging the tendon sheath and thus allowing it to elongate.

Once the correction has been completed, it is necessary to maintain it with boots that should be worn continuously for a few months initially, and then at night for up to 3 years.

Metatarsus adductus

Metatarsus adductus is the most common foot deformity in the newborn, with an incidence ranging from 1 to 6.1 cases per 1,000 live births. It may be bilateral in up to 50% of cases. It is more common in the female population and the side most affected is the left. Associated pathologies should be sought, especially hip dysplasia, which can be found in up to 10% of patients with metatarsus adductus.

The natural history in most cases is spontaneous correction, in up to 85% of cases by 3 months of age, although this will depend on the degree and initial flexibility. **Metatarsus varus,** however, consists of the same deformity but enlarged, with the presence of a medial crease at the level of the tarsometatarsal joint, indicating some degree of medial subluxation. It is a more severe form of adductus in which there is no spontaneous correction and the deformity is fixed.

According to the degree of forefoot abduction flexibility, it can be classified as follows:

- **Category A:** light or flexible.
- **Category B:** moderate or fixed.
- **Category C:** severe or severe.

On examination, the forefoot is found to be medially deviated. In the normal foot, the medial knoea of the sole runs from the middle of the heel to the third toe. In metatarsus varus, the medial line runs lateral to the third toe. The lateral border of the foot is convex and the medial border is concave. The foot becomes bean-shaped and the base of the fifth metatarsal becomes slightly prominent.

The prognosis, as well as the treatment, depends on the degree of flexibility of the patient. Group A is most likely to improve during the first 3 months of life and parents should only be advised to perform stretching by abduction of the forefoot, as well as stimulating the newborn's eversion of the foot.

Category B patients require evaluation by a paediatric orthopaedic surgeon, but correction by serial casting (every 1 to 2 weeks and up to 3-4 casts) or the use of a forefoot abduction brace to maintain correction will be the norm.

The more nigid feet will require serial casts in the first weeks of life, taking advantage of the ligamentous laxity of neonates. Rarely, surgical treatment will be necessary and is usually delayed until 2 years of age.

Talus valgus foot

Radiographically, these are feet with normal bone structure. There is no dislocation or subluxation of the tarsal bones. This type of deformity is the most frequent in breech births (young mothers and primiparous).

The causes can be various, for example: defective foetal positioning, compression of the foetus by a small uterus or a strong abdominal musculature.

In flexible feet, treatment begins with manipulations and, in most cases, the musculature acquires tone and the foot becomes spontaneously balanced. This deformity is practically always resolved without problems, with the use of serial plaster casts being necessary on rare occasions.

Congenital vertical astragalus

In some cases, it can be diagnosed before birth, thanks to ultrasonographic studies, occurring in 1 in 10,000 live births, with no sex predilection, and bilaterally in 50% of neonates.

The aetiology is unknown, although a hereditary influence has been detected in some patients, in whom there is a marked familial association (mutation of the *HOXD10* gene). In addition, it is often associated with other pathologies such as: arthrogryposis, spina fida and neurofibromatosis.

Treatment in the vast majority of cases is surgical, with a multitude of techniques for reduction and subsequent stabilisation of the astragalus in its correct position.

It should be borne in mind that, if they do not receive adequate treatment, these patients are predisposed to painful deformities, which result in significant disability and functional limitation.

Hip dysplasia

Developmental dysplasia of the hip can be defined as a clinical picture of variable onset, defined as the abnormal formation of the coxofemoral joint between the date of organogenesis and maturation. The clinical manifestations of the process can be considered as a spectrum in time and intensity.

Until recently this process known as congenital hip dislocation has been replaced by the current term developmental hip dysplasia. The term congenital has been replaced by developmental, as sometimes the normal hip at birth may have more severe abnormalities. In addition, it is accepted that changes occur over time, so that a subluxated hip may be dislocated over time.

Within the instability spectrum we must distinguish:

- Subluxed or lax hips: the femoral head slides in the acetabulum, and at rest is resting on the floor of the acetabulum.
- Subluxed hips: the femoral head is displaced within the acetabulum, but unlike above, the resting femoral head is displaced away from the floor of the acetabulum.
- Dislocatable hips: The femoral head is inside the acetabulum if at rest, but it is possible to manually move it out of the acetabulum cavity with a palpable clunk.
- Dislocated hips: are in an abnormal position, even at rest.

Epidemiolog^a

Incidence of hip dysplasia:

- Paediatric screening: 8.6/1000 NBs
- Ultrasound: 25/1000 NB

Incidence of hip dislocation: 0.1%.

Coexisting natal factors:

- Breech presentation.
- Tortfcolis.
- Clubfoot.
- Metarsus adductus.
- Firstborn.
- Male: 4.1/1000; Female: 19/1000 RN

Multifactorial familial predisposition:

1-2% Biological parents.

2-10% siblings.

Pathogenesis

Three teonas:

1. Mechanical. It denotes abnormal intrauterine positioning as the cause.
2. Primary acetabular dysplasia. Advocated by Faber and Whinne-Davis.
3. Ligamentous laxity. These same patients have also observed increased ligamentous laxity in hip dysplasia patients and their first-degree relatives.

Evolution

The changes begin in the capsule of the coxofemoral joint, its laxity allows the femoral head to begin to protrude from the acetabulum. As the laxity progresses, the psoas tendon crossing the front of the joint capsule causes a narrowing of the isthmus. At this point the dislocation becomes fixed.

Barlow, noted that 1 in 60 neonates showed hip instability at birth, but that after 4 days 50% of them showed stability.

Diagnosis

Ortolani manoeuvre: the manoeuvre aims to put the hip back in place, thus assessing that the hip is not in place. Barlow manoeuvre: detects if the hip is subluxated, a clunk is perceived.

The presence of asymmetna in the skin folds is a sensitive but unspecific sign of abnormality. This finding, which may be observed in 30 % of all infants if not accompanied by other signs, is of no importance.

Initial table

Before ambulation the diagnosis is based on physical examination, until 4-6 months of age the detection depends on the Barlow and Ortolani manoeuvres. From the age of 6 months onwards, a difference in the arc of movement may be noticed and there is difficulty in changing diaphragms. Differences in the length of the limbs or asymmetry of the folds may be noticed.

At the beginning of ambulation, the assimilation in gait, at this time pain may appear or the assimilation of gait may become more noticeable.

As time goes by, the limitation of abduction, the asymmetry of the skin folds and Galeazzi's sign (relative shortening of the femoral segment) become more important.

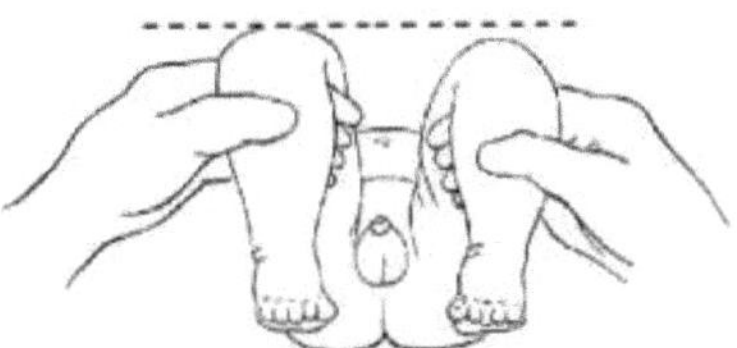

Figure 31.5. Galeazzi's sign.

Radiographic signs

X-rays before the age of 4 months may not detect any abnormal relationship between the upper end of the femur and the acetabulum, as secondary ossification centres have not developed.

Hilhenreiner's Knea is the horizontal line drawn through the triradiate cartHago. Perkin's Knea is the perpendicular drawn with it at the level of the lateral edge of the acetabulum. These two Kneas divide the area into four quadrants. The ossification nucleus of the femoral head or the medial peak of the metaphysis should fall in the inferointernal quadrant.

The best diagnostic method prior to ossification of the femoral head is ultrasonography.

Above the age of 6 months the usual exploratory sign of hip dysplasia will consist of limited abduction of the hip. In children who have already started to walk, hip dysplasia is identified, not by systematic examinations, but by a parent who notices abnormalities in gait. Often they notice the deviation of one foot outwards on the normal side, and think that this is the abnormal side. In hip dysplasia the foot is deviated to a more neutral position.

Treatment

Whatever the age at which the diagnosis is made, the treatment targets are:

1. Reduce the femoral head, the cartilage on the surface of the femoral head should contact the acetabulum, there should be no space between them.

2. It must remain stable in the reduced position.

3. Must show resolution of all dysplastic signs of bone and cartilage.

Bibliograffa

1.   Subcommittee on Developmental Dysplasia of the Hip American Academy of Pediatrics Committee on Quality Improvement. Clinical Practice Guideline: Early Detection of Developmental Dysplasia of the Hip. *Pediatrics* 105 (4):896-905, 2000.

2.   B. K. Foster. Initial screening, diagnosis and referral of patients with developmental dysplasia of the hip. *Current Opinion in Pediatrics (ed.esp.)* 1 (7):186-188, 1995.

3.   C. Jimenez Jimenez, M. Delgado Rodnguez, M. Lopez Moratalla, M. Sillero Arenas, A. Bueno Cavanillas, and R. Galvez Vargas. Risk factors for congenital hip dysplasia and immature hip at birth. A case-control study. *An.Esp.Pediatr.* 43 (3):191- 196, 1995.

4.   *Information from Mangurten HH. Birth injuries. In: Fanaroff AA, Martin RJ, eds. Neonatal-perinatal medicine: diseases of the fetus and infant. 6th ed. St. Louis:Mosby-Year Book, 1997:425-54.*

5.   *Orthopaedic problems in the newborn.* J. Carlos Abril, P. Bonilla, C. Miranda. *Pediatr Integral 2014; XVIII(6): 375-383*

6.   Fundamental of Pediatric Orthopedics. Lynn T. Staheli. Raven Press 1992.

7.   Lowell and Winter's Pediatric Orthopaedics. Edited by R.T. Morrissy and S.L. Weinstein. Lippincott Williams and Wilkins. Fifth Edition.

8.   Manual of Paediatric Orthopaedics. Paul D. Sponseller and Heidi M. Stephens. Ed Masson 1995.

32. Fever in infants and children

Dr. Esther Ocete Hita

Normal body temperature is maintained between 36.5° C and 37.5° C. In children, a fever is considered to be present when the temperature is higher than:

- 38° C measured in the rectum.
- 37.5° C measured in the mouth.
- 37.2° C measured at the armpit.

Fever is one of the most frequent reasons for consultation in primary care. Between 19 and 30 % of patients consult for this reason. High fever in children may be accompanied by headache, shivering, sweating, malaise, drowsiness or irritability. In very young children, it may be associated with weakness, lack of mobility and the possibility of developing febrile convulsions. In addition, the heat loss associated with fever is accompanied by fluid loss, both through increased sweating and through loss of fluid through respiration, and can lead to dehydration if the fluid is not replenished.

Normal body temperature varies from person to person and throughout the day. Normal body temperature is highest in preschool children. Several studies have documented that the peak temperature tends to be in the afternoon and is highest around 18 to 24 months of age. The significance of fever depends on the clinical context rather than the peak temperature; some minor illnesses cause high fever, while some serious illnesses cause only a slight rise in temperature.

Physiopathology

Fever is a response to the release of endogenous pyrogenic mediators called cytokines.

Cytokines stimulate the production of prostaglandins by the hypothalamus; prostaglandins reset and raise the temperature regulation point. Fever plays an integral role in the fight against infection and, although it can be bothersome, does not require treatment in an otherwise healthy child. However, fever increases metabolism and places demands on the cardiopulmonary apparatus. It may therefore be deleterious in children with pulmonary or cardiac involvement or neurological impairment. It may also be the catalyst for febrile convulsions, a usually benign condition in childhood.

Body temperature results from the balance between heat production and heat loss; this balance is controlled by the thermoregulatory centre located in the anterior hypothalamus. Heat is generated through endogenous production in metabolic processes and also when ambient temperature exceeds body temperature; heat loss takes place through body surfaces, in particular the skin and lungs.

It is accepted that the onset of fever is a consequence of stimulation of the production of endogenous pyrogens, polypeptides produced by various cells, mainly monocytes and macrophages. The prototypical endogenous pyrogen is interleukin-1, although there are many substances considered as such (tumour necrosis factor, interferon, etc.). Exogenous pyrogens are constituted by various agents, such as bacteria and their endotoxins, viruses, fungi, protozoa, immune reactions, tumours, drugs and others; exogenous pyrogens have the capacity to trigger the release of endogenous pyrogens by macrophages and other sources.

The pathogenesis of fever has the same pathophysiological mechanism for processes of very different aetiology, making fever a totally unspecific sign.

Fever represents the disruption of the balance between the thermogenic and thermoprophic systems, which can be caused by infectious and non-infectious processes. Raising body temperature by a few degrees can increase the efficiency of macrophages in destroying invading micro-organisms, thereby also hindering the replication of different micro-organisms, thus giving an adaptive advantage to the immune system.

Finally, the mechanism of action of antithermals is based on inhibiting prostaglandin synthesis, which leads to reduced cAMP production, which in turn prevents the increase in threshold temperature.

Etiolog^a

The causes of fever differ depending on whether the fever is acute (< 14 days), acute recurrent or periodical (episodic fever separated by afebrile periods) or chronic (> 14 days), which is more commonly known as fever of unknown aetiology. Response to antipyretics and temperature level are not directly related to aetiology or severity.

Acute: Most acute fevers in infants and young children are due to infections. The most frequent are respiratory or digestive viral infections (generally speaking, the most frequent causes). Certain bacterial infections (otitis media, pneumonia, urinary tract infection). However, the possible infectious causes of acute fever vary with the age of the child. Neonates (newborns < 28 days) are considered functionally immunocompromised because they often fail to contain infection locally and, as a result, are at increased risk for serious invasive bacterial infections most commonly caused by organisms acquired during the perinatal period. These organisms can cause bacteraemia, pneumoma, pyelonephritis, meningitis and/or sepsis. Most febrile children aged 1 month to 2 years without an obvious focus of infection on examination (fever without focus) have a self-limiting viral illness. However, a small number (perhaps <1% in the post-pneumococcal conjugate vaccine era) of these patients are initiating a serious infection (e.g., bacterial meningitis). Therefore, the main concern in a patient with fever without focus is whether occult bacteraemia (pathogenic bacteria in the bloodstream, but without focal signs and symptoms on examination) is present. The most common causative organisms of occult bacteraemia are *Streptococcus pneumoniae* and *Haemophilus influenzae*. The widespread use of vaccines against these two organisms has made occult bacteraemia much less frequent.

Kawasaki disease, heat stroke or heatstroke and some toxics (anticholinergics) are non-infectious causes of acute fever. Some vaccines can cause fever, either in the first 24-48 hours after administration of the vaccine (e.g., with pertussis vaccination) or 1-2 weeks after receiving the vaccine (e.g., with measles vaccination). These fevers usually last from a few hours to a day. If the child is otherwise well, an evaluation is not necessary.

Tooth eruption does not cause significant or prolonged fever.

Acute recurrent/periodic: Acute relapsing or periodical fever are episodes of fever alternating with periods of normal temperature.

Chronic: Fever that occurs daily for > 2 weeks and for which initial cultures and other investigations fail to produce a diagnosis is considered fever of unknown aetiology. Potential categories of causes include localised or generalised infection, connective tissue disease and cancer.

Fever of unknown origin: In children, despite the many possible causes, true fever of unknown origin is more likely to be a rare manifestation of a common illness, rather than a rare disease; respiratory infections account for almost half of the cases of fever of unknown origin associated with infection.

Temperatures 5°C higher than the individual's normal temperature (41-42°C) are life-threatening, as major metabolic changes occur, including changes in nucleic acid and protein synthesis, changes in cell permeability and intracellular pH. In practice, the main complication relates to depolarisation, probably due to intracellular potassium depletion, of excitable tissue, including the cardiac and cerebral conducting system. Most deaths from hyperthermia or hyperpyrexia are due to cardiac arrhythmias.

Conditions under which hyperthermia occurs include intense exercise, malignant hyperthermia, malignant neuroleptic syndrome, hyperthyroidism, overheating and heat stroke, among others.

Evaluation

Anamnesis: History of current illness should record the degree and duration of fever, the method of measurement, and the dose and frequency of antipyretics (if any were administered).

Important associated symptoms suggestive of severe disease are lack of appetite, irritability, lethargy, and change in crying (e.g., duration, character). Associated symptoms that may suggest the cause are vomiting, diarrhoea (including the presence of blood or mucus), coughing, respiratory distress, protection of a limb or joint, and concentrated, foul-smelling urine.

Drug history should be reviewed to assess the possibility of drug-induced fever. Predisposing factors for infection should be identified. In newborns, these factors are prematurity, prolonged rupture of membranes, maternal fever, and positive prenatal tests (usually for group B streptococcal infections, cytomegalovirus infections or sexually transmitted diseases). In all children, predisposing factors include recent exposure to infection (including infection of family members and caregivers), indwelling medical devices (e.g., catheters, ventnculo-peritoneal shunts), recent surgery, travel and environmental exposures (e.g., to endemic regions, ticks, mosquitoes, cats, farm animals or reptiles), and known or suspected immunodeficiencies. The review by apparatus and systems (in the anamnesis) should ask for symptoms suggesting possible causes, such as rhinorrhoea and congestion (viral upper respiratory tract infection), headache (sinusitis, meningitis), otalgia or waking up at night with signs of malaise (otitis media), cough or wheezing (pneumonia, bronchiolitis), abdominal pain (pneumonia, strep throat, gastroenteritis, urinary tract infection, abdominal abscess), low back pain (pyelonephritis) and any history of joint swelling or redness (Lyme disease, osteomyelitis). Personal history should include fever or previous infections or diagnosed illnesses predisposing to infection (e.g. congenital heart disease, sickle cell anaemia, cancer, immunodeficiency). Family history of an autoimmune disorder or other inherited diseases (e.g., familial dysautonomia, familial Mediterranean fever) is inquired. Vaccination history is reviewed to identify patients at risk for vaccine-preventable infections.

Physical examination: Vital signs should be explored and changes in temperature and respiratory rate recorded. In a child who appears compromised, blood pressure should also be measured. In infants, a rectal temperature should be taken for accurate recording. Any child with cough, tachypnoea or respiratory distress requires pulse oximetry. The child's general appearance and response to examination are important. An overly compliant or apathetic febrile child is of greater concern than an uncooperative one. However, an irritable or inconsolable infant is also of concern. The febrile infant who appears quite compromised, especially when the temperature has dropped, is of great concern and requires close assessment and continued observation. In any case, a child who appears relieved after antipyretic treatment does not always have a benign disorder.

The following findings are of particular importance:

- Age < 1 month
- Lethargy, apathetic or toxic appearance
- Respiratory distress
- Petechiae or purpura
- Lack of comfort

Interpretation of findings: While severe illness does not always cause high fever and many high fevers are due to self-limiting viral infections, a temperature > 39°C in children < 2 years indicates a higher risk of occult bacteraemia. Other vital signs are also significant. Hypotension should raise concern for hypovolaemia, sepsis or myocardial dysfunction. Tachycardia in the absence of hypotension may be caused by fever (10 to 20 beats per min per degree increase above normal) or hypovolaemia. An increased respiratory rate may be a response to fever, sometimes indicating a pulmonary origin of the disease. Acute fever is of infectious origin, most cases are of viral aetiology. Anamnesis and physical examination are adequate to reach a diagnosis in children over 2 years of age who otherwise appear well and without toxic appearance. They usually present a viral respiratory disease (recent contact with sick people, rhinorrhoea, wheezing or coughing) or digestive disease (contact with sick people, diarrhoea and vomiting). In contrast, in infants < 24 months, the possibility of occult bacteraemia, plus the frequent absence of local findings in newborns and young infants with severe bacterial infection, require a different approach. Acute recurrent or periodical fever and chronic fever (fever of unknown origin) require a high index of suspicion for many possible causes. However, certain findings may suggest the disorder in question: aphthous stomatitis, pharyngitis and adenitis (PFAPA syndrome); intermittent headaches with rhinorrhoea or congestion (sinusitis); weight loss, high-risk exposure and night sweats (tuberculosis); weight loss or difficulty gaining weight, palpitations and sweating (hyperthyroidism); weight loss, anorexia and night sweats (cancer).

Complementary studies

Further investigations depend on the age, the appearance of the child and whether the fever is acute or chronic. In acute fever, further investigations for infectious causes depend on the age of the child. In general, children < 36 months, even those who do not appear very ill and those with an apparent source of infection (e.g., otitis media), require a thorough work-up to rule out serious bacterial infections (e.g., meningitis, sepsis). In all febrile children < 1 month, additional tests (blood count, blood culture, urine culture...) should be performed.

Chest X-ray is done in those with respiratory manifestations and stool cultures are done in those with diarrhoea.

Febrile infants between 1 and 3 months are differentiated according to their temperature, clinical appearance and laboratory findings. Febrile infants with a poor appearance, abnormal crying, or a rectal temperature > 38.5°C are at high risk of severe bacterial infection, regardless of initial laboratory results, and will require hospital admission. If children are sent home with a febrile episode they should be observed in the home environment.

Treatment

Treatment focuses on the underlying disease. Fever in an otherwise healthy child does not necessarily require treatment. Although antipyretics may provide relief, they do not change the course of an infection. In fact, fever is part of the inflammatory response to infection and may help the child fight it. However, most physicians use antipyretics to help relieve discomfort and reduce physiological stress in children who have cardiopulmonary or neurological disorders or a history of febrile seizures. The commonly used antipyretic drugs are Paracetamol and Ibuprofen. Paracetamol tends to be preferred, because ibuprofen reduces the protective effect of prostaglandins in the stomach and, if administered chronically, may cause gastritis. Non-pharmacological methods of fever relief include placing the child in a warm or lukewarm bath, using cool compresses and undressing. Caregivers should be cautioned not to use a bath of cold water, which is unpleasant and, by causing shivering, may paradoxically raise body temperature. As long as the water temperature is slightly lower than the child's, a bath induces temporary relief.

Measures to avoid: Cleaning the body with an isopropyl alcohol wipe should be discouraged, as alcohol can be absorbed through the skin and cause toxicity. There are numerous home remedies, ranging from the innocuous (e.g. placing onions in socks) to the annoying (e.g. placing coins on the skin, cupping).

Febrile convulsions

Seizures in children with high fever are very common episodes, especially between the first and fifth year. In general, they are very benign and do not require treatment, especially if they occur in healthy children and do not occur repeatedly.

A febrile seizure is a phenomenon of infancy or childhood, usually occurring between the ages of 3 months and 5 years, related to fever, but without evidence of intracranial infection or identified cause. Seizures with fever in children who have previously experienced an afebrile seizure are ruled out. Febrile seizures must be distinguished from epilepsy, which is characterised by recurrent afebrile seizures.

A seizure is always an episode of sudden onset, caused by an excessive neuronal discharge, which provokes alterations in movements and consciousness. In the case of febrile convulsions, it is the fever of extracerebral origin that conditions the neuronal discharge, through physiopathological mechanisms that are not well known, but which seem to be related to haemodynamic disturbances and metabolic alterations which, by affecting an immature brain, such as that of the child, which may also be genetically predisposed (if there is a family history), thus increases neuronal excitability, triggering the convulsion.

Key concepts

-     Most cases of acute fever are due to viral infections. - The causes and evaluation of acute fever differ according to the age of the child.

-     A small but real number of children < 24 months with fever without signs of localisation (especially those who are incompletely immunised) may have pathogenic bacteria in their bloodstream (occult bacteraemia) and be starting a potentially serious infection.

-     Teething does not cause significant fever.

-     Antipyretics do not change evolution, but can make children feel better.

Bibliograffa

1.   Gonzalo de Liria CR, Mendez Hernandez M. Fever without focus. Diagnostic and therapeutic protocols of the Spanish Association of Paediatrics. Infectolog^a. 2008. http://www.aeped.es

2.   Garrido Romero R, Luaces Cubells C. Infant with fever without focality. In: Benito J, Luaces C, Mintegi S, Pou J (eds). Tratado de Urgencias en Pediatna, 2^ edicion; Madrid:

Ergon. 2010. p. 247-58.

3.   Baraff LJ. Management of infants and young children with fever without source. Pediatr Ann. 2008; 37: 673-9.

4.   Mintegi Raso S, Gonzalez Balenciaga M, Perez Fernandez A, Pijoan Zubizarreta JI, Capape Zache S, Benito Fernandez J. Infant aged 3-24 months with fever without focus in the emergency department: characteristics, treatment and subsequent evolution. An Pediatr (Barc). 2005; 62: 522-8.

5.   Jhaveri R, Byington CL, Klein JO, Shapiro ED. Management of the non-toxic-appearing acutely febrile child: a 21st century approach. J Pediatr. 2011; 159: 181-5.

6.   Manzano S, Bailey B, Gervaix A, Cousineau J, Delvin E, Girodias JB. Markers for bacterial infection in children with fever without source. Arch Dis Child. 2011; 96: 440-6.

7.   Soult Rubio JA, Lopez Castilla JD. Smdrome febril sin focalidad. Pediatr Integral. 2006; 10: 255-61.

8.   Sherman JM, Sood SK. Current challenges in the diagnosis and management of fever. Curr Opin Pediatr. 2012; 24: 400-6.

33. Childhood diabetes

Dr. Jose Uberos Fernandez

Diabetes is defined as a syndrome, resulting from an absolute or relative insulin deficiency, leading to a disorder primarily of carbohydrate metabolism, with hyperglycaemia and glycosuria, and resulting in polyuria and polydipsia.

Epidemiology^a of type 1 diabetes

The estimated frequency is 11 cases per 100,000 population. In its various forms it affects 1-2% of the population; the childhood form is most frequent in the age range between 5-6 years and 11-12 years. It affects both genders equally and is most often seen in families with parents with diabetes.

Aetiopathogenesis of type 1 diabetes

There is a clear familial association, with the risk of diabetes in siblings of patients with diabetes being close to 7%, this increased susceptibility has been linked to the presence of specific genetic spetffic loci (6p21.3.) and the presence of certain histocompatibility antigens HLA DR3, DR4, DQB1.

Triggers for type 1 diabetes include dietary, infectious and some toxic factors, such as nitrosamines and nitrates. In all cases, an autoimmune response to pancreatic beta cells has been identified, with destruction of the pancreatic islets of insulin production. The reduction of pancreatic beta-cells is a progressive process leading initially to impaired fasting blood glucose levels, impaired oral glucose tolerance test and finally to diabetes.

Although, as indicated at the beginning of this topic, the absence of insulin mainly affects carbohydrate metabolism, the metabolism of proteins and proteins is also affected. With regard to carbohydrate metabolism, the absence of insulin reduces cellular uptake of glucose and therefore its use as an energy substrate, initiating the mobilisation of stored carbohydrates in the form of glycogen, which is known as glycogenolysis. Both factors, i.e. decreased glucose utilisation and increased glucose production from stores, are responsible for hyperglycaemia. Kpid metabolism is also affected by the absence of insulin, in particular lipolysis is increased in an attempt to utilise fatty acids as an energy substrate at the cellular level. The preferential use of fatty acids as an energy source leads to an increase in ketone bodies, which are responsible for the vomiting that can dominate the clinical course of these patients. The alteration of protein metabolism takes the form of a decrease in protein synthesis and an increase in protein proteolysis. It should be remembered that insulin, among other effects, enhances the cellular uptake of glucose, but also of amino acids in the process of protein building.

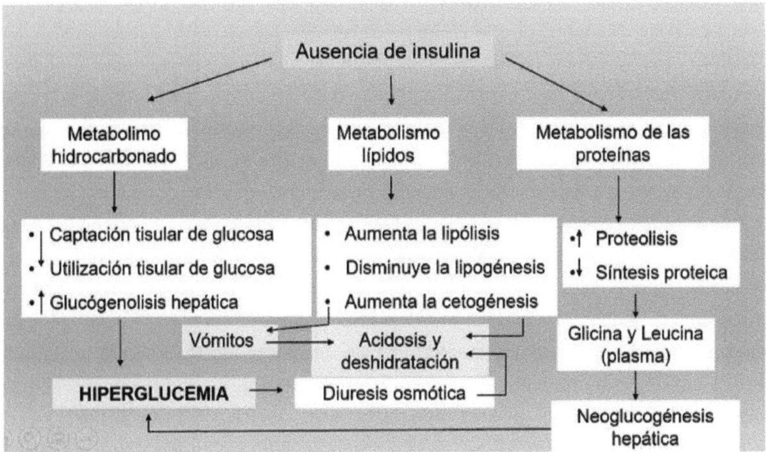

Figure 33.1. Pathogenesis of type 1 diabetes.

Chemical manifestations

At its onset, type 1 diabetes manifests with polyuria with nocturia, polydipsia, weight loss; the latter is often a consequence of anorexia, asthenia and abdominal pain which develop in response to increasing ketonemia. If these clinical manifestations go unnoticed, a severe ketoacidotic form with dehydration may develop.

After initiation of insulin treatment, and in dehydrated forms with adequate water and electrolyte replacement, there is a complete remission of symptoms and initially of insulin requirements, a period known as the "honeymoon", which is due to the endogenous production of insulin by the remaining pancreatic beta cells that persist. Subsequently, with the slow elimination of these cells, exogenous insulin requirements will increase again.

Diagnosis

The diagnosis of diabetes is made when fasting blood glucose levels are above 126 mg/dL and there are also clinical symptoms. We speak of impaired glucose tolerance, which can be considered as pre-diabetes, when basal glucose values are between 110 and 126 mg/dL.

Complications

Poorly controlled diabetes leads to a number of long-term complications, mostly vascular. Disruption of the small vessels leads to microangiopathy, responsible for retinopathy, nephropathy and cardiomyopathy. Disruption of larger blood vessels leads to macroangiopathy, responsible for coronary, cerebral or peripheral angiopathy, neuropathy (central, peripheral, autonomic). Hyperglycaemia is the cause of cataracts.

Typical forms of childhood diabetes

In recent decades, an increase in the number of diabetes cases has been detected at the expense of forms considered atypical in childhood such as type 2 diabetes (MODY - Maturity Onset Diabetes of the Young), forms associated with mitochondrial DNA mutations and Wolfram syndrome. According to various series, type 2 diabetes accounted for 1-2% of new cases of diabetes in past decades, however, it is recently reported that 8-45% of new cases of diabetes will be of this form. Different ethnic groups have shown a high incidence; thus, certain ethnic groups such as the Pima Indians (Arizona), native populations of Canada and the African-American population in general have been reported to show a prevalence far above that described among the Caucasian population; in all these cases a high association with obesity has been observed (1).

Classically, type 2 diabetes is characterised by resistance to the peripheral action of insulin and an inability of plasma beta cells to maintain an adequate level of insulin secretion. Insulin resistance is characterised by a decreased ability of insulin to stimulate glucose utilisation by muscle cells and adipose tissue, altering lipase suppression and generating an increase in plasma free fatty acids, which themselves alter glucose transport in muscle tissue and function as a potent inhibitor of insulin action. At the liver level, resistance to insulin action results in a further increase in blood glucose levels. Initially, hyperglycaemia is compensated by an increase in pancreatic insulin secretion which is soon insufficient to maintain a balanced situation. The fact that most cases of type 2 diabetes in childhood are diagnosed around the age of 13 years, in particular it seems to be related to Tanner stage III, indicates that puberty-related factors may be involved. It is known that in normal situations puberty is associated with relative insulin resistance, partly due to increased levels of GH and IGF-1, which is partly compensated by increased insulin secretion, without resulting in changes in blood glucose.

Obesity is associated with increased fasting insulin levels and increased insulin secretion response to intravenous glucose infusion. Low birth weight is also shown to be a major factor in the development of insulin resistance, obesity and type 2 diabetes in adulthood. In 50% of cases the diagnosis is made by the finding of glycosuria and hyperglycaemia in a routine blood test; in other cases (5-25%) it may debut as ketoacidosis, in these cases the differential diagnosis should be made with type 1 diabetes, from which it can be differentiated in principle by finding that the daily insulin requirements are lower than usual in type 1 diabetes (2).

Obesity is a constant fact in type 2 diabetes, between 70-90% of these young people are obese and in 40% of cases obesity can be considered morbid. Dermatological manifestations of diabetes and in particular acanthosis nigricans, related to peripheral insulin resistance, can be detected in about 90% of patients with type 2 diabetes, which seems to be due to a local stimulation of the skin by increased growth factors in these patients.

Treatment goals include maintaining blood glucose levels in the normal range and promoting peripheral insulin utilisation, including regular exercise, maintaining a balanced diet and trying to control obesity. Oral antidiabetic drugs such as sulphonylureas, which promote insulin secretion and can be used in MODY type diabetes, are of little use in these patients; it should be remembered that these patients are often hyperinsulinaemic. Metformin may be useful as it decreases hepatic glucose production, increases hepatic sensitivity to insulin and increases glucose uptake by muscle tissue, without exerting direct effects on pancreatic beta cells.

Treatment of type 1 diabetes

The goal of treatment is to maintain blood glucose levels between 80-180 mg/dL. Treatment is based on the following pillars:

- Insulin therapy.
- Diet.
- Physical exercise.
- Psychological support and education.

Diet

The aim of the diet is to provide sufficient calories to maintain growth, which is achieved with 1000 Kcal + 100 Kcal per year. The distribution of macronutrients should be 50-60% carbohydrates, 25-30% fats and 12-15% proteins. Cholesterol intake should be less than 300 mg^a. The distribution of meals should be 5 meals a day. The diabetic diet is organised in portions, a portion is understood to be the quantity of any food that provides 10 carbohydrates. The daily calorie distribution for each meal is as follows: breakfast 20%, mid-morning 5-10%, lunch 30%, afternoon snack 5-10%, dinner 25% and afternoon snack 10%.

Physical Exercise

Physical exercise aims to promote a normal life and increase muscle glucose consumption. Physical exercise lowers blood glucose levels, reduces insulin requirements, improves lipid levels, and increases the sense of well-being and quality of life. Among the risks of excessive physical exercise is to induce hypoglycaemia or reactive hyperglycaemia.

Insulin

The first commercial insulin preparations, of porcine or bovine origin, contained many impurities and a variability in potency that could vary by up to 25%, making dose adjustment difficult. In the 1930s, the first long-acting insulin was developed, a zinc protamine insulin that was used alone without the addition of regular insulin. The combination of slow acting insulin (zinc insulin) and NPH (Neutral Protamine Hagedom) came into use in the 1950s. Until this time one of the major drawbacks following insulin treatment was the development of immune-mediated lipoatrophy and insulin allergy. These two complications became less frequent with the introduction in the 1980s of purified porcine insulin and recombinant human insulin. The commercialisation of this constant potency insulin allowed refinement of the control of the diabetic subject, which led the Diabetes Control and Complications Trial and the United Kingdom Prospective Diabetes Study to publish in the 1990s the optimal ranges of control of the diabetic subject to avoid the long-term complications that are described in: Diabetes Control and Complications Trial Research Group (3). Criteria considered as good control of the diabetic patient and minimising long-term complications include:

- Pre-prandial blood glucose between 70-120 mg/dl
- Postprandial blood glucose: less than 180 mg/dl.
- Blood glucose at 3 a.m. greater than 65 mg/dl.
- HbA1c in normal range: less than 6%.

Insulin analogues, i.e. partially modified insulin molecules, have gradually been introduced on the market which, while maintaining their hypoglycaemic effect, allow more flexible glycaemic control with a lower incidence of hypoglycaemic complications. The following table from the article by Irl B. Hirsch reproduces the duration of the treatment. Hirsch reproduces the duration of action of standard insulin and insulin analogues:

Rapid acting insulin analogues

Insulin in monomer or d^er conformation is absorbed much more rapidly than regular insulin which, having zinc in the molecule, results in the formation of much slower absorbing hexamers. Insulin Lispro, the first fast-acting analogue developed, differs from regular insulin in its ability to dissociate into monomers in subcutaneous tissue. The inversion of the lysine chain at position 29 and the proline chain at position 28 are the structural changes responsible for its faster tissue dissociation. On the other hand, the immunogenic profile of insulin lispro is similar to that of recombinant insulin.

Another fast-acting analogue introduced on the market is aspartic insulin, which replaces lysine in position 28 of the beta chain with aspartic acid.

Both types of insulin analogues have similar pharmacokinetics and their doses are bioequivalent in potency to regular insulin. The main indication for insulin analogues would be postprandial replacement therapy in situations of marked hyperglycaemia, in which they have been shown to be superior to regular insulin, improving glycated haemoglobin values and reducing the incidence of hypoglycaemia.

Both insulin lispro and insulin aspartic are suitable for use in deep subcutaneous infusion, and their advantages over regular insulin include a lower incidence of hypoglycaemia.

Long-acting insulin analogues

The first long-acting insulin analogue, insulin glargine, was marketed in 2001, the result of a modification involving the substitution of a glycine for asparagine at position 21 of the alpha chain and the addition of two arginine molecules at position 30 of the beta chain.

These changes cause the insulin molecule to precipitate at the injection site, making it less soluble. Among the advantages that treatment with this type of insulin appears to offer, a reduction in the risk of nocturnal hypoglycaemia is described, and in fact this is one of the main indications for those subjects who repeatedly experience nocturnal hypoglycaemia episodes with NPH insulin.

Another recently developed long-acting insulin analogue is insulin detemir, an acylated derivative of human insulin which binds to albumin, with less variability in values due to more regular absorption and release. The duration of its effect appears to be shorter than that of insulin glargine, requiring two daily doses to maintain adequate average levels.

Childhood diabetes intervention programmes

They focus on the organisation of workshops for parents and patients and their objectives include:

- Assessment of diabetes knowledge (surveys)
- Glucometer monitoring
- Diabetes management: insulin, diet and exercise
- Techniques and skills for self-monitoring and correct insulin administration

Occupational therapy can be used to treat diabetes in the following ways:

- Teach the patient a routine of: insulin regulation, mealtimes, sleep and exercise schedules.
- To have a means by which the patient can demonstrate the type of diet he/she has to follow through the preparation and planning of the diet.
- Continually assess the patient's skills and teach compensatory activities when complications arise throughout the course of the disease, e.g. diabetic foot, amputation, vision loss, etc.
- Provide psychological support, as treatment may give the patient feelings of depression, dependency or anger, among others.

Bibliograffa

1. Gabbay M, Cesarini PR, Dib SA. [Type 2 diabetes in children and adolescents: literature review.] J Pediatr (Rio J) 2003 May;79(3):201-8.

2. Odeleye OE, de Court, Pettitt DJ, Ravussin E. Fasting hyperinsulinemia is a predictor of increased body weight gain and obesity in Pima Indian children. Diabetes 1997 Aug;46(8):1341-5.

3. The Diabetes Control and Complications Trial Research Group. The Effect of Intensive Treatment of Diabetes on the Development and Progression of LongTerm Complications in Insulin-dependent Diabetes Mellitus. N Engl J Med 1993;329:977-86.

4. Hirsch IB. Insulin analogues. N Engl J Med 2005;352:174-83.

34. Accidents and poisoning in childhood

Dr. Esther Ocete Hita

In the last two decades, we are seeing a significant decline in the infant mortality rate. In most European countries it has been in the range of 6 to 15 per thousand. Thanks to advances in preventive medicine, mortality during childbirth and in the first weeks of life, as well as mortality related to infectious and oncological diseases, has decreased significantly. However, it is striking that while mortality due to disease is falling, there is a significant increase in morbidity, mortality and disability due to accidents. In industrialised countries, childhood accidents are the leading cause of death in children over 1 year of age. It seems that our society is getting better and better prepared to cope with diseases and yet it does not find solutions to act against accidents.

Before going any further, the word accident must be defined: "is an event independent of the will of the subject, caused by an external agent acting rapidly and manifested by an injury to the body or mind". This definition is intended to dismiss the idea that accidents happen by chance and are therefore unavoidable.

Children, with their special way of being, always exploring everything and without fear of danger, and the environment in which they usually move, mean that accidents have a recognised epidemiological pattern. We therefore know the causes of these accidents: 53.6%, falls and blows; 12.2%, traffic; 10.7%, poisoning; 7.3%, burns; 4.5%, drowning; 10.7%, other). In the face of this, the only means available to society to better protect children and reduce accidents is prevention.

Epidemiolog^a

Looking at the incidence we observe several features:

- Gender: accidents are much more frequent in boys (71 %) than in girls (29 %), irrespective of age.

- Age: the highest incidence of accidents in childhood occurs between 5 and 9 years of age. At this age, they tend to play on their own, and are no longer as vigilant as at younger ages. They also start to go to school, shopping, etc. on their own. However, intoxications are more frequent in children between 1 and 4 years of age due to the fact that at this age they start to walk and lose control when we are at home.

Prevention

Children's bedroom. The child's bedroom is the place in the house where safety measures must be taken to the maximum, as it is where the child will spend most of the time and where we can find an infinite number of dangers.

The carrycot is a large wicker, fabric or wooden basket that can be used in the first 3 months of life, before the baby learns to roll over. It must comply with a series of safety measures such as: it must be wide enough, with high edges to prevent it from falling over and padded to prevent it from being knocked. The bottom of the bed should be flat and flat with a breathable mattress and quilts. Sheets and quilts should be fastened with clips, never with straps or ropes.

Cot: This is the most frequently used piece of children's furniture and therefore the most important element in the room. From the age of three months to three years the child will sleep in it. The distraction of parents or caregivers, leaving the child alone, is one of the main causes of TBI (traumatic brain injury) after the child climbs over the rail and falls. When purchasing a cot, it must meet a number of requirements: - The cot must be stable and safe. - The bars must have an adequate separation, neither too wide so that the child can put his head in (never more than 15 cm), nor too narrow, as feet or hands can get trapped. The safety distance is between 6 and 7.5 cm apart. The height of the handrail must not be less than 60 cm from the lower support. Ë1 bed base should be a flat, solid and ventilated wooden or latex slatted bed base. The mattress should fit snugly to the bed base and the sides of the cot, there should be no gaps for the child to put his head through. The ideal height of the mattress is between 8 and 15 cm. It is very common for babies to sleep with dummies. We should never place elements such as chains, cords, etc. on the dummies to put around the child's neck, especially when putting the child to bed. Changing table: the changing table should be stable, not wobbly, slightly concave and with a handrail. It should not be too small (minimum 60-80 cm), if it is too small the baby should never be left unattended. Most accidents from the changing table are caused by carelessness.

Drawers. Furniture drawers are a temptation and are often used as a ladder. They should be kept closed and with a safety stop.

Lamps. Lamps can tip over, striking the child or causing a short circuit and subsequent fire or electrocution. Floor or table lamps should be replaced by wall lamps.

Plastic bags. We must also keep all types of plastic bags out of their reach; children often play by putting their heads in them and can suffocate. Use perforated plastic bags for storing toys, so that if they put their heads in them, they can breathe.

Walker or "taca-taca". Walking frames have been in use since at least the 17th century, but the dangers associated with their use have only been highlighted in the last two decades. Many parents, when their child starts to walk, often think of buying a baby walker, so that the child can wander freely around the house without the danger of falling. Nothing could be further from the truth. The most important injuries were caused by falls down the stairs. The American Academy of Pediatrics has now totally discouraged their use.

Bedside table in the parents' bedroom. The child, as a curious being, tends to explore everything within reach. Bedside table drawers are often one of the child's weaknesses and a place of maximum risk, as this is where adults tend to keep the most frequently used drugs. Medicines are at the top of the statistics for acute poisoning in children.

Banera. The bath is a great danger. The daily bath is a moment of relaxation and pleasure, even at a very young age. Babies should never be left alone for a moment. It only takes a second for a child, who is always playing sitting down without getting up, to drop a toy, stand up, slip or hit his head, lose consciousness and drown.

Small electrical appliances. Such as cooker, hairdryer, radio, etc., should never be in the bathroom to prevent them from inadvertently falling into the water. Children should not be allowed to handle them as soon as they come out of the water, as they could get wet and receive an electric shock.

Wet floor. All children, in their play, throw water on the floor, and care should be taken to place a mat or towel on the floor or to catch the water before the child goes outside, to prevent the child from slipping and falling.

Cosmetics. Poisonings by these products are the most frequent in children under 6 years of age. Although the components of cosmetics in the proportions present are not dangerous, it is essential to have an idea of the potential toxicity of some of them, such as alcohol, acetone, solvents and glycols or hydrogen peroxide. Hair straightening and curling products may contain potassium bromate, which can cause vomiting and collapse in children, or perborate and borate which, after systemic absorption, lead to hypotension, disturbance of water and electrolyte balance, metabolic acidosis, convulsions, coma and apnoea. In the case of fixing and polishing products containing ethyl alcohol (20-30%), hypoglycaemic coma may occur in young children at doses of 1 ml/kg body weight; the same may occur with certain perfumes, scented waters, lotions and colognes, some of which have alcohol percentages of 50-95%. Nail polish removers contain acetone in concentrations of 50-95%, which can cause CNS depression similar to etheric intoxication in children. Other cosmetics, such as shampoos, skin creams, sunscreens, suntan lotions, deodorants, toothpastes, etc., do not usually pose a risk of PCR.

Kitchen. The kitchen is another room in the house with many dangers and where children sometimes spend many hours while carrying out daily household chores (cooking, washing, washing up, etc ...). Fire. One of the main problems we encounter are burns. The place where most burns occur is in the home and in the kitchen; this is why we will try to keep the child away from the kitchen and, if this is not possible, we will always keep him away from the fire, also preventing him from playing with matches, lighters (danger of ignition of clothes) or with the oven. When it comes to cooking, we should place great emphasis on using, if possible, the back burners and, if we need to use the front burners, place the handles of the frying pans towards the inside to prevent children from reaching them and tipping them over. If we have a low oven, we should protect the glass, especially if there are children who are crawling or starting to walk, as they need their hands to stabilise their walk, as they could lean on the glass and burn their hands. Kitchen utensils. They are very dangerous, as is the case with knives and scissors. They must be well hidden and out of reach. Household cleaning products. They are second only to medicines as a cause of toxic accidents. Any products used in the home for cleaning, plant maintenance or DIY have toxic chemical components and are therefore dangerous for children. The general rule is that no child should have access to them. In most households, however, the most common place to store these products is in the cupboard under the sink. Nowadays, the containers are often brightly coloured and very attractive to children, yellow, green, red, blue, even with mummies or drawings on them. The most common products involved are dishwashers, dish polishes, detergents and fabric softeners, stain removers, floor cleaners, window cleaners, toilet bowl cleaners, drain cleaners, hypochlorite (le_na), etc. As a precaution we should keep the cleaning products perfectly labelled and packaged, stored in locked cupboards.

Fires. In fires the main cause of death is produced, not by the fire itself, but by the inhalation of smoke and toxic gases. Only 5% of deaths are caused by clothes catching fire. There are many ways to prevent fires. First of all, avoid fast burning materials in the house and place fire and smoke detectors in all rooms of the house, preferably in the bedrooms, as most fires occur while we are sleeping. It is advisable to place fire detectors and sprinkler systems in the most dangerous places in the house, such as kitchens, fireplaces, etc. Water heaters, cookers, cookers, gas installations, etc. should be checked periodically by specialised personnel. Never smoke in bed. Do not allow children to play with matches, lighters, etc.

Dining room-lounge. In the dining room and especially at mealtimes, we must observe certain safety measures such as: do not use tablecloths that are too long, as the children can pull them off and spill hot food, glasses, plates, etc. If we are drinking hot Kquido, do not hold the children in your arms, as they can stretch out their hand in an unguarded moment and throw it over them (be very careful with fondues). Do not walk around with hot liquids (soups, coffees, milk, etc.) while the children are around, they can trip and spill it all over themselves. The living room is usually the family meeting point. In this room there are many possibilities for accidents such as electrical sockets, which should have special protectors when not in use, and other household appliances such as television, music equipment, etc., which should be well attached to the wall so that the child cannot reach the back of them, which is where the electrical connections are located. As a precautionary measure, all electrical appliances should be switched off and unplugged when not in use, and the television table should be safe and stable so that it does not tip over easily. Another point of risk is the display cabinets with glassware (cups, glasses, etc.), make sure that the child does not play with them, due to the possibility of breakage and the consequent risk of serious injury. Falls from the sofa are also frequent in infants, either by letting them fall asleep on the sofa or by using it as a changing table. If there is a fireplace, it should be well protected, preventing children from getting close to it. Many houseplants, both indoor and garden grown, can be highly dangerous. Some are dangerous because of their leaves, others because of their bulbs and others because of their fruits.

Dispatch. The growing number of electrical appliances in the home has increased the risk of electrical accidents when used incorrectly or without taking the appropriate precautions. Nowadays, with the use of computers and the Internet, in any house there is already a room for these devices (computer, scanner, printer, modem, etc.). Each of these devices needs its own electrical connection, which is why it is very common to find an infinity of cables dragging under tables, chairs or in the corners of the room. Accidents caused by electricity account for only 1.8% of accidents, but they can cause serious injuries. Two types of electrical accidents are the most frequent in the home; those caused by direct contact with the current and those caused by incorrectly insulated appliances. As a preventive measure, any electrical appliance that is not in perfect conditions of use should be rejected. Accidents due to direct contact are the most frequent in children and occur when children directly touch the terminals of a plug that is not fully inserted or the metal part of a lamp holder or an uncovered cable. Another frequent situation is when the child handles or touches a poorly insulated electrical appliance; this can occur, for example, when leaving the bathroom and touching the hairdryer with wet hands, bare feet or wet floor; it can also occur in summer, when leaving the swimming pool and opening a refrigerator.

Windows, balconies and stairs. When a child starts to wander around, it is a very dangerous time, as he or she will enter places previously unknown to him or her. It is now advisable to assess the possible dangers in the house and take appropriate preventive measures before any damage is done. The greatest danger is to be found on windows, balconies and terraces. Windows. They are a temptation for children, especially when they have learned to walk and can freely approach them. Through them they can observe the street, the people, the cars, everything that fascinates them when they go for a walk. That is why they are a real danger. All low windows should be excluded. We should never place toys or objects that could attract their attention near them. We must avoid placing pushchairs, large toys, toy chests, etc., under the windows, as they can use them to climb. The right thing to do is to place security locking systems, which prevent children from opening them but at the same time facilitate ventilation and allow us to open them in case of fire. For example, safety chains can be installed that allow us to open them only 15-20 cm. The glass of the windows is also an issue to be taken into account, it should not break easily and, in case it does, it should not break and fall on the child. Ideally, double-glazed windows

glass or those with a metal mesh inside. It is also worth remembering that there are transparent films which, when applied to the glass, prevent the glass from coming loose in the event of breakage. The same care should be taken with glass doors and, above all, with sliding balcony doors. Accidents happen every year, both to children and adults, with this type of door. Stickers should be applied at different heights to mark the glass and the type of glass should be selected carefully. "What may seem expensive at first may turn out to be cheap in the long run". Balconies and terraces. It is advisable to place a net (e.g. plastic) on the inside of the railing, well fixed to prevent the child from climbing or passing through the bars. In the case of excessively low railings, it is advisable to extend them with a piece of this netting. It is very important on terraces or balconies not to leave objects on which the child can climb (small chairs, large flowerpots, baby walkers, clotheslines, etc.). Stairs. This section covers both internal and external staircases. It is advisable to place a compact safety gate at the entrance to the staircase with bars close together like those of cots, where it cannot jump, and with a secure locking system. These gates are also recommended in areas of the house where there may be dangers: garages, storerooms, etc.

Outside the home In children, it has been observed that from the age of 2 years onwards there is an increase in accidents outside the home. This is due to the fact that children spend more and more time outside the home in parks, kindergartens, schools, etc. Our mission as parents is to educate them and progressively give them greater autonomy and responsibility, so that they see that we trust them, without ever losing our vigilance. "The best prevention is a good education". We are going to review these out-of-home accidents according to the place where they can occur. Street. It is statistically proven that the most frequent extra-domiciliary accidents in children occur at the time of entry and exit of the school and in the spring and summer months. In the first situation, children are usually in a hurry or playing with their friends, so they do not pay adequate attention to road safety rules such as walking on the pavement, crossing at zebra crossings, waiting for the traffic light to be green, etc. The increase observed in the spring and summer months is due to the fact that with the better weather and more hours of sunshine, children spend more time outdoors, playing in the street or parks, playing outdoor sports, etc.... In this aspect we must instil in the population in general and children in particular a good road safety education and a series of safety rules such as:

Children should not use the street as a playground. They should get used to playing in playgrounds or play areas. Urge the municipal authorities to create these areas with good safety measures and isolated from traffic, with well signposted entrances and exits. If the child is small, he/she should be accompanied by an adult and held by the hand. A child should not be allowed to use the street to run, even if it is on a wide pavement, as he/she will do the same in narrower places, with lots of people or traffic. As soon as the child's maturity allows (around 3 years of age), he/she should be taught the rules of road safety and behaviour. They should be taught the meaning of zebra crossings and pedestrian crossings, when to cross and when not to cross, always look both ways, be taught the different symbols and colours of traffic lights, how to drive, etc. Remember that children learn much better if walking in the street is not a series of orders but a pleasant moment when they discover new things. It is essential to teach by example (it is no use telling them to cross at the zebra or pedestrian crossing, if they then see us crossing in the middle of the street).

Accidents as a pedestrian on the street/road. According to studies by the Direccion General de Trafico, in 66% of the cases the pedestrian was committing an offence when he/she was hit, mainly crossing the road in an inappropriate place or walking on a road without taking sufficient precautions. The highest percentage of victims are among those over 60 and under 18 years of age. One third of children killed in road traffic accidents are pedestrians and in recent years 75% of children killed in road traffic accidents in cities were pedestrians. Prevention. 1. Children should not be allowed to use the road as a play area or at least under adult supervision. 2. Pedestrian areas and open spaces should be created and used for play. These should be separated from traffic. Parents should make it a habit for children to play in playgrounds or playgrounds located for this purpose. 3. If there is no playground, neighbours should organise themselves and apply to the relevant municipality. 4. If the child is small, he/she should always hold the hand of an adult and not be allowed to run freely on the pavement. 5. Teach them the possible dangers, but teach them well. Let us not forget that children learn by imitation, therefore, let us cross the street at pedestrian crossings when the traffic lights are green, zebra crossings, etc., always looking before crossing in both directions. The instructions we give to children should be clear and concrete. 6. From the age of 3, children should be taught these basic safety rules. On roads or streets without pavements, teach them to walk in the opposite direction to the direction of traffic, in order to better see oncoming cars and avoid being run over.

Accidents as a bicycle or moped driver. It has been shown that the majority of injuries resulting from bicycle or moped accidents are due to: 90% from falling, 20% from uneven pavement: 20% from more than one rider on the bicycle or moped; 10% from inability to use the brakes in an emergency or failure to brake in time. Of these accidents, 90% were male, only 20% were wearing helmets and, in the case of bicycles, none were wearing other protection, either on their knees or elbows. Preventive measures on bicycles. Teach your child to ride a bicycle correctly. Choose a suitable place with smooth pavement and away from traffic. It is advisable to wear comfortable (sports) clothing for cycling, which is clearly visible both during the day and at night (reflective material).

Children under 5 years of age should not be allowed to ride alone on the streets, especially at dusk, when light conditions make visibility difficult (250% of accidental deaths on bicycles occur at the end of the day). A bicycle should always be purchased according to the size of the child. The child should be able to touch the ground with the tip of his foot when sitting on it, and there should be 3 centimetres of space between the bar and his crotch when standing with his feet on the ground. The use of a helmet is essential. The chance of suffering a head injury in cyclists who wear helmets is 20:1 for those who do not. When falling off the bike, the first thing to hit the ground is the head. In most developed countries, helmets are compulsory for cycling, regardless of the age of the rider. Here again we remind you that the best education is by example and parents should also protect themselves with helmets. It is important to ensure that the helmet used also protects the chin. It is also advisable to protect the child with suitable elbow and knee pads. On the road, they should ride on the hard shoulder or the "cycle lane", if there is one, or otherwise as close as possible to the right-hand edge of the road, giving vehicles the right of way. Teach them to indicate in advance the manoeuvres to be carried out and not to execute them until they are sure that there is no danger. If travelling in a group, ride in a line and not side by side. Point out to them the dangers of letting their hands off the handlebars, "holding on" to other vehicles, riding on pavements or between vehicles, etc. Preventive measures on mopeds. The use of helmets on motorbikes and mopeds reduces head injuries by 85% and brain injuries by 88%. And fatalities have been reduced by 51% with helmet use. 2. For it to be effective, it must be correctly positioned, avoiding it being tilted forwards or backwards, given that its function, in addition to withstanding blows, is to absorb them. 3. The safety strap fastened, otherwise it will be thrown off in the event of a fall. 4. Tight, but without constricting any part of the head. Do not use one that has already suffered a severe blow. 6. Since the Traffic Regulations came into force (1992), their use has been compulsory on all types of roads, for both drivers and passengers.

Car accidents as a passenger. Children travelling in a car are exposed to a myriad of dangers if they are not properly restrained, such as being thrown out of the vehicle or being thrown into the vehicle in any direction, hitting the windscreen or other passengers and suffering serious injury or trauma. It has been shown that under heavy braking or in a frontal collision, occupants are propelled forward with a force equal to the speed of the vehicle and the intensity of the brake pedal pressure. Thus, at 60 km/h the impact force against the front windscreen is equivalent to 30 times the weight of the driver or passenger (e.g. a child weighing 20 kg x 30 = 600 kg). The consequences in terms of personal injury are more severe if it is the rear seat passenger who is thrown out, as he/she will impact with the above-mentioned force against the front seat occupants. Never think that an infant or child in the arms of an adult is safer, because at speeds above 5 km/h they cannot be restrained in the event of an accident or braking, and will be thrown out of their arms. The safest option for children is to use a seat belt and a child safety seat specifically designed for such use and correctly fitted (child restraint system). These systems are ideal for protecting children in the event of an accident as well as contributing to the child's comfort during the journey. Child safety systems (seat belts, safety seats). It is estimated that of the 1,400 children killed in road accidents in Europe, 1,000 could have been saved if a restraint system had been used correctly. For this reason it is essential that parents are made aware of the importance of these devices and their proper use, as they must be adapted to the child's weight and size, as well as to the vehicle in which they are installed, in order to be useful. It is forbidden to drive with children under 12 years of age in the front seats of the vehicle, unless they are using devices approved for this purpose (Art. 10 of the Road Traffic Regulations). In general, the simple act of fastening seat belts has been shown to reduce the number of fatalities and injuries by more than 40 per cent. Overall, the use of seat belts is widespread. Seventy-eight per cent of the users use it when travelling in the front seats. However, this figure drops significantly when rear seat users (usually children) are counted and when it comes to buckling up for short journeys in urban areas. The maximum number of persons that can be transported may not exceed the number of seats for which the vehicle is authorised, all of which are located and stowed in the designated space. The second pillar of child restraint systems (ISS) is the child restraint seat. These are not all the same, but vary according to the weight and age of the children, and there are several different groups. Other safety systems (airbags). The fitting of airbags in cars has led to a decrease in fatalities in road accidents, in fact, approximately 1,500 lives are saved each year. When a collision occurs, the airbag is deployed at a speed of 300 km per hour, in hundredths of a second, and remains inflated for a short time, just long enough to prevent the body from hitting the glass or dashboard, for example. But this protective system can become a dangerous weapon if the adult is not fastened with a seat belt, in which case at the moment of collision he is thrown forward, meeting an airbag that is coming out with brutal force, which causes the passenger to be thrown against the seat and then, due to inertia, to bounce back towards the dashboard at a higher speed. This sudden movement causes loss of head control, which can lead to cervical spine injuries capable of causing death or lifelong paralysis. If this happens to a child, who is lighter, shorter, has a proportionately larger head and less muscle control than an adult, the results will be disastrous. But even when the child is seated in the car seat and wearing a seat belt, the airbag can explode, due to the proximity of the seat to the dashboard, and can hit the child sharply and cause irreversible injury or even death. It has been proven that these bags are not as dangerous when the child is facing forward. Therefore, up to the age of 12, the safest place for a child is in the centre of the rear seat to avoid any side impact. Also, in the back, the child will be further away from the front impact of an accident and, therefore, will have more mass to protect him or herself. If it is not possible to place it in this position in the car, place it forward facing and move the front seat as far back as possible, i.e. as far away from the airbag as possible, and exercise extreme caution when driving. This issue has caused such serious concern that, since 1 January 1997, all vehicles fitted with a passenger-side airbag must display a warning prohibiting children from travelling in the front seat. In short, remember: Never carry a child in your arms. Children must always be restrained when travelling in a car. Up to the age of 12 months (9 kg) children can travel in their car seat in the front seat in the rearward-facing position, unless the car is fitted with an airbag. From this age onwards, they should sit in the back seat, with the seat belt fastened, with a special seat or cushion, at least until the seat belt passes over the shoulder, always avoiding rubbing the neck. Use the seat belt on urban and interurban roads. Its use is compulsory for both the driver and the occupants. Teach your child to fasten and unfasten the seat belt. Never clamp the seat belt. Children should be properly restrained to avoid disturbing the driver. Children should be seated in the car, it is not a place to jump out of the car. Remember that child safety systems must be appropriate for the age and weight of your child. If you do not have a child restraint system at the time, it is better to have an incorrectly fitted seat belt than to carry your child without any restraint at all. Teach your child to always get out of vehicles from the door near the curb or shoulder. Remember to lock the child safety locks on the back doors of cars. If the child is very excited and causes nervousness in the driver, the best thing to do is to stop the car and "calm the nerves".

Playgrounds, theme parks - fairground attractions. Playgrounds facilitate psychomotricity, physical exercise and interaction with other children, but they should not endanger their safety. When entering a playground, we must look at the different apparatus that compose it, if they are appropriate for the age of our child and if their state of maintenance is correct. Reject all those made of metal or plastic that have sharp or splintered edges. The floor of the playground should be made of cork or other material that will cushion the blow in the event of a blow, so that injuries are less severe. Discard those public playgrounds that are dirty or have deficiencies that do not comply with European Union safety standards and in the event of an accident, report it to the corresponding Town Hall so that it can be repaired or replaced. Dress the child in suitable clothing for playing in the playground, avoiding all clothing that can get caught, and above all, hats or hoods with drawstrings tied around the neck. If the playground is suitable for play, we must explain to the child how to use the play equipment and the dangers to avoid. Swing. According to a study carried out in our country, the swing accounts for 59.1% of accidents in playgrounds. Children should be taught from a very early age how dangerous it is if it is not used correctly. They should be told not to "get off while it is moving", but to wait for it to stop. Do not stand in front of it, nor run through the area of the swings. Slide. In the same study, the slide accounts for 40.9% of accidents. Children should be taught to go up one behind the other, without pushing each other. They should hold on tightly to sit down, go down slowly and, above all, not jump off until the previous child has gone down. Metal structures. "Monkey bars" (suspended parallel rings or bars) on which children play by swinging and "climbing frames" (metal structures) on which children climb. They are extremely dangerous if one is overconfident, as the falls are often from a considerable height and can result in significant head trauma. According to several studies, the risk of accidents on these devices is seven times higher than on swings. It has also been observed that three times as many accidents occur in schools and kindergartens than in public playgrounds, possibly due to a greater number of children and less control. Theme parks. These attractions are becoming more and more popular. They are attended by adults and children of different ages and not all of them are suitable for all children. We must know how to explain to the youngest children that the safety rules are there to be complied with and that we, the adults, should not be the first to break them, using little tricks so that the children can access them (stretching to give their size, indicating that they are older, etc.). Make them see that when they are older they will be able to go on the other attractions. In the popular festivals of all the cities and towns in Spain, fairground attractions are usually installed. They attract many visitors, including children. We must know how to distinguish between safe and dangerous ones and not let children go on them, especially if they do not meet the highest safety standards.

Beach, sea, sea, lakes, swimming pools. When the good weather arrives, we all want to go out to the beach, the sea or the lake to enjoy a happy day. What we have to make sure is that at the end of the day we can still say the same thing. Submersion accidents in water, known as drowning and semi-drowning, are child accidents that deserve special attention, not so much because of their incidence as because of their high mortality rate and the tremendous after-effects they leave behind. There are studies that show that they are the 7th cause of child accidents but they occupy the 2nd place in deaths by accident. According to other studies, for every 30 children who suffer a submersion accident, only 1 child is saved, which indicates their seriousness. Submersion accidents tend to have a higher incidence in the summer months (June, July, August, September) with 68% of the cases and a peak in July. The number of occurrences varies according to the place where the bathing takes place: 5% in the sea, 20% in rivers, 28% in lakes, and 39% in swimming pools. This difference in percentages is due to the fact that in the most dangerous places, we take extreme vigilance or precautions (sea); however, when the waters are calmer, we think that there are fewer dangers and we neglect prevention (in the sea and lakes). The number of accidents in swimming pools is striking, with the highest number of accidents occurring in private pools where there is less surveillance. Water parks are places which, despite the large number of visitors they receive, do not have too many accidents due to extreme vigilance. Preventive measures: when children are small, we must not let them out of our sight for a single moment. At bath time we will be close to them, keeping an eye on them, even if they are in small swimming pools or inflatable pools that we place on terraces or in gardens. Never trust them, even if they are wearing "cuffs" or floats, as they can deflate, break or come off, and the supervision of a responsible adult is always more effective. Older children should be taught about the risks they may encounter and learn to swim as soon as possible. In the sea, explain the currents, the strength of the waves and teach them to respect the signals and recommendations of the lifeguards (colour of the flags: green = good sea; yellow = caution; red = danger). Advise them not to dive alone in case of problems, and not to dive in unknown or dangerous places. Do not dive in headfirst without knowing the depth of the place because of possible injuries to the cervical spine by colliding with stones hidden under the water, with tragic consequences (paraplegia or tetraplegia). Be careful when diving in the vicinity of boats, especially with older children. If they are involved in water sports, make them wear life jackets at all times. Avoid excessive exposure to the sun, and use sunscreen. Make the child take a shower before going into the water and do not bathe while digesting. Avoid dangerous games such as prolonged diving. In case of children with tympanic perforation, force them to wear protective earplugs as they may suffer from dizziness. All public and private swimming pools should be fenced, with a fence high enough so that it cannot be climbed over by children and with a locked gate to prevent access by children without the presence of an adult or lifeguard.

Bibliograffa

1. En Familia web pages of the Spanish Paediatrics Association, revision date 10/09/2022. Available at: http://enfamilia.aeped.es/prevencion.

2. Valdes Rodnguez E, Gonzalez Luque JC. http://www.dgt.es/Galerias/seguridad-vial/ formacon-vial/cursos-para-profesores-y-directores-de-autoescuelas/doc/XIV Curso31ComportamientoPrimerosAuxilios.pdf.

Manrique Martmez I; Pons Morales S. Accidentes infantile. In "Tratado de Urgencias en pediatna". Benito J, Luaces C, Mintegui S, Pou J. 2^ edition. Editorial Ergon. Madrid 2011 pp 947963.

3. Manrique Martmez I; Pons Morales S. Accidentes infantile. In "Tratado de Urgencias en pediatna". Benito J, Luaces C, Mintegui S, Pou J. 2^ edition. Editorial Ergon. Madrid 2011 pp 947-963.

4. Sastre Paz Marta, Clara Zoni Ana, Esparza Olcina M.^ Jesus, Cura MJ Isabel del. Prevalence and factors associated with unintentional injuries. Rev Pediatr Aten Primaria [Internet]. 2016 Sep [cited 2022 Sep 05] ; 18(71): 253-258. Available from: http://scielo.isciii.es/scielo.php?script=sci_arttext&pid=S1139-76322016000300006&lng=es.

35. Immunoprophylaxis in paediatrics

Dr. Jose Uberos Fernandez

In the prevention of communicable diseases, it is essential to break the epidemiological chain at any of its three links:

*   Source of infection.
*   Transmission mechanisms.
*   Healthy susceptible individual.

At the source of infection, the sanitary actions that can be undertaken are: isolation, specific treatment and elimination of the carrier of the infection (e.g. rabid dog).

On the transmission mechanisms, possible actions include general sanitation (waste disposal, water supply, etc.) or specific (disinfection, disinsection, disinfestation, rat extermination, etc.) and mechanical barriers.

The susceptible healthy individual can be targeted by chemoprophylaxis, passive immunisation and active immunisation.

*   Chemoprophylaxis is the set of measures taken to protect or preserve healthy individuals from disease, consisting of the administration of chemical substances.

*   Passive immunity is the transfer of active immunity, in the form of antibodies, from one individual to another. Passive immunity can occur naturally, e.g. when maternal antibodies are transferred to the foetus through the placenta, and it can also be

artificially induced, when high amounts of human (or animal) antibodies specific to a pathogenic micro-organism or toxin are transferred to susceptible individuals. Passive immunisation is used when there is a high risk of infection and insufficient time for the body to develop its own immune response. Passive immunity provides immediate protection, but the body does not develop immunological memory, therefore, the patient is at risk of being infected by the same pathogenic microorganism once the transferred antibodies have been eliminated. Maternal passive immunity is a type of naturally acquired immunity, and refers to immunity transmitted by antibodies to a foetus by its mother during pregnancy. Immunoglobulin G is the only antibody isotope that can pass through the placenta. Passive immunity is also provided through the transfer of immunoglobulin A antibodies found in breast milk that are transferred to the infant's digestive tract, protecting it against infection, until the newborn can synthesise its own antibodies.

Artificially acquired passive immunity is a short-term immunisation induced by the transfer of antibodies, which can be administered in various forms; as human or animal blood plasma, as human bank immunoglobulin for intravenous or intramuscular use, and in the form of monoclonal antibodies.

• Active immunity. When B and T lymphocytes are activated by a pathogenic micro-organism, they give rise to memory B and T lymphocytes. Throughout life these memory lymphocytes will "remember" each specific micro-organism they have come into contact with, and will be able to mount a specific immune response. This type of immunity is both *active* and *adaptive*. Active immunity often involves cellular and humoral immunity, as well as the innate immune system. The *innate system* is present from birth and protects an individual from pathogenic microorganisms regardless of immunological recall, whereas adaptive immunity occurs only after infection or vaccination and is therefore "acquired" during life. Naturally acquired active immunity occurs when a person is exposed to a live pathogenic micro-organism, and develops a primary immune response, which leads to an immunological memory. Artificially acquired active immunity can be induced by a vaccine, a substance containing an antigen. A vaccine stimulates a primary response against the antigen without causing the symptoms of disease. The term vaccination was coined by Edward Jenner and adapted by Louis Pasteur for his pioneering work on vaccination. The method Pasteur used involved treating infectious agents for those diseases in such a way that they had the capacity to cause serious illness. Pasteur adopted the name vaccine as a generic term in honour of Jenner's discovery.

Classification of vaccines

Vaccines can be classified according to three points of view: microbiological, according to their composition; technological, according to the way they are obtained; and sanitary, according to the objectives to be achieved by their application to individuals or communities.

From a **microbiological point of view,** vaccines are classified as vmc or bacterial; each of them is further classified as live or attenuated and killed or inactivated. The latter are further classified into whole vaccines (containing the whole virus or bacterium) and subunit vaccines (containing antigens or fractions of the micro-organism). Attenuated vaccines are achieved by selection of avirulent or virulence-attenuated mutants, and must be stable and maintain stable immunological properties. This type of vaccine results in an inapparent or symptomless infection that confers immunity similar to that of natural infection. Killed or inactivated vaccines are prepared by inactivating suspensions of viruses or bacteria by physical (heat) or chemical (formalin or beta-propiolactone) methods. In some cases these vaccines are prepared from toxins, i.e. antigens secreted by the micro-organism (tetanus, diphtheria), from viral fractions (Hepatitis B) or from bacterial fractions (pneumococcal capsular polysaccharides, *Haemophilus influenzae*); in the latter type of vaccines the immunity generated is mainly humoral and the cellular immunity is of lesser intensity.

From a **technological point of view**, vaccines are classified into live, inactivated and genetic vaccines. In genetic vaccines, it is not the micro-organism or its immunogenic fractions that are injected, but the gene encoding the immunising protein. New methods of vaccine production use recombinant DNA technology for the production of immunising proteins. Some authors classify live vector-based gene vaccines among live vaccines and DNA plasmid-based vaccines among inactivated vaccines.

Technological classification is based on the epidemiological objectives to be achieved, and to understand this classification it is essential to differentiate between individual and herd immunity. The protection conferred on the individual varies according to the vaccine; for some vaccines the protection is absolute and lasts for life; for others it is very high but only lasts for a limited period.

In relation to the **epidemiological objectives**, it is necessary to consider the reservoir: infections with a human reservoir and inter-human transmission and those with a non-human reservoir (zoonosis). In both groups, vaccination protects the vaccinated individual. But in diseases with a human reservoir and human-to-human transmission, vaccination not only provides individual protection but also a collective or community protection (herd immunity) that helps to break the chain of transmission. Herd or "herd" immunity is defined as the resistance of a group or population to the invasion or spread of an infectious agent as a result of the resistance to infection of a high proportion of the individual members of the group or population. Resistance is a function of the number of susceptible individuals and the likelihood that they will come into contact with an infected person.

Systemic and non-systemic vaccines

In order to protect susceptible individuals and also to obtain herd immunity, public health services in all countries have recommended the routine administration of vaccines which have been shown to be effective against communicable diseases of human reservoir and inter-human transmission. The tetanus vaccine has also been included among the systemic vaccines, even though tetanus is neither a human reservoir nor inter-human transmissible disease, but in this case the objective is only the protection of the individual, not of the community. On the other hand, the influenza vaccine has not been included among the systemic vaccines, even though it has a human reservoir and inter-human transmission, because the protection conferred by the vaccine is very limited in duration and there is a large antigenic variation between seasons.

Table 35.1. Classification of vaccines.

Types of vaccines		Attenuated (live) vaccines	Inactivated vaccines
Vfricas	Whole	• Oral Poliomyelitis (not available in Spain) • Yellow fever • Rotavirus • Sarampion-rubeola-mumps (VT or PRRS) - chickenpox (varicella)	• Poliomyelitisinyectable • Tick-borne encephalitis • Japanese encephalitis • Hepatitis A • Rabia
	Sub-units		• Fractional influenza of subunits • Hepatitis B • Human papillomavirus
Bacterial	Acellulars		- Acellular pertussis
	Polysaccharide + protein conjugates		• *Haemophilus influenzae* type b • Meningococcus C and ACWY • Pneumococcus 10 and 13 valent
	Whole	• Tuberculosis or BCG (not available in Spain) • Oral typhoid fever	- Oral cholera
	Capsular polysaccharides		• Parenteral typhoid fever • Pneumococcal 23 valent
	Surface proteins		- Meningococcal B
	Toxoids		- Diphtheria - Tetanus

The systematic vaccines, which are included in the respective vaccination schedules, are of great individual and community interest and are therefore indicated for the entire population, with the exception of specific contraindications.

Non-systemic vaccines, on the other hand, are not administered as part of a public health programme as is the case with systemic vaccines. They are administered on an individual basis. From a health point of view, non-systemic vaccines can be grouped as follows:

•   Indicated in Spain in certain individual or environmental circumstances: anti-rabies, antityphoid, BCG, anti-influenza.

•   Mandatory or required for certain international travel: yellow fever, cholera.

General characteristics of vaccines

The two main properties that a vaccine must have are safety and protective efficacy.

Safety. Vaccines must be safe, although no vaccine is free of side effects; the degree of safety is related to the severity of the disease to be prevented. The evaluation of safety, together with efficacy, is carried out in studies with volunteers (clinical trials). Post-marketing studies are important in this respect, as they allow the detection of possible rare effects by increasing the size of the investigated sample. Two observations are examples of such studies: the possible association proposed between hepatitis B vaccination and multiple sclerosis, which was discarded; and the association between rotavirus vaccination and intestinal intussusception in infants, which was confirmed.

Efficacy. This refers to the capacity of a vaccine to protect vaccinated individuals, but all of this in the context of an experimental study, therefore, in a selected sample. If this circumstance is extrapolated to the population as a whole, we should speak of effectiveness. If we refer to the cost-benefit ratio, we must talk about the efficiency of a vaccine. The efficacy of a vaccine is related to its immunogenicity, i.e. the specific immune response generated.

The specific immune response following natural (infection) or artificial (vaccination) exposure of the susceptible host to antigens involves two types of lymphocytes, marrow-dependent B-lymphocytes and thymus-dependent T-lymphocytes. The main characteristic of B-lymphocytes is their ability to produce antibodies or immunoglobulin (Igs). B-lymphocytes after antigenic stimulation differentiate and replicate producing different types of isotypes (IgM, IgA, IgG, IgE). T-lymphocytes are produced in the bone marrow and migrate to the thymus where they mature. There are two main types of T cells, cytotoxic T cells (CD8) and helper (Th) T cells (CD4). Th lymphocytes are further subdivided into Th1 and Th2. The main function of Th2 lymphocytes is to help B lymphocytes proliferate and secrete antibodies. The Th2 response is involved in the allergic-type immune response. The main function of Th1 lymphocytes is the activation of macrophages.

First exposure to an immunogenic antigen (primary response) activates virginal B cells. Re-exposure to the same antigen (secondary response) activates clones of memory cells. The ability of T and B cells to remember the identity of an antigen and produce faster, stronger and longer-lasting responses to the next or successive exposures is called immunological memory. It is important to note that all immunogenic agents can trigger a primary response. can trigger a primary response, but only T-dependent antigens can trigger immunological memory. T-independent antigens (capsular polysaccharides) do not induce immunological memory, which is why some vaccines conjugate them to a protein transporter to induce immunological memory.

Vaccination schedules

A vaccination schedule is the chronological sequence of **routine** immunisations for a given geographical area, intended to **protect its population** against those **infections of potential local prevalence** against which a **safe vaccine is available**.

There are several types of vaccination schedules depending on the target population and the way in which they are implemented. Thus, depending on the age of implementation, we can distinguish between children's or adult calendars; depending on the time of administration of the vaccines, we speak of a systematic or catch-up calendar; depending on the state of health of the recipients of the vaccines, we speak of a calendar for the immunodepressed, for the chronically ill, for premature babies, for pregnant women; depending on the occupation of the recipient of the vaccines, we speak of a vaccination calendar for travellers, for health workers, for public services, etc.

Table 35.2. Andalusia vaccination schedule (2022).

Vaccination Schedule 2021-2022

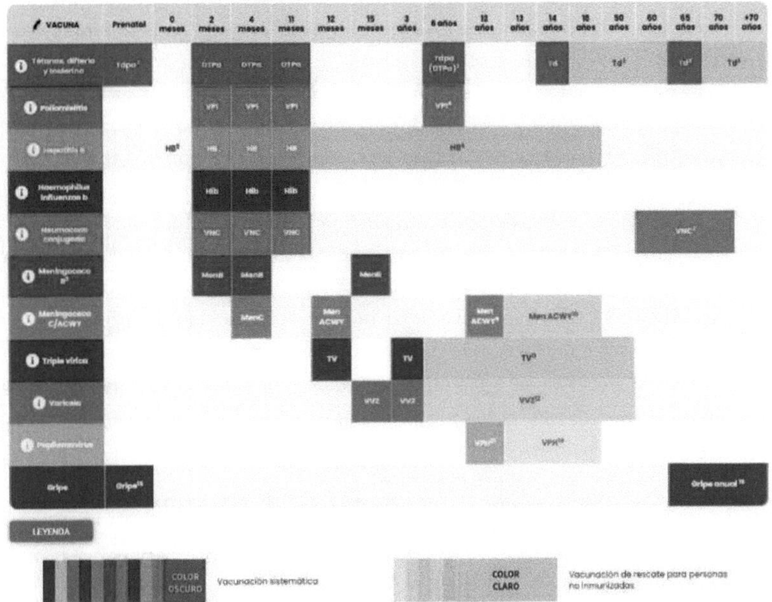

The history of vaccination schedules is relatively recent, the first official vaccination schedule in our country dates from 1972 and included a small number of compulsory vaccinations such as smallpox, polio and DTP. After the various smallpox vaccination campaigns carried out in the 1920s, vaccination against smallpox and diphtheria became compulsory in 1944, followed by various vaccination campaigns against poliomyelitis (1963) and DTP (1965). Vaccination against measles and rubella began in 1978. In 1980, following the declaration of the global eradication of smallpox, smallpox vaccination was discontinued, and a year later (1981) systematic MMR vaccination was introduced. In 1984, vaccination against Hepatitis B was introduced. The first unified systematic vaccination schedule dates from a relatively recent date (1996); so as we can see, the history of vaccination schedules is relatively recent. After this date, new vaccines have been added to the vaccination schedule, such as the vaccine against *H. influenzae* type b in 1998, against meningococcus C in 2000, against chickenpox in 2005 and the recent addition of the vaccine against human papillomavirus or meningococcus ACWY.

When drawing up or modifying a vaccination schedule, criteria derived from the disease, the vaccine available and the target society must be taken into account. On the disease side, we need to know data on mortality, morbidity, incidence and burden of disease in the vaccine-eligible population. On the vaccine side, we are interested in knowing its immunogenicity, efficacy, effectiveness and safety. On the part of the society to which the vaccination schedule is addressed, we must take into account the efficiency of the vaccination programme, the population's perception of the vaccine and its impact on the population. In short, a vaccination schedule must have a series of characteristics that can be summarised in the following aspects: dynamic and up-to-date, adapted and flexible, clear and simple, safe and effective, unified and accepted, useful and possible. If we analyse some of the calendars currently in force in Spain, we will understand that these characteristics are not always present.

It should be borne in mind that a series of events always occur after the introduction of a vaccination programme or a specific vaccine, as shown in the following figure, where the decrease in the incidence of the disease after the implementation of the vaccine is reproduced. The decrease in the incidence of the disease leads to a situation of false security that causes a relaxation in vaccination efforts, resulting in decreases in vaccination coverage and the risk of epidemic outbreaks. This leads to intensified vaccination efforts and the re-establishment of a low prevalence of the disease.

Strategies to be considered to improve vaccination coverage include the following:

•   Reducing missed opportunities for vaccination, which means taking advantage of any medical event to update the vaccination schedule and using accelerated or rescue vaccination schedules.

•   Overcoming public reluctance to vaccinate.

•   Identify false contraindications to vaccination.

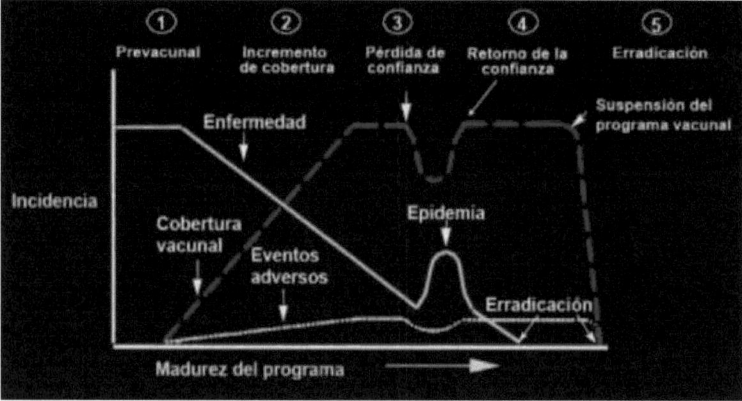

Figure 35.1. *Evolution of any vaccination programme.*

False contraindications to vaccine administration include the following:

○ Mild to moderate fever and moderate diarrhoea.

o Antibiotic treatment (except for BCG and oral typhoid vaccine).

○ Convalescence from acute illness.

○ Personal or family history of non-anaphylactic reaction to a vaccine dose.

○ Prematurity.

○ Breastfeeding.

○ Family history of seizures.

○ Malnutrition

○ Allergic desensitisation treatment.

Vaccination in pregnancy and lactation

The risk from the administration of vaccines during pregnancy is mostly theoretical, as a general rule live vaccines should be avoided, and given the possibility of miscarriage, vaccination in the first trimester of pregnancy should be avoided. Inactivated or toxoid vaccines are generally safe. Cohabitants of a pregnant woman can be vaccinated without restriction and there appears to be no risk to the foetus in administering Igs to the pregnant woman. There are a number of vaccines that are not contraindicated for administration during pregnancy:

- Influenza vaccine.
- Tdpa: If the pregnant woman has been immunised during childhood and more than 10 years have elapsed since the last dose, she should receive 1 dose. If she has not been vaccinated during infancy, she should receive the accelerated vaccination schedule, with at least two doses in the 2nd-3rd trimester of pregnancy. This ensures that the newborn has adequate protection against tetanus in the first 2 months of life.

In special circumstances, vaccination may be indicated against:

- Hepatitis A and B.
- Yellow fever vaccine (avoid first trimester).
- Rabies vaccine (post-exposure).

Contraindicated vaccines:

- Triple vfrica.
- Chickenpox.

Vaccination in preterm infants

BCG vaccination is safe in infants older than 34 weeks gestational age, however, vaccination should be performed once the newborn has left the neonatal unit. Vaccination against hepatitis B should be performed according to the general vaccination schedule in newborns weighing more than 2000g. In newborns weighing less than 2000 g, if the mother is HBsAg negative, vaccination should be deferred until 2000 g; if the mother is HBsAg positive or HBsAg unknown, 0.5 ml of hyperimmune Ig (IM) and the first dose of vaccine should be administered. Vaccination is continued at 1-2 and 6 months with a booster (4^ doses) at 15-18 months of age. Vaccination with DTaP, Hib, Pneumococcal, Meningococcal C and polio should be started at 2 months of chronological age. Influenza vaccination is recommended from 6 months of age, especially in newborns with bronchodysplasia.

Simultaneous administration of vaccines

There is no contraindication to the simultaneous administration of vaccines; however, non-combination vaccines should not be mixed in the same syringe. It should be noted that simultaneous administration leads to an accentuation of the possible side effects described. If not administered simultaneously, live injectable vaccines should be separated by a minimum of 4 weeks. Oral live vaccines do not interfere with each other when administered simultaneously, while the combination of live and inactivated vaccines can be administered at any interval.

Contraindications to vaccines

A contraindication is a condition of the individual that significantly increases the risk of a serious adverse effect if a particular vaccine is administered:

Permanent contraindications

• Anaphylactic allergic reaction to a previous dose of a vaccine or to a vaccine component.

• Encephalopathy of unknown aetiology appearing within 7 days after the administration of a pertussis vaccine component.

Both situations contraindicate the administration of new doses.

Temporary contraindications

• Temporary contraindications allow the administration of a vaccine once they have been resolved:

• Pregnancy. In general, the administration of live vaccines is contraindicated.

• Immunosuppression. Attenuated vaccines are also generally contraindicated.

• Any moderate or severe illness (asthmatic crisis, decompensated cardiopathy, acute diarrhoea...), with or without fever.

• Patient age. It has already been mentioned that there are minimum ages for receiving different vaccines with guaranteed safety and efficacy and, in some cases, there are also maximum age limits.

In any case, after vaccination, the child should be observed for 20-30 minutes at the vaccination site. Adequate equipment should be available to treat any adverse reactions that may occur.

Vaccine components

The types of components included in a vaccine are as follows:

Immunising antigen.

Suspension liquid. Saline solution, distilled water or sometimes culture by-products necessary for the production of vaccines.

Preservatives, stabilisers and antibiotics. These are substances used to stabilise the various components of the vaccine or to prevent contamination by other micro-organisms or degradation of the vaccine. In rare cases, they may cause allergic or toxic reactions (gelatins, aminoglycosides, polymyxin B, formaldehyde).

Adjuvants. Adjuvants are substances or procedures which, when incorporated into the antigen or injected simultaneously with it, make the immune response more effective. Adjuvants are intended to increase the immunogenicity of highly purified or recombinant antigens in order to reduce the amount of antigen and the number of immunisations required. In this way they can increase the efficacy of vaccines in newborns, the elderly and immunocompromised persons. They can promote the induction of mucosal immunity and enhance cellular immunity, increasing functional antibody titres (bactericidal, neutralising, etc.). Adjuvants are nowadays very present in the development of new vaccines.

The use of the term adjuvant is due to Ramon Gaston, who in 1925 observed that the immunological response to antitoxins can be increased by adding substances such as agar, lectins, tapioca, etc. Later Glenny et al. observed in 1926 that diphtheria toxoid associated with aluminium hydroxide is more immunogenic than diphtheria toxoid alone. Later, in 1936, Thibault and Richou discovered the adjuvant properties of Quil A, a saponin extracted from the bark of a South American tree, the *Quillaja saponaria*. The most extensive work on the importance of adjuvants is undoubtedly due to Freund, who in 1937 discovered the immunopotentiating effects of inactivated tubercle bacillus combined with paraffin oil. The use of adjuvants in vaccines at the present time is not free of controversy, under a theoretical framework the ideal adjuvant should not be toxic, should stimulate the immune response both cellular and humoral, should promote long-term immune response, what we call immunological memory, should not induce autoimmunity, should not be mutagenic, carcinogenic or teratogenic, should not be pyrogenic and should be stable in conditions of temperature, pH and time.

Types of adjuvants.

• Mineral salts:

₀Aluminium hydroxide

₀Aluminium phosphate

₀Calcium phosphate

• Lipid particles: ₀Liposomes ₀Immune-stimulating complexes.

• Immunostimulatory adjuvants:

₀Saponins.

₀Muramyl dipeptide (MPD).

₀Bacterial DNA (oligo CpG).

₀Lipopolysaccharides (LPS).

₀MPL and synthetic derivatives.

₀Lipopeptides.

• Microparticles:

₀Biodegradable microspheres of biodegradable particles.

₀Virus like particles.

• Mucosal adjuvants: ₀Choleric toxin. ₀Toxin from mutants: LTK63 and LTR72. o *E. coli* labil toxin.

• Interleukins:

₀IL-2, IL-12, GM-CSF, INF-Y.

• Genetics:

₀Genes encoding co-stimulatory molecules.

Mechanism of action of adjuvants

They can act through two main mechanisms:

1. By acting through the antigen release system, increasing the availability of antigen in antigen presenting cells. Delayed antigen clearance and increased response to antigen at specific physiological sites is achieved. Included in this group of adjuvants are insoluble aluminium salts, liposomes, virosomes, microparticles (PLG), emulsions and virusLike particles.

Immunopotentiators: directly activate cellular receptors and induce cytokine release. MPL and derivatives, MDP and derivatives, oligonucleotides (CpG), double-stranded RNA, pathogen-associated alternative molecular patterns, quils, resiquimod act as immunopotentiators.

Aluminium salts

Aluminium hydroxide is commonly used as crystalline aluminium oxyhydroxide which adsorbs negatively charged antigens. Aluminium phosphate is used as a hydroxyphosphate which adsorbs positively charged antigens. The depot effect of aluminium salts was described by Glenny in 1931. Aluminium salts convert soluble antigens into particles with a diameter of less than 10 mcm, which are taken up by antigen-presenting cells. In addition, aluminium salts induce eosinophilia, activate complement, stimulate B-lymphocytes, DCs and macrophages, regulate co-stimulation signals in monocytes and promote IL-4 release. In addition, the administration of aluminium salts induces inflammation at the injection site, attracts antigen-presenting cells and thus enhances the immune response.

Emulsions

Emulsions are liquid dispersions of two immiscible phases, usually oil and water, each of which can be either the dispersed or the continuous phase, resulting in a hydro-oily or oleo-aqueous emulsion respectively.

• Freud's complete adjuvant: hydro-oily solution with paraffin oil and dead mycobacteria.

• Freud's incomplete adjuvant: No mycobacteria. Causes local reactogenicity, accumulation in organism and tumour induction in mice.

• SAF: Oleo-aqueous emulsion with squalene and threonyl-MDP (mycobacterial cell wall peptidoglycan derivative). Causes unacceptable adverse effects: uveitis in rabbits, very pyrogenic.

• MF59: Non-viscous emulsion, easy to inject. Squalene is a natural component of cell membranes. Synthetic precursor of cholesterol. It is biodegradable and biocompatible and stable for at least 3 years. No depot effect. Generates a local immunostimulatory environment at the injection site, which locally activates monocytes and granulocytes. Induces the production of cytokines that increase the recruitment of immune cells from the blood to peripheral tissues. They are responsible for increased uptake of androgen by monocytes at the injection site, increased differentiation of monocytes into dendritic cells and potent induction of the CCR7 host receptor found on maturing dendritic cells. Evidence with MF59 in influenza vaccine showed higher antibody rates than with virosome or subunit vaccines. MF59 has also been used in other investigational vaccines: cytomegalovirus, herpesvirus, HIV, hepatitis B and hepatitis C.

Liposomes

They are hollow microspheres with 1 or more lipid bilayers. The membrane is made up of cholesterol and phosphoKpids similar to cell membranes, so that when introduced into the host there is no rejection. They prolong the contact time of androgens with the immune system, which results in a longer exposure time to androgen-presenting cells. They enhance cellular and humoral immunity for protein and androgens and polysaccharides. There are two types of liposomes: proteosomes and cochleates; the former are small vesicles of bacterial origin in association with viral prothemes that induce a Th1 immune response, the latter are non-vesicular lamellar bilayers. Calcium ions are added to them, causing them to coil up and leave a space where prothymes or DNA are loaded.

Virosomes

They are tiny spherical vesicles, which contain viral prothemes embedded in their membrane. These prothemes allow the virosome membranes to fuse with cells of the immune system, releasing their contents (the specific androgens of the vaccine) directly to their targets. Once the androgens are released, the virosomes are completely degraded inside the cells. The main advantage of virosomes is that they mimic the natural form of androgen presentation and stimulate both the humoral and cellular pathways of the immune system by releasing the androgens at the specific targets and amplifying the immune response. They are delivery systems with wide applications as they can be administered parenterally or nasally. Currently, the hepatitis A vaccine (Hepaxal) or the influenza vaccine (Inflexal) use virosomes and are commercially available.

Combined vaccines

They contain more than one antigenic component of one or different micro-organisms and are administered together in a single injection. Their formulation requires ensuring the absence of physical, chemical or biological instability between their components.

The main advantages of using combination vaccines are as follows:

- Decrease the number of injections, which provides a better acceptance in general and also by healthcare personnel.
- The reduction of side effects.
- Reduction of exposure to excipients.
- Facilitate vaccination opportunities.
- Improve vaccination coverage.
- Allow simultaneous vaccination against several diseases.
- Enable the incorporation of new vaccines.
- Simplify vaccination programmes.
- Facilitate the standardisation of vaccination guidelines.
- Savings in material and administration time.
- Ease of transport, storage and preservation.

They must meet a number of conditions, such as stability for a reasonable period of time under appropriate storage measures (36-48 months), immunogenicity and efficacy similar to that of their individual components, same age of administration for each of them, minimal local and general reactogenicity, absence of immunological interference between the antigens they contain, possibility of integration into the vaccination schedule, and a tolerable and adequate volume to be injected.

They may contain different antigens of the same micro-organism (called poly- or multivalent), such as oral (attenuated) and parenteral (inactivated) poliovirus vaccines, pentavalent rotavirus vaccines, human papillomavirus (HPV) vaccines, pneumococcal vaccines (polysaccharide and conjugate) or tetravalent meningococcal vaccines, pneumococcal (polysaccharide and conjugate) or tetravalent meningococcal vaccines, or be composed of antigens from different micro-organisms, be they viruses (measles, rubella and mumps), bacteria, such as DTaP, or bacteria and viruses, such as pneumococcal pneumococcal pneumococcal pneumococcal vaccine; or bacteria and viruses, such as pentavalent (DTPa-VPI-Hib) and hexavalent (DTPa-VPI-Hib-HB) vaccines. No combination vaccine mixes attenuated and inactivated components in the same preparation.

The MMR vaccine (measles, mumps and rubella) and the varicella vaccine are licensed in many countries from the age of 9-12 months. The possibility of combining the three vaccines in a single injection improves the vaccination rate and reduces unnecessary health care costs. Some laboratories have developed a tetravalent combined measles, rubella, mumps and varicella vaccine (Priorix-Tetra) which has been licensed in many European countries, the US and Australia. There is little information on the safety and efficacy of co-administration of Priorix-Tetra with hepatitis A and pneumococcal vaccines in children older than 12 months. MM. Blatter et al (1) study the immunogenicity of the tetravalent vaccine when co-administered with hepatitis A or pneumococcal conjugate vaccines. They conducted a phase II clinical trial in which the tetravalent vaccine (GSK or Merck) was administered at 4°C or -20°C together with the hepatitis A and pneumococcal conjugate vaccine. The authors determine immunogenicity by analysing the production of antibodies against each of the vaccine diseases. Reactogenicity is determined by recording symptoms occurring from days 0-42 after vaccination. The authors were able to recruit 1850 patients of whom 1783 were vaccinated and demonstrate non-inferiority of the tetravalent vaccine co-administered with hepatitis A or pneumococcal conjugate vaccine when stored at 4°C or -20°C for both GSK and Merck tetravalent vaccines. All vaccines show acceptable reactogenicity when co-administered with hepatitis A or pneumococcal conjugate vaccine.

Bibliograffa

1.   Blatter MM, Klein NP, Shepard JS, Leonardi M, Shapiro S, Schear M, et al. Immunogenicity and safety of two tetravalent (measles, mumps, rubella, varicella) vaccines coadministered with hepatitis a and pneumococcal conjugate vaccines to children twelve to fourteen months of age. Pediatr Infect Dis J 2012 Aug;31(8):e133-e140.

2.   American Academy of Pediatrics. Active and passive immunization. In: Kimberlin DW, Brady MT, Jackson MA, Long SS, eds. Red Book: 2015 Report of the Committee on Infectious Diseases. 30^ ed. Elk Grove Village, IL: American Academy of Pediatrics; 2015. pp. 1-107.

3.   Australia Government. Department of Health. Fundamentals of immunisation. In: The Australian Immunization Handbook. 10th ed., 2013. Available at: https://immunisationhandbook.health.gov.au/

4.   Centers for Disease Control and Prevention. Vaccine Recommendations and Guidelines of the Advisory Committee on Immunization Practices [online]. Available at: https://www.cdc.gov/vaccines/hcp/acip-recs/index.html [accessed 23/1/2018].

5.   L. Salleras. *Vacunaciones preventivas*, Barcelona:Masson, 2003. 1063 pages.

36. Basic cardiopulmonary resuscitation in paediatrics

Dr. Esther Ocete Hita

Causes of cardiorespiratory arrest in paediatrics

Both the causes and treatment of cardiorespiratory arrest in paediatric patients differ from what occurs in adult patients due to anatomical and physiological differences; and even throughout the paediatric age from the neonatal period to adolescence they also change. In children, cardiac disease, unlike in adults, is not the primary cause of cardiorespiratory arrest. In children the arrest is usually secondary to another serious non-heart disease. This is why the most frequent rhythm in infant cardiorespiratory arrest (CRA) is bradycardia progressing to asystole and not ventricular arrhythmias (the most frequent cause in adult patients).

In general, the prognosis for resuscitation when the cause is not acute is worse than in children and although paediatric CPR outcomes have improved significantly in recent years, morbidity and mortality remain very high. The anatomical and pathophysiological characteristics of children that should be considered for resuscitation are listed in table 36.1.

As the age of the child decreases, all these differences with the adult are accentuated; while in the adolescent they have practically disappeared.

Table 36.1. Anatomical and pathophysiological differences in children.

V^a aerial	Proportionally larger head, prominent occiput and tendency to flex on the neck when supine. Small face and mouth, large tongue which can obstruct the airway and can be difficult to control with the laryngoscope blade. In the first 6 months of life, breathing is mainly nasal; obstruction can lead to respiratory failure. The larynx is elevated, at the level of c_i whereas in the adult it is at C5-C6. The epiglottis is large and lax Short vocal cords Physiological stenosis at the level of the cricoid cartilage which makes the larynx funnel-shaped in young children, in adults it is cylindrical and the risk of foreign body obstruction at this level is higher.
Breathing	The main respiratory muscle in infants is the diaphragm, the rib cage is still very elastic and the intercostal muscles are weak. Respiratory rate increases with increasing age of the child
Circulation	Volemia decreases with age, in a newborn it is 80 ml/kg and in an adult 60-70 ml/kg. Normal heart rate is higher the younger the age of the child Blood pressure is lower the younger the age of the child.
Neurological	The younger the age of the child the greater the inability to communicate

	what is happening to him/her Use for neurological assessment Glasgow scale adapted for children under 5 years of age
Exhibition	Increased risk of hypothermia

Causes and prevention of death

The causes of death differ in the different age groups: while in the first year of life, in addition to sudden infant death syndrome, congenital malformations are the most frequent; in the rest of the paediatric age groups and in our environment it is trauma.

De aM the importance of accident prevention measures through primary, secondary (to reduce the effect of accidents) and tertiary prevention measures (to reduce the consequences of accidents, e.g. promoting training in paediatric life support).

The importance of recognising a serious paediatric patient is fundamental to prevent the situation from progressing to cardiopulmonary arrest, the prognosis of which, as we have already mentioned, is poor.

Respiratory failure occurs in any process in which the entry of air into the lungs is difficult. In these cases, compensatory mechanisms are activated, such as increased respiratory frequency, increased heart rate and the use of accessory respiratory muscles (intercostal, suprasternal, nasal...). Progressively, central cyanosis (due to failure to maintain adequate arterial oxygen saturation) and hypercapnia (increased $paCO_2$) may appear.

The whine is often heard in infants and young children when there is a pathology predisposing to alveolar collapse and is usually an indicator of severe disease.

Table 36.2. ABCDE rapid assessment of the severe child.

A. V^a aerial	Safe and permeable/obstructive
B. Breathing	Frequency, work of breathing, oxygenation/ventilation
C. Circulation	Heart rate, blood pressure, peripheral perfusion
D. Neurological status	Consciousness, convulsions, glycaemia test, focality or abnormal posture
E. Exhibition	Body temperature, injuries

Cardiocirculatory failure or shock is a clinical situation in which organ perfusion is compromised and its aetiopathogenesis is diverse (hypovolaemic, distributive, cardiogenic, obstructive or dissociative). Initially, the child will try to maintain adequate oxygen supply to the tissues by compensatory mechanisms such as tachycardia, vasoconstriction and increased cardiac contractility. Hence hypotension is a late and poor prognostic finding. Signs of hypoperfusion of the different systems include alterations in peripheral perfusion, decreased level of consciousness, hypotoma and oliguria. In the case of any patient with clinical illness, it is recommended to use the paediatric assessment triangle and to act according to the ABCDE sequence of action (Table 36.2), performing continuous re-evaluation of the patient, especially each time treatment measures are taken.

These initial recognition measures can provide the information necessary to detect the cause of the patient's severe condition in order to provide appropriate aetiological treatment. The most common causes of severe illness and their initial management in paediatrics are listed in table 36.3.

Table 36.3. Most frequent causes of severe illness in the paediatric patient and initial treatment measures.

Status asthmaticus	Supplemental oxygen titrated for SpO2 of 94 to 98 %. **Salbutamol** 2.5-5 mg (0.15 mg/kg) spacer/nebulised oral or intravenous **systemic corticosteroids** (prednisolone IV 1-2 mg/kg, max 60 mg/day) **Magnesium IV** (severe asthma). Single dose of 50 mg/kg over 20 min (max. 2 g).
Anaphylaxis	**IM adrenaline** 0.01 mg/kg; can be administered with a syringe (1 mg/ml solution), or self-injectable adrenaline (0.15 mg (<6 years) - 0.3 mg (6-12 years) - 0.5 mg (>12 years) y)). If symptoms do not improve rapidly, administer a second dose of IM adrenaline after 5 to 10 minutes. In cases of refractory anaphylaxis, consider the use of IV or intraosseous (IO) adrenaline. **Inhaled SABA** (salbutamol) and/or inhaled adrenaline for bronchospasm. Intravenous or oral **H1 and H2 antihistamines** to relieve subjective symptoms (especially skin symptoms). **Glucocorticosteroids** (methylprednisolone 1-2 mg/kg) only for children requiring prolonged observation.
Cardiocirculatory shock	Cannulation of a peripheral line, if not successful after 5 minutes, cannulation of an intraosseous line. **Balanced crystalloids** 10 ml/kg up to 60cc/kg. Re-evaluate after each bolus for signs of fluid overload (crackles, oedema, hepatomegaly). In this case, therapy should be stopped. In cases of haemorrhagic shock, consider early **blood products**, or if available, whole blood, in children with severe trauma. **Tranexamic acid** (TxA) in all children requiring transfusion following major trauma - as soon as possible within 3 hours of injury - and/or major bleeding. Start **vasoactive drugs** early, in continuous infusion, in children with circulatory failure when there is no improvement after multiple fluid boluses or if their infusion has been stopped due to fluid overload. **Hydrocortisone** stress dose (1 to 2 mg/kg) in children with septic shock, unresponsive to fluids and vasoactive drugs. Broad spectrum **antibiotics as** soon as possible in septic shock (first hour).
Convulsive status	**Midazolam** IM 0.2 mg/kg (max. 10 mg) or pre-filled syringes: 5 mg for 13-40 kg, 10 mg >40 kg); intranasal/buccal 0.3 mg/kg; IV 0.15 mg/kg (max. 7.5 mg) or **Diazepam** 0.2-0.25 mg/kg IV (max. 10 mg)/rectal 0.5 mg/kg (max. 20 mg). If seizures persist after 5 minutes, administer a second dose of benzodiazepine and prepare a long-acting second-line drug for administration: **Levetiracetam** 40-60 mg/kg IV max. 4,5g, over 15') **Fenitofna** 20 mg/kg IV (max. 1.5 g, over 20 min) **Valproic acid** 40 mg/kg IV (max 3g; over 15 min; avoid in cases of suspected liver failure or metabolic disease - which can never be ruled out in infants and young children - as well as in pregnant adolescents). **Phenobarbital** (20 mg/kg over 20 min) IV if none of the three recommended therapies are available. If seizures persist: consider additional second-line drug. After 40 minutes, if seizures persist, consider **third-line drugs**: midazolam at anaesthetic doses, ketamine, pentobarbital/thiopental or propofol; preferably under continuous EEG monitoring (with adequate oxygen, ventilation and perfusion support).
Severe hypoglycaemia (<50mg/dl) with ne urological	IV bolus **glucose 0.3 g/kg**; preferably as a 10 % (100 mg/ml; 3 ml/kg) or 20 % (200 mg/ml; 1.5 ml/kg) solution. When IV glucose is not available, **glucagon** can be given as a temporary rescue, either IM or SC (0.03 mg/kg or 1 mg >25 kg; 0.5 mg <25 kg) or intranasally (3 mg; 4-16 years).

symptoms	Measure blood glucose 10 minutes after treatment and repeat if response is inadequate. Reasonable targets are an increase of at least 50 mg/dL (2.8 mmol/L) and/or a blood glucose target of 100 mg/dL (5.6 mmol/L).

Paediatric Basic Life Support

A set of manoeuvres which, without the use of devices, makes it possible to recognise a child in a situation of cardiorespiratory arrest and to provide sufficient oxygenation to protect the brain and other organs until advanced resuscitation is possible.

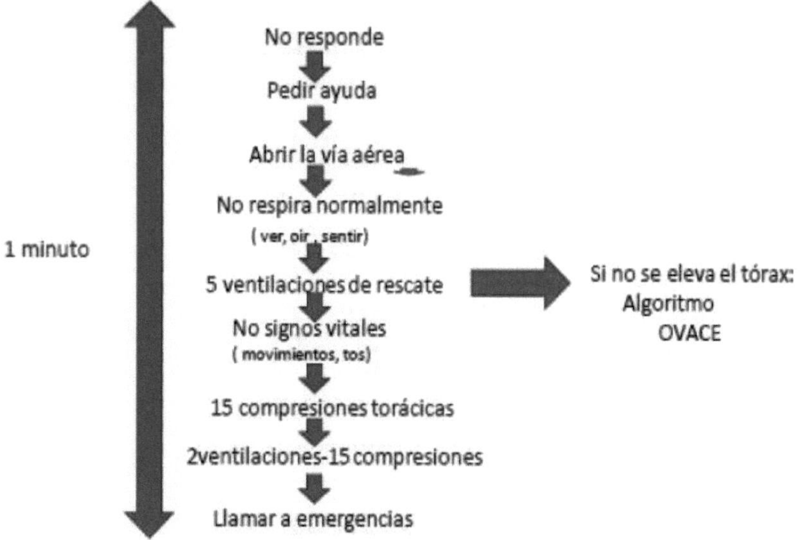

Figure 36.1. *Basic Paediatric Life Support Algorithm*

These measures should be implemented immediately and in the following sequence:
- Ensure first and foremost the safety of both the rescuer and the child.
- Check if he/she responds to verbal and tactile stimulation and ask for help aloud.
- If the child does not respond, open the airway and assess breathing for no more than 10 seconds. If there is any doubt as to whether breathing is normal, act as if it is not normal. If there is effort but no air movement, the airway is not open. In unconscious trauma victims, open the airway using the jaw thrust manoeuvre to prevent rotation of the spine.
- In cases where there is more than one rescuer, a second rescuer should call for emergency help after recognising unconsciousness, preferably using the speakerphone function of a mobile phone. If there is only one rescuer, with a mobile phone, he/she should first call for help (and activate the speakerphone function) immediately after the initial rescue breaths. If no phone is available, perform 1 minute of CPR before leaving the child to call for emergency help.
- In the unconscious child, if breathing is abnormal, 5 initial rescue breaths will be administered.

300

- For infants, ensure a neutral head position. Perform mouth-to-nose insufflations on the infant.
- In older children, a greater extension of the head may be required. Perform mouth-to-mouth insufflations by manually plugging the nose.

Insufflations should last about 1 second, long enough for the chest to rise visibly.

If insufflations do not raise the thorax, it is possible that the airways are obstructed (we will follow the algorithm below).

- In cases where rescuers are unable or unwilling to begin ventilations, they should proceed with compressions and add ventilations to the sequence as soon as they can be performed.
- 15 chest compressions should be given unless there are clear signs of circulation (e.g. movement, coughing). Compressions should be of good quality:
  - 100-120 per minute
  - Depth: depress the lower half of the sternum to at least one third of the anteroposterior dimension of the thorax. Compressions should never be deeper than 6 cm Kmite for adults (approximately the length of an adult thumb).
  - Retraction: Release all pressure between compressions allowing the thorax to fully retract.
  - When possible, perform compressions on a firm surface.
  - In infants, the two-thumb circular technique is preferred for chest compression, but if there is only one rescuer, the two-finger technique may also be used. In children older than 1 year, depending on the size and breadth of the hand, the one- or two-handed technique may be used.
- After 15 compressions, 2 rescue breaths should follow and then alternate (duty cycle 15:2). CPR should not be interrupted at any time unless there are clear signs of circulation (movement, coughing) or if the rescuer is exhausted.
- Two or more rescuers should exchange frequently to perform chest compressions.
- If there are clear signs of life, but the child remains unconscious and is not breathing normally, ventilation shall be continued exclusively.

-Recovery position: Unconscious children who are not in cardiorespiratory arrest and who are breathing normally can be placed laterally in the safety position.

Use of an Automated External Defibrillator (AED)

In paediatrics, the only situation in which we should initially suspect that the cardiorespiratory arrest is of cardiac origin is in the case of witnessed subito collapse. In this case, the probability that the arrest is due to an arrhythmia and in particular to a primary defibrillable rhythm is very high, therefore, it is justified that if there is only one rescuer the first manoeuvre is to ask for help so that an AED can be provided as soon as possible. If there is more than one rescuer, it will be the second rescuer who will immediately call for help and then collect and apply an AED (if feasible).

As soon as the AED is available, the stickers are applied, chest compressions are stopped for rhythm analysis, and if the device recognises a shockable rhythm, it indicates that a shock should be delivered. Immediately after shock delivery or a decision not to shock, chest compressions shall be restarted immediately.

If available with the defibrillator, paediatric dose attenuators shall be used for infants and children under 8 years of age. If not available, a standard AED will be used for all ages.

Pediatric airway obstruction by foreign body (OVACE)

OVACE should be suspected, in the absence of witnesses, when the onset of respiratory symptoms (coughing, retching, stridor, distress) is very abrupt and there are no other signs of illness; or when there is a history of ingestion of risky foods (such as nuts) or playing with small objects just prior to the onset of symptoms.

There are three possible situations, from the least to the most life-threatening:

1.) If **the child is coughing effectively** (coughing forcefully, breathing before coughing, still crying or talking), no manoeuvre is necessary. Except encourage the child to cough and monitor the child's condition.

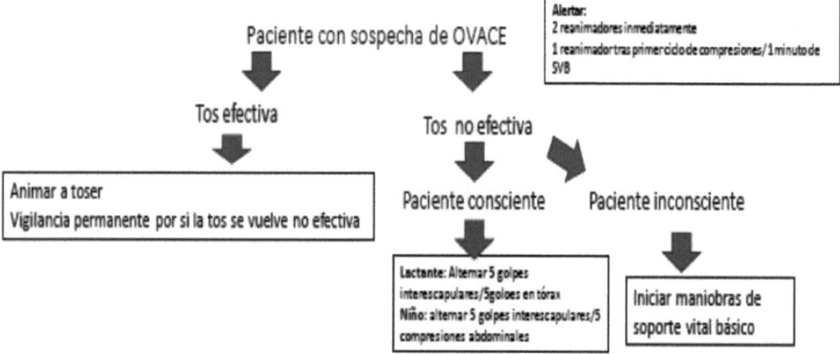

Figure 36.2. Treatment algorithm for foreign body airway obstruction.

) **If the child's cough becomes ineffective** (decreased consciousness, weak cough, inability to breathe or vocalise, cyanosis), shout for help and if there are two rescuers, one of them should alert the emergency services, preferably by mobile phone (loudspeaker function). If only one rescuer is present, he/she will initiate rescue manoeuvres unless he/she can also use the loudspeaker function of the mobile phone to alert the emergency services.

2.1) If coughing is ineffective but **the child is still conscious**, give 5 sharp blows with the heel of the hand to the interscapular area. If back blows do not relieve the OVACE, give 5 chest thrusts to infants or 5 abdominal thrusts to children (Heimlich manoeuvre). If the foreign body has not been expelled and the victim is still conscious, continue the sequence of back blows and chest thrusts (for infants) or abdominal thrusts (for children).

2.2)) If coughing is ineffective and **the child is unconscious**, the basic life support algorithm will be instituted: opening of the airway, administration of 5 ventilations and in the absence of signs of vitality, start chest compressions following the sequence of 15 chest compressions and 2 ventilations.

Conclusions

Preventing the possible causes of cardiorespiratory arrest in children, as well as the early detection and subsequent implementation of measures to ensure that a serious patient progresses to cardiorespiratory arrest is fundamental, since the prognosis once it occurs is poor and the subsequent risk of sequelae, mainly neurological, is high.

Once cardiorespiratory arrest has been recognised, basic life support manoeuvres must be started immediately and, if a mobile phone is available, the call to emergency services must be activated simultaneously through the handsfree system.

Bibliograffa

1. Van de Voorde P, Turner NM, Djakow J, de Lucas N, Martinez-Mejias A, Biarent D, Bingham R, Brissaud O, Hoffmann F, Johannesdottir GB, Lauritsen T, Maconochie I. European Resuscitation Council Guidelines 2021: Paediatric Life Support. Resuscitation. 2021 Apr;161:327-387. doi: 10.1016/j.resuscitation.2021.02.015. Epub 2021 Mar 24.PMID: 33773830 2. Lopez-Herce J, Manrique I, Calvo C, Rodnguez A, Carrillo A, Sebastian V, del Castillo J; on behalf of the Grupo Espanol de Reanimacion Cardiopulmonar Pediatrica y Neonatal. Novedades en las recomendaciones de reanimacion cardiopulmonar pediatrica y Kneas de desarrollo en Espana. Annals of Paediatrics. Vol. 96. Num. 2. pages 171-175 (February 2022. DOI: 10.1016/j.anpedi.2021.05.020

3. Gavin D. Perkins , Graesner JT, Semeraro F, Olasveengen T, Soar J, Lott C, Van de Voorde P , Madar J, Zideman D, Mentzelopoulos S , Bossaertmetro L, Greif T, Monsieurs K, Svavarsdo'ttir H ,Nolan JP, name of the European Resuscitation Council Guidelines Contributors. European Resuscitation Council Guidelines 2021: Executive summary.Resuscitation.Volume 161, April2021   ,   Pages-1-60.https://doi.org/10.1016/j.resuscitation.2021.02.003.

4. Long E, Duke T. Fluid resuscitation therapy for paediatric sepsis. .J Paediatr Child Health. 2016 Feb;52(2):141-6. doi:10.1111/jpc.13085.PMID: 27062617 Review.

5. Topjian AA, Raymond TT, Atkins D, Chan M, Duff JP, Joyner BL Jr, Lasa JJ, Lavonas EJ, Levy A, Mahgoub M, Meckler GD, Roberts KE, Sutton RM, Schexnayder SM; Pediatric Basic and Advanced Life Support Collaborators. Part 4: Pediatric Basic and Advanced Life Support: 2020 American Heart Association Guidelines for Cardiopulmonary Resuscitation and Emergency Cardiovascular Care. .Circulation. 2020 Oct 20;142(16_suppl_2):S469-S523. doi: 10.1161/CIR.0000000000000901. Epub 2020 Oct 21.

37.Bioethics and paediatrics. Children's rights

Dr. Francisco Moreno Madrid

What is bioethics? What is it for? Is it useful?

Bioethics is the ethics of the medical sciences: medicine and biology. There are several definitions, although the initial one remains the discipline that unites:

- Biological knowledge
- With the knowledge of human values (Potter).

Its development runs parallel to the great scientific and technological revolution in biomedicine which:

- It has changed our way of life.
- It is also changing, overflowing the basic concepts of ethics and law on a daily basis.

Difficult questions are being asked which were unthinkable in the past. The answers we give will influence our lives and the generations to come. eIs it legitimate to clone a human being? eCan a terminally ill patient be helped? eHow far should manipulation of the human being be allowed? eWhere is the limit to biomedical research set? eWhat role does human dignity play in the debate about new technologies? Etc.

eIn the end, they are nothing more than the great questions that man has asked himself throughout his existence: eWhat is life? eWho does it belong to? eWhat is freedom? eWhat is human dignity?

A classic definition of bioethics is that it is seen as a **bridge to the future, between:**

- Science and the humanities
- Law and morality
- Ideas and beliefs
- Climate and technology
- Professionals and patients
- Between the patients' reality (which will be everyone's at some point) and our own).

Ethics, morals, law

Ethics comes from Greek: ethos; Moral from Latm: mos/ mori. Although etymologically they have the same meaning: way of being, character. Their meaning has been separated:

1. Moral

Set of personal, individual values. Everyone bases them as they wish. It is impossible to organise a society, as there can be as many morals as there are people. It is usually linked to a particular religion or belief.

2. Ethics

A set of minimum values that a society accepts for peaceful coexistence and mutual respect. They are demanded of citizens in conscience, but are not imposed. They can be identified with the universal declaration of human rights. E.g.: truth, freedom, solidarity, justice, solidarity, honesty, etc.

3. Law

Some of the values of ethics are considered so important that they are coercively enforced: laws, laws of the land, laws of the state, and laws of the people.

Principles of bioethics

Bioethics has 4 main principles that can be considered as the basic values that help us to assess whether a clinical decision can be considered ethical.

1. Autonomy

Respect for the patient's decisions. Unlike the traditional or paternalistic view, predominant for centuries: seeking the best interests of the patient as understood by the health professional, regardless of the patient's opinion and whatever the cost.

2.   Charity

Moral obligation to do good for the patient. Do no harm, maximising the possible benefits and minimising the possible risks. Assessment of the risk/benefit ratio.

3.   Justice

Equitable distribution of health resources

4.   Non-maleficiency

Protect the patient from the potential harms of medicine.

In these principles lies the modern view of the ethics of the health professions. The pursuit of the greatest possible well-being for the patient must take into account the patient's opinion and the efficient management of resources.

Bioethics, paediatrics and value-based medicine

Bioethical conflicts are always conflicts of values. Clinical practice confronts the professional with problems that are disconcerting because they are neither measurable nor evaluable. They have to do with the intangible world of values where bioethics has its field of action. Bioethics offers a theoretical framework with some contents, some principles that order what would otherwise be a chaos of subjective beliefs.

Ethics points to general principles that guide our actions and reflects on the rational foundations of conduct. Morality refers to concrete norms, and is more related to orientations of a private nature, linked to a particular religion or belief.

Bioethics must necessarily be secular, rational, dialogical, pluralistic, critical and guided by broad principles, not by individual principles or ideas.

The four main principles of bioethics (autonomy, beneficence, justice and non-maleficence) can be considered as basic values that serve to frame the ethical correctness of a clinical decision.

The first moral duty of the professional is to have good scientific and technical competence. But a new profile of excellence requires combining these three aspects:

1.   Training and working from the best scientific evidence.
2.   Respect for and inclusion of patients' values in the clinical relationship.
3.   Active militancy in professional values.

In addition to scientific and technical competence, in order to aspire to excellence, values, attitudes and behaviours oriented towards the benefit of the patient and society, rather than self-interest, are required.

Professionals obtain external goods such as money, prestige, power, etc., which are Hcitos, but when these external goods constitute our main objective over the internal ones, such as vocation and caring for people who are in a situation of vulnerability with respect to us, many bioethicists argue that we are abandoning in a certain way the ^z, the essential meaning of our profession.

The American Academy of Paediatrics lists a series of principles among which it emphasises the commitment to teamwork and to the defence of children's rights by assuming the role of <u>advocates for children</u>. **The Spanish Association of Paediatrics (AEP)** has established an ethical framework, a commitment to the ethics of organisations. It has highlighted a series of **values** that should permeate all paediatric activities in a transversal manner.

1. Personal. Transparency, tolerance, empathy, honesty, trust, credibility, confidentiality, respect for human rights, loyalty and responsibility.

2. Professionalism. Quality, scientific competence, responsible research, commitment to human and ethical training, patient-centred professionalism.

3. The specifics of the child's relationship with minors: the child's right to information, commitment to promoting the moral autonomy of the child, respect for cultural diversity.

4. Social: Technical commitment, defence of children's rights, solidarity with the most disadvantaged, sustainable and efficient management of health resources.

It has also defined the aims inherent in paediatrics:

1. Disease and injury prevention and health promotion.

2. Relief from pain and suffering.

3. The care and cure of the sick and the care of the incurable, putting cure and care on the same level.

4. The avoidance of premature death and the pursuit of a peaceful death, avoiding the temptation to prolong life unduly.

5. The defence of children in all areas.

Children's rights

Laws reflect the values of society at a given moment or time. In the case of minors, strange as it may seem, it was not until the end of the last century that States began to recognise the existence of the specific needs of children: the right of all children, simply because they are children, to receive care, giving priority to their rights as persons.

Sometimes we forget that we were born and live on the "good side of the world", that democracy and with it the economic and social development of peoples is a rare commodity in time and in the number of people it reaches. Unfortunately, the exploitation of children is not something from the past that we see in the movies or read about in books, but it is suffered and suffered today in a large part of the world.

UNICEF estimates that 150 million children are exploited, most of them in Asia and the Pacific, Africa, South America, the Middle East. Most of them work in the agricultural sector, especially in the mining industry, or are recruited as soldiers. Girls are used for domestic work, forced into marriage or prostitution.

The consequences are devastating:

- Poverty is perpetuated^ both cause and consequence
- Dropping out of school^ Prevents access to better jobs
- Its full development is prevented^ game
- Physical and psychological health
- Their dignity is undermined

Declaration of the Rights of the Child

Adopted in 1959 by the United Nations General Assembly. This recognition was the first major international consensus on children's rights. It establishes a series of principles for the protection of children, but these principles were not sufficient to protect children's rights because, legally, this declaration was not legally binding.

United Nations Convention on the Rights of the Child. 1989

It has become the most ratified human rights treaty in history. It has transformed the lives of children. It has been signed by practically all the countries of the world, unlike the previous one, they incorporate it into their laws, into their law, which implies the **obligation** to comply with them. Children's rights have 4 key principles:

1.	Non-discrimination. All children have the same rights, regardless of skin colour, religion, background or ideas of their parents.

2.	Best interests of the child. Set of actions and processes aimed at guaranteeing an integral development and a dignified life, as well as the material and affective conditions that allow minors to live fully and achieve the maximum possible wellbeing. It is a guarantee that minors have the right to have, before any action is taken with respect to them, those that promote and protect their rights and not those that violate them.

3.	Right to life, survival and development.

4.	Participation. The right to be consulted on situations affecting them and to have their views taken into account It is significant that this is a convention rather than a declaration. This means that participating States are obliged to ensure compliance.

In practice, these principles translate into actions that have a great impact on children's well-being:

•	In early childhood care, a rights-based approach implies more integrated programmes that address problems on several fronts (nutrition, vaccines, neonatal care, etc.).

•	In education, this approach implies a greater focus on equal access to education for boys and girls in order to avoid school drop-out.

•	In child protection, the rights-based approach means the development of a protective environment that identifies and reinforces the main components that can protect children (families, communities, laws, media...).

This treatise contains a profound insight: Children are not simply objects belonging to their parents and on whose behalf decisions are made, nor are they adults in the process of being formed. They are human beings and individuals with their own rights. The Convention says that childhood is separate from adulthood, which ends at the age of 18, and that it is a special and protected stage during which children should be helped to grow, learn, play, develop and thrive in dignity.

The Preamble recalls the fundamental principles of the United Nations and the specific provisions of certain treaties and declarations relating to human rights; it reaffirms the need to provide children with special care and assistance in view of their vulnerability; underlines in particular the primary responsibility of the family for protection and care, the need for the child's protection before and after birth, the importance of respect for the cultural values of the child's community and the crucial role of international co-operation in the realisation of the rights of the child.

"Children have the right to the enjoyment of the highest attainable standard of health and to have access to medical and rehabilitation services, with special emphasis on those related to primary health care, preventive care and the reduction of infant mortality. It is

the obligation of the State to take the necessary measures aimed at the abolition of traditional practices harmful to the health of the child".

Since its adoption, there has been considerable progress in the world in fulfilling children's rights to survival, health and education through the provision of essential goods and services, as well as a growing recognition of the need to establish a protective environment that shields children from exploitation, abuse and violence.

"No cause deserves higher priority than the protection and development of the child, on whom depend the survival, stability and progress of all nations and, indeed, of human civilisation".

Rights of hospitalised children

In 1986 the European Parliament adopted the European Charter for Hospitalised Children, which sets out the rights of minors in this situation.

* The right of the child not to be hospitalised unless he/she is unable to receive the necessary care at home or in a health centre.
* Be accompanied by his or her parents or a person standing in for them.
* To receive information adapted to their age.
* Being hospitalised with other children
* Continuing their school education during their stay in hospital
* The right of parents or a person standing in loco parentis to express their agreement with
the treatments applied to the child
* Not to receive useless medical treatment and not to endure avoidable physical and moral suffering.
* To be provided with age-appropriate toys, books and audiovisual media during their stay in hospital.
* To be treated with tact, courtesy and understanding and to have their privacy respected.

BIBLIOGRAPHY

1   Camps V. The excellence of the health professions. Medical Humanities. 2007;2:1- --13.

2   . Gracia D. New challenges in the ethics of health professions. In: Como arqueros al blanco. Estudios de bioetica. Madrid: Triacastela; 2004. p. 279-99.

3   Horton R. The coming decade for global action on child health. Lancet. 2006;367:3--5

4   The Goals of Medicine. New York: The Hastings Center, 1996 (Spanish translation, Los fines de la medicina. Barcelona: Fundacion Vfctor Grifols i Lucas, 2004).

5   . Martmez Gonzalez C. Sanchez Jacob M. Bioethics, paediatrics and value-based medicine. An Pediatr Contin. 2011;9(6):397-402

6   . Sanchez Jacob M. The ethical framework of the Spanish Association of Paediatrics: a commitment to organisational ethics. An Pediatr (Barc). 2011;75 (6): 355-57.

7   Riano Galan I. Bioethics in the training of paediatricians. An Pediatr (Barc). 2014; 80:69- 70

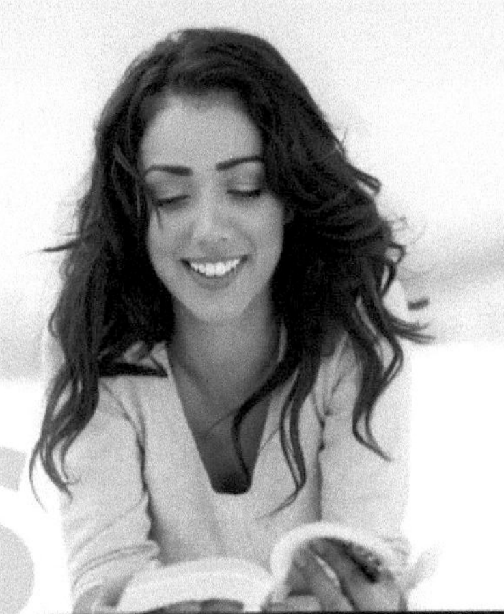

yes **I want** morebooks!

Buy your books fast and straightforward online - at one of world's fastest growing online book stores! Environmentally sound due to Print-on-Demand technologies.

Buy your books online at
www.morebooks.shop

Kaufen Sie Ihre Bücher schnell und unkompliziert online – auf einer der am schnellsten wachsenden Buchhandelsplattformen weltweit! Dank Print-On-Demand umwelt- und ressourcenschonend produzi ert.

Bücher schneller online kaufen
www.morebooks.shop

info@omniscriptum.com
www.omniscriptum.com

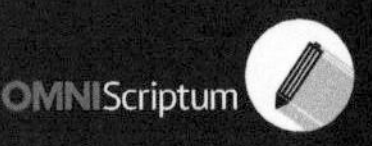

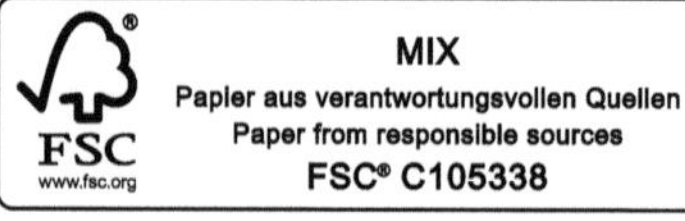

Printed by Books on Demand GmbH, Norderstedt / Germany